Canine and Feline Behavior

Editor

CARLO SIRACUSA

VETERINARY CLINICS OF NORTH AMERICA: SMALL ANIMAL PRACTICE

www.vetsmall.theclinics.com

January 2024 • Volume 54 • Number 1

ELSEVIER

1600 John F. Kennedy Boulevard • Suite 1800 • Philadelphia, Pennsylvania, 19103-2899
http://www.vetsmall.theclinics.com

VETERINARY CLINICS OF NORTH AMERICA: SMALL ANIMAL PRACTICE Volume 54, Number 1
January 2024 ISSN 0195-5616, ISBN-13: 978-0-443-12997-1

Editor: Stacy Eastman
Developmental Editor: Varun Gopal

Veterinary Clinics of North America: Small Animal Practice (ISSN 0195-5616) is published bimonthly by Elsevier Inc., 360 Park Avenue South, New York, NY 10010-1710. Months of issue are January, March, May, July, September, and November. Business and Editorial Offices: 1600 John F. Kennedy Blvd., Ste. 1800, Philadelphia, PA 19103-2899. Customer Service Office: 3251 Riverport Lane, Maryland Heights, MO 63043. Periodicals postage paid at New York, NY and additional mailing offices. Subscription prices are $391.00 per year (domestic individuals), $100.00 per year (domestic students/residents), $503.00 per year (Canadian individuals), $544.00 per year (international individuals), $100.00 per year (Canadian students/residents), and $220.00 per year (international students/residents). For institutional access pricing please contact Customer Service via the contact information below. To receive student/resident rate, orders must be accompanied by name of affiliated institution, date of term, and the *signature* of program/residency coordinator on institution letterhead. Orders will be billed at individual rate until proof of status is received. Foreign air speed delivery is included in all *Clinics* subscription prices. All prices are subject to change without notice. **POSTMASTER:** Send address changes to *Veterinary Clinics of North America: Small Animal Practice*, Elsevier Health Sciences Division, Subscription Customer Service, 3251 Riverport Lane, Maryland Heights, MO 63043. Customer Service (orders, claims, online, change of address): Elsevier Periodicals Customer Service, Elsevier Health Sciences Division Subscription **Customer Service 3251 Riverport Lane Maryland Heights, MO 63043. Tel: 1-800-654-2452 (U.S. and Canada); 314-447-8871 (outside U.S. and Canada). Fax: 314-447-8029. E-mail: journalscustomerservice-usa@elsevier.com (for print support); journalsonlinesupport-usa@elsevier.com (for online support).**

Reprints. For copies of 100 or more of articles in this publication, please contact the Commercial Reprints Department, Elsevier Inc., 360 Park Avenue South, New York, NY 10010-1710. Tel.: 212-633-3874; Fax: 212-633-3820; E-mail: reprints@elsevier.com.

Veterinary Clinics of North America: Small Animal Practice is also published in Japanese by Inter Zoo Publishing Co., Ltd., Aoyama Crystal-Bldg 5F, 3-5-12 Kitaaoyama, Minato-ku, Tokyo 107-0061, Japan.

Veterinary Clinics of North America: Small Animal Practice is covered in *Current Contents/Agriculture, Biology and Environmental Sciences, Science Citation Index, ASCA, MEDLINE/PubMed (Index Medicus), Excerpta Medica,* and *BIOSIS.*

Contributors

EDITOR

CARLO SIRACUSA, DVM, MS, PhD
Diplomate, American College of Veterinary Behaviorists; Diplomate, European
College of Animal Welfare and Behavior Medicine; Associate Professor of Clinical
Animal Behavior and Welfare, Department of Clinical Sciences and Advanced Medicine,
School of Veterinary Medicine, University of Pennsylvania, Philadelphia, Pennsylvania,
USA

AUTHORS

MARIANGELA ALBERTINI, DVM, PhD
Associate Professor, Department of Veterinary Medicine and Animal Sciences, University
of Milan, Via dell'Università, Lodi, Italy

MARTA AMAT, DVM, PhD
Diplomate, European College of Animal Welfare and Behavioural Medicine; School of
Veterinary Medicine, Universitat Autónoma de Barcelona, Spain

DANIELLE BERGER
The Penn Vet Working Dog Center, Philadelphia, Pennsylvania, USA

JONATHAN BOWEN, BVetMed, MRCVS, Dip (AS)CABC
Queen Mother Hospital for Small Animals, Royal Veterinary College, North Mymms,
Hertfordshire, United Kingdom

MAYA BRAEM, DR MED VET
Diplomate, European College of Animal Welfare and Behavioural Medicine (Behavioural
Medicine); Veterinary Hospital, University of Zürich, Zürich, Switzerland

FERGUS M. COUTTS, BVM&S, MSc, MRCVS
Pain Management and Rehabilitation Centre, Broadleys Veterinary Hospital, Stirling,
United Kingdom

LETICIA M.S. DANTAS, DVM, MS, PhD
Diplomate, American College of Veterinary Behaviorists; Certified Fear Free Professional,
Member of the Fear Free Advisory Board, Clinical Assistant Professor, Department of
Biomedical Sciences, Behavioral Medicine Service, University of Georgia Veterinary
Teaching Hospital, Athens, Georgia, USA

SAGI DENENBERG, DVM, MRCVS
Diplomate, American College of Veterinary Behaviorists; Diplomate, European College of
Animal Welfare and Behaviour Medicine; Recognised Specialist in Veterinary Behavioural
Medicine, North Toronto Veterinary Behaviour Specialty Clinic, Richmond Hill, Ontario,
Canada

DANA EBBECKE, BA
The Penn Vet Working Dog Center, Philadelphia, Pennsylvania, USA

JAUME FATJÓ, DVM, PhD
Diplomate, European College of Animal Welfare and Behaviour Medicine (Behaviour Medicine); Affinity Foundation Chair for Animals and Health, Autonomous University of Barcelona and Institut Hospital del Mar d'Investigacions Mèdiques, Barcelona, Spain

HAGAR HAUSER, DVM
Diplomate, American College of Veterinary Behaviorists; Metropolitan Veterinary Associates, Norristown, Pennsylvania, USA

DEBRA HORWITZ, DVM
Diplomate, American College of Veterinary Behaviorists; Veterinary Behavior Consultations, St Louis, Missouri, USA

GARY M. LANDSBERG, DVM
Diplomate, American College of Veterinary Behaviorists; Diplomate, European College of Animal Welfare and Behaviour Medicine; CanCog Inc, Fergus, Ontario, Canada

SUSANA LE BRECH, DVM, MSc, PhD
School of Veterinary Medicine, Universitat Autónoma de Barcelona, Spain

AMY LEARN, VMD
Diplomate, American College of Veterinary Behaviorists, Animal Behavior Wellness Center, Richmond, Virginia, USA

M. LEANNE LILLY, DVM
Diplomate, American College of Veterinary Behaviorists; Assistant Professor-Clinical, Department of Clinical Sciences, College of Veterinary Medicine, The Ohio State University, Columbus, Ohio, USA

KAREN L. MACHIN, DVM, PhD
Department of Veterinary Biomedical Sciences, Western College of Veterinary Medicine, University of Saskatchewan, Saskatoon, Saskatchewan, Canada

XAVIER MANTECA, DVM, PhD
Diplomate, European College of Animal Welfare and Behavioural Medicine; School of Veterinary Medicine, Universitat Autónoma de Barcelona, Spain

KEVIN J. MCPEAKE, BVMS, PGDip(CABC), PhD, AFHEA, CCAB, MRCVS
Diplomate, European College of Animal Welfare and Behavioural Medicine (Behavioural Medicine); The Royal (Dick) School of Veterinary Studies, Midlothian, United Kingdom

DANIEL S. MILLS, BVSc, PhD, CBiol, FRSB, FHEA, CCAB, FRCVS, RCVS
Diplomate, European College of Animal Welfare and Behavioural Medicine (Behavioural Medicine); Animal Behaviour Cognition and Welfare Group, Department of Life Sciences, University of Lincoln, Lincoln, United Kingdom

NIWAKO OGATA, BVSc, PhD
Diplomate, American College of Veterinary Behaviorists; Certified Fear Free Professional, Member of the Fear Free Advisory Board, Associate Professor, Veterinary Behavior Medicine, Department of Clinical Sciences, Purdue University, West Lafayette, Indiana, USA

CYNTHIA OTTO, DVM, PhD
Diplomate, American College of Veterinary Emergency and Critical Care; Diplomate, American College of Veterinary Sports Medicine and Rehabilitation; The Penn Vet Working Dog Center, Philadelphia, Pennsylvania, USA

LUDOVICA PIERANTONI, DVM
Diplomate, European College of Animal Welfare and Behavioural Medicine (Behavioural Medicine); Veterinary Behaviour and Consulting Services at CAN Training Centre, Naples, Italy

PATRIZIA PIOTTI, DVM, MSc, PhD
Department of Veterinary Medicine and Animal Sciences, University of Milan, Lodi, Italy

FEDERICA PIRRONE, DVM, PhD
Associate Professor, Department of Veterinary Medicine and Animal Sciences, University of Milan, Lodi, Italy

LENA PROVOOST, DVM
Diplomate, American College of Veterinary Behaviorists; Lecturer of Animal Behavior and Welfare, Clinical Sciences and Advanced Medicine, University of Pennsylvania, Philadelphia, Pennsylvania, USA

LISA RADOSTA, DVM
Diplomate, American College of Veterinary Behaviorists; Florida Veterinary Behavior Service, West Palm Beach, Florida, USA

CARLO SIRACUSA, DVM, MS, PhD
Diplomate, American College of Veterinary Behaviorists; Diplomate, European College of Animal Welfare and Behavior Medicine; Associate Professor of Clinical Animal Behavior and Welfare, Department of Clinical Sciences and Advanced Medicine, School of Veterinary Medicine, University of Pennsylvania, Philadelphia, Pennsylvania, USA

VALARIE V. TYNES, DVM
Diplomate, American College of Veterinary Behaviorists; Diplomate, American College of Animal Welfare; SPCA of Texas, Dallas, Texas, USA

CLARA WILSON, BSc, MSc, PhD
The Penn Vet Working Dog Center, Philadelphia, Pennsylvania, USA

Contents

 Video content accompanies this article at http://www.vetsmall.
theclinics.com.

> Sickness is a normal response to infections or stress triggered by proin-
> flammatory cytokines that drive local and systemic inflammatory re-
> sponses. Proinflammatory cytokines act on the brain causing the so
> called "sickness behavior,"which is thought to improve recovery but can
> become maladaptive in the long term. Chronic inflammation characterizes
> many diseases and there is some evidence that dogs and cats experience
> age-associated increases in inflammation, a condition named "inflammag-
> ing." A complex and multifactorial relationship exists between these in-
> flammatory mechanisms, pain, and psychological illness that may
> complicate veterinary diagnosis and affect the outcome.

> Like many physical disorders, the clinical signs associated with metabolic
> diseases affecting thyroid, adrenal, and pancreatic function are reflective
> of nonspecific changes in behavior. Additionally, patients who have under-
> lying disorders associated with fear, anxiety, stress, conflict, and/or panic
> may be under treatment with medications that alter basal thyroid, glucose,
> and cortisol levels. Through reinforcement and punishment of behaviors
> associated with clinical signs caused by organic or iatrogenic endocrine
> disease, behaviors can be perpetuated and become persistent patterns.
> Screening all patients presenting with a primary behavior complaint or
> those with behavioral clinical signs of endocrine diseases is essential. Al-
> leviating stress immediately while working up or treating metabolic disease
> reduces suffering and may stave off the adoption of behavior patterns
> more permanently.

 Video content accompanies this article at http://www.vetsmall.
theclinics.com

> The condition of separation-related problems (SRPs) is common in com-
> panion dogs and clinicians should be comfortable diagnosing it. There
> are numerous diagnoses related to physical disease that have clinical
> signs similar to SRP, that exacerbate SRP, or may cause regression in
> treatment of SRP. Common examples include conditions affecting the

following systems: musculoskeletal, neurologic, gastrointestinal, and dermatologic. Therefore, it is important for clinicians to rule out causes of physical disease and address them accordingly. The signalment of the patient, medications they are receiving, and other behavioral comorbidities should also be considered.

significant influence on their overall health, behavior, and ability to perform their working role effectively.

Behavior changes may indicate primary physical disease or primary behavioral disorders in veterinary patients. It is imperative to recognize that secondary behavioral problems can develop due to medical causes. The incidence of systemic disease increases with age and behavior manifestations can be similar to those expected with cognitive dysfunction syndrome. In this article, we review basic concepts of cognition, aging, and cognitive dysfunction syndrome. Additionally, we provide information regarding factors that influence cognition, and the role medical conditions have on the behavior of aging pets.

Inappropriate elimination or behavioral periuria/perichezia is likely the most reported feline behavioral problem worldwide. A change in behavior is often one of the early signs of physical disease and in addition can aggravate an existing behavioral response. An initial determination of causation is essential; is it medical or behavioral, or a combination of both? Stress activates both the sympathetic adrenomedullary system for short-term responses and the hypothalamic pituitary adrenal axis for long-term responses. Once medical problems have been treated or ruled out, attention should shift to minimizing and using various therapeutic options to help improve and/or resolve undesirable elimination problems.

The health of the skin and coat of a cat is connected to the behavioral health of the animal. Stressed animals can cause lesions to their skin and coat such as alopecia, ulcers, and self-mutilation. On the other hand, localized or systemic health problems can cause stress, or pain, and therefore can increase overgrooming and poor skin health. When treating overgrooming and related skin lesions, all the physical and behavioral causes must be addressed through a multimodal approach.

In cats, age-related pathologic condition and neurologic degeneration can produce changes in activity, vocalization, appearance, appetite, litter box use, sleep–wake cycle, personality, and cognitive ability. These changes can influence the relationship between owner and pet. Although cognitive dysfunction syndrome (CDS) can cause altered behavior later in life, other medical or behavioral causes may mimic these clinical signs or complicate diagnosis. Management and treatment of CDS can be accomplished through pharmacologic intervention, diet and nutritional supplementation, and environmental enrichment aimed at slowing the progression of the disease.

Valarie V. Tynes

Behavioral and physical health are intricately interconnected in most animals, and the rabbit is no different. Medical or physical conditions can lead to anxiety and stress, and anxiety and stress can lead to physical illness. Rabbits are very prone to fear, anxiety, and stress, especially when their husbandry is not appropriate and their environmental and behavioral needs are not met. Any rabbit presenting for acute behavior changes should be examined thoroughly for underlying medical conditions and the appropriateness of their environment examined equally closely. Physical health is unlikely to exist without behavioral and/or emotional health and vice versa.

Maya Braem

Sensory processing sensitivity (SPS) is a personality trait described in humans and dogs that mediates how individuals are affected by experiences. It involves being aware of subtle stimuli, high emotional intensity and empathy, and deeper processing of information. Recognizing individuals scoring higher in SPS is likely to help better diagnose, treat, and prevent both psychological (behavioral) and physical problems, leading to increased welfare and quality of life of the animal and its surroundings.

Leticia M.S. Dantas and Niwako Ogata

The stress response affects the central nervous system and multiple other systems in the body. Chronic mental and behavioral pathologies are associated with inflammation, dysfunctions in the immune response and an increased risk for other chronic inflammatory and metabolic diseases. Psychiatric treatments alleviate fear, stress and anxiety, increase the quality of life and lifespan for dogs and cats. Multiple safe psychoactive medications that can be used in association are available to help veterinary patients. Clinicians should understand the function of neurotransmitters and hormones on emotional processing, cognition and behavior, and drug mechanism of action so medication selection is appropriate for each individual patient.

VETERINARY CLINICS OF NORTH AMERICA: SMALL ANIMAL PRACTICE

SERIES OF RELATED INTEREST

Veterinary Clinics: Exotic Animal Practice
https://www.vetexotic.theclinics.com/
Advances in Small Animal Care
https://www.advancesinsmallanimalcare.com/

THE CLINICS ARE NOW AVAILABLE ONLINE!
Access your subscription at:
www.theclinics.com

Preface

The False Dichotomy Between Medical and Behavioral Problems

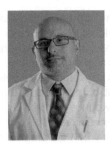

Carlo Siracusa, DVM, PhD
Editor

Approaching veterinary behavior problems as diagnoses of exclusion is unfortunately not rare. In such cases, after having ran multiple diagnostic tests and not having found any remarkable results, the veterinary clinician concludes "there is nothing medical… it has to be behavioral!" I envisioned this issue of *Veterinary Clinics of North America: Small Animal Practice* to help resolve this false dichotomy.

Medicine is the practice of preventing, diagnosing, and treating disease, and behavior is an integral part of medicine rather than an alternative to medicine. Changes in behavior are always among the signs of disease, and often they are the signs that induce caregivers to bring their pet to the veterinary clinic. The branch of veterinary medicine that diagnoses and treats disease manifesting primarily through behavioral signs is behavior medicine. Therefore, we have elected in this issue to differentiate between behavioral and physical or organic signs of disease, rather than between behavioral and medical signs of disease, when appropriate.

Although diseases always manifest through both behavioral and physical signs, behavioral signs are more salient than physical signs in some cases and vice versa. Like physical signs, behavioral signs are caused by underlying anatomical and physiological changes. As much as physical signs, behavioral signs of disease must be taken into account in the clinical reasoning process.

The articles in this issue review some clinical presentations common in general practice, discuss their etiopathogenesis, and describe both their behavioral and their physical signs. Part of these presentations, such as separation-related problems or aggression, fall commonly under the umbrella of behavior medicine, because very salient behavior signs characterize them. Others, like pain or metabolic disease, are commonly ascribed to other branches, like orthopedics or internal medicine.

Vet Clin Small Anim 54 (2024) xiii–xiv
https://doi.org/10.1016/j.cvsm.2023.09.005
0195-5616/24/© 2023 Published by Elsevier Inc.

Going through this collection of articles, the reader will first explore how the immune system regulates the behavioral and physical phenomena associated with animal health and disease. Field experts will then guide the reader through a series of clinical presentations of dogs, cats, and rabbits, including metabolic diseases, separation-related problems, aggression, pain and discomfort, abnormal repetitive behaviors, inappropriate elimination, skin disease, and cognitive changes associated with physical disease and aging. An article on the popular topic of veterinary psychopharmacology follows.

To close this issue, the reader will explore how individual animals process internal and external stimuli in very different ways, and why these individual differences are relevant in our daily clinical practice. Traditional western veterinary medicine taught us that animal disease is an objective phenomenon that all animals experience in a similar way. Entire experiments on animal disease, often used as translational models for human disease, rely on the assumption that animals are input-output models that process disease with negligible differences. A growing body of evidence on the differences in how individual animals experience internal and external stimuli, and therefore disease, is developing. We must never discount this individuality when we diagnose and treat our patients.

In conclusion, the goal of this issue of *Veterinary Clinics of North America: Small Animal Practice* is to foster an understanding of behavior as an integral part of medicine, in which disease is considered as a whole phenomenon with integrated behavioral and physical signs, which are regulated by underlying common pathophysiological processes. I hope readers will enjoy the issue and the valuable contributions of our authors.

CONFLICT OF INTEREST/DISCLOSURES

The author has no conflicts of interest to disclose.

Carlo Siracusa, DVM, PhD
Department of Clinical Sciences
and Advanced Medicine
School of Veterinary Medicine
University of Pennsylvania
3900 Delancey Street
Philadelphia, PA 19104, USA

E-mail address:
siracusa@vet.upenn.edu

Inflammation and Behavior Changes in Dogs and Cats

Patrizia Piotti, DVM, MSc, PhD[a,1],
Ludovica Pierantoni, DVM, ECAWBM (Behavioural Medicine)[b,1],
Mariangela Albertini, DVM, PhD[a,*], Federica Pirrone, DVM, PhD[a]

KEYWORDS

- Inflammation • Behavior changes • Aging • Domestic dogs • Domestic cats

KEY POINTS

- Inflammation is a series of complex response events caused by the host system facing infection or injury.
- Inflammation responses are driven by proinflammatory cytokines that are released peripherally but also act centrally on the brain causing the behavioral symptoms of sickness.
- Sickness behavior results both from peripheral (eg, infection) and central (eg, psychological) pathways.
- Proinflammatory cytokines play a major role in inflammation that represents a significant risk factor for morbidity and mortality in the elderly animals.

 Video content accompanies this article at http://www.vetsmall.theclinics.com.

INTRODUCTION

It is noticeable that behavior changes are among the first and most important issues related to inflammatory activity. Proinflammatory cytokines are known to be cell signaling molecules that guide an organism's response to illness, injury, and infection.[1] Therefore, inflammation is traditionally perceived as associated with acute or chronic medical disorders.[1] Nevertheless, potent broad-spectrum inflammogens, such as the bacterial endotoxin lipopolysaccharide (LPS), have been shown to induce in rodents depressive-like symptoms, often known as "sickness behaviors" (SB), potentially arisen from an interaction between the immune system and the serotonine (5-HT) system.[2] Cytokines, such as interferon-alpha, tumor necrosis factor alpha,

[a] Department of Veterinary Medicine and Animal Sciences, University of Milan, Via dell'Università, 6, Lodi 26900, Italy; [b] Veterinary Behaviour & Consulting Services at CAN Training Centre, Via Camaldolilli, 79, Naples 80128, Italy
[1] These authors contributed equally to this article.
* Corresponding author.
E-mail address: mariangela.albertini@unimi.it

Vet Clin Small Anim 54 (2024) 1–16
https://doi.org/10.1016/j.cvsm.2023.08.006
0195-5616/24/© 2023 Elsevier Inc. All rights reserved.

interleukin (IL)-1 and IL-2, signal to the brain the presence of an infection in the periphery[3] eliciting the sickness behavior through an endocrine mechanism or direct neural transmission.[4] Originally described by Hart,[5] cytokine-induced SB occurs in birds and mammals, including dogs and cats, as part of an adaptive, motivational response to preserve energy and help in recovery from infection.[4]

Inflammation-induced SB refers to both nonspecific clinical and behavioral signs that include fatigue, sleepiness, vomiting, diarrhea, anorexia, or decreased food and/or water intake, fever, decreased general and body-care activities (ie, grooming), social withdrawal or loss of interest in social activities, and altered cognition. In addition, enhanced pain-like behaviors are often observed, although these can be followed by hypoalgesia during the latest stages of sickness. In humans, proinflammatory cytokines have been reported to induce not only symptoms of sickness, but also true major depressive disorders in vulnerable subjects, even without previous history of mental disorders.[6] All these signs have been shown to be independent of the febrile response.[7] In fact, not only infections but also the chronic activation of the stress response system can overtax homeostatic regulatory systems, resulting in SB.[8] In dogs and cats, the hypothalamus-pituitary–adrenal (HPA) axis and the stress response may be activated by external environmental events such as sudden changes, unknown or loud noises, novel and unfamiliar places and objects, and the approach of strangers, or even by psychological stressors.[9,10] Similarly to infection, environmental and psychological stressors may be linked to immune activation and proinflammatory cytokine release[11,12] as well as to changes in mood and pathologic pain (**Fig. 1–3**).[8,9,13]

INFLAMMATION AND THE BRAIN

The brain monitors the peripheral innate immune response using different immune-to-brain communication pathways[14–18] that act in parallel and, when activated, lead to the production of proinflammatory cytokines by central nervous system (CNS) parenchymal macrophages, called local microglial macrophages. The receptors for these mediators are expressed by both neuronal and non-neuronal brain cells,[12] but the brain circuitry that mediates the behavioral effects of cytokines remains mostly unclear. It seems highly probable that different behaviors observed in cytokine-induced SB are controlled by different brain areas: this means that, for example, the social withdrawal observed in case of infection likely involves different areas than those involved in the loss of appetite[19] or in the activation of the HPA axis.[20]

Many SB-related abnormalities, such as states of anxiety and feeding difficulties, have been reported in family dogs and cats after the exposure to unusual external events, including changes in caretaking and daily routine, or psychological stress, regardless of the presence of physical disease (**Table 1**).[31] Therefore, veterinary clinicians should consider the possibility of exposure to environmental and/or psychological stressors in dogs and cats assessed for SB signs.

The view of this behavioral complex as the expression of a motivational state has important implications in terms of allostasis, which represents the ability of the individual of balancing a whole of internal and external stimuli (allostatic load) before there are negative effects on its welfare (allostatic overload)[32] homeostasis. Different motivational states of SB, such as fear, hunger or thirst, or fighting infectious pathogens, have different physiologic requirements and their own regulatory systems, but they can act together and each combination will exert a different pressure on the behavioral and physical health of an animal. Therefore, the clinician will have to strive to individuate the possible causes behind SB and how their interaction is affecting the health and welfare of the patient.

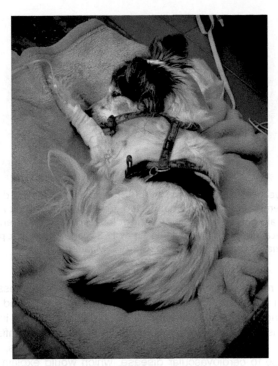

Fig. 1. Sickness behavior in a 17-year-old dog with acute pyelonephritis. The dog's reactivity, feeding, and social behavior are reduced, resting, and apathy increases. (*Courtesy of* Patrizia Piotti DVM, MSc, PhD, MRCVS. Milan, Italy).

From an evolutionary perspective, the behavioral effects of cytokines in response to acute stressors are beneficial for an organism. In response to an infection, individuals seek rest and care, which is advantageous as it favors recovery, therefore allowing shifting to a state of increased arousal and readiness for action when they are

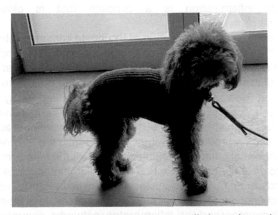

Fig. 2. Cowering behavior and painful posture in a poodle brought to the behavior consult for fear and anxiety. The history and further examinations revealed an old fracture of the right foreleg and dysplasia of the left knee. (*Courtesy of* Ludovica Pierantoni DVM, ECAWBM - Behavioral Medicine. Naples, Italy).

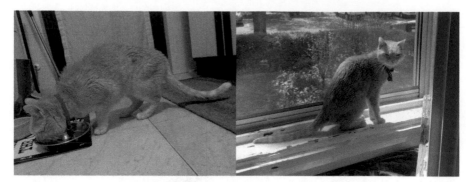

Fig. 3. Left: A 16-year-old cat with hyperthyroidism and chronic kidney disease (CKD)International Renal Interest Society (IRIS) 3 manifested an increased activity levels and decreased appetite (behavioral signs) associated with weight loss, moderate to severe sarcopenia, and dehydration (physical signs). Right: the same cat at 17.5 years. An antalgic posture is evident. (*Courtesy of* Patrizia Piotti DVM, MSc, PhD, MRCVS. Milan, Italy).

confronted with a real or potential threat favors. Conversely, if sickness is prolonged or exaggerated with respect to the causal factors that have triggered it, the sickness response is no longer adaptive, as it typically occurs during chronic inflammatory disease. In these cases, inappropriate, prolonged activation of proinflammatory cytokines may be involved in brain and systemic disorders, ranging from Alzheimer'sdisease to cardiovascular disease, which would explain changes in the mental state and cognition of affected-individuals.[3] Moreover, chronic inflammation is involved in the pathogenesis of many diseases associated with aging. Aging is reported as potentially increasing the risk for SB also in non-human animals, one example is cats with interstitial cystitis.[31] Given the exceptional growth in the worldwide dogs and cats population age, recognizing the effects of inflammation on behavior changes of elderly pets has broad animal health implications.

INFLAMMATION AND AGE (INFLAMMAGING)

Low-grade sterile inflammation is a process that is closely related to immunosenescence.[33]

Immunosenescence is the dysregulation of the innate immune system that occurs in elderly individuals[34] and predisposes them to increased morbidity and mortality due to infection and age-related pathology.[35] In human medicine, the most consistent findings of recent studies show an age-related impairment of the cell-mediated immune function.[36] Moreover, decreased T cell proliferation has been recognized as a peculiarity of immunosenescence in cats[37] dogs,[38] horses,[39] and humans.[40] Reduced blood CD4(+) T cells (with imbalance in Th1 *versus* Th2 functional activity), elevation in the CD8(+) subset, and reduction in the CD4:CD8 ratio are also reported in senior dogs and cats. Conversely, the dysregulated activity of the innate immune system at brain level leads to an enhanced production of proinflammatory cytokines, such as IL-6, and a decreased production of anti-inflammatory cytokines, such as IL-10.[41] A large part of the aging phenotype, including immunosenescence, is explained by an imbalance between inflammatory and anti-inflammatory networks, occurring in the absence of overt infection, which results in a status of chronic, low-grade inflammation, called inflammaging.[41] Initially defined by Franceschi and colleagues in 2000,[42] inflammaging became the focus of many subsequent studies, which in the last decade have

Table 1 Most common and evidence-based indicators of conditions associated with behavioral changes[21–30]		
Medical Conditions and Behavior Changes		
Medical conditions[a,b]	Behavioral changes	
Pain	Loss of normal behavior	Development of new behavior
	Decreased ambulation or activity Decreased interaction with other pets and people Lethargy Loss of appetite Decreased resting behavior/ decreased sleep	Aggressive behavior House-soiling Fearful behavior Vocalization Altered posture and facial expressions Restlessness and repetitive behavior
Endocrine conditions		
Hypothyroidism		Aggressive behavior (dogs)
Hyperthyroidism		Aggressive behavior (cats), typically above the age of 13 years
Neurologic conditions	Absence of neurologic changes in imaging or laboratory examinations (caused by tumors of frontal regions of the brain)	Absence of neurologic, imaging, or laboratory examinations (caused by idiopathic epilepsy, mild traumatic brain injury[TBI], transient ischemia)
Behavioral changes typically associated with age-related cognitive dysfunction[c] but present an earlier age of onset compared to that associated with typical age-degeneration (below 10 years)		Fear and anxiety and cognitive (associated with epilepsy) Unknown association between TBI and behavior changes Unknown association between transient ischemic attacks and behavior changes

As a general rule, if there is a sudden change in the behavior of an adult animal, which is not justified by causes in the social or physical environment, then a medical cause should be suspected and investigated.

[a] All cases of aggressive behavior in dogs should be checked for hypothyroidism (elevated serum thyroid-stimulating homone (TSH) and reduced free-T4) due to all described cases in the literature having normal patterns and contextualized behavior.

[b] Neurologic conditions can be associated with behavioral changes and a) changes in the neurologic examination, with changes in the laboratory and/or imaging work-up (eg, brain tumors, brain ischemia, traumatic injuries); b) and changes in the neurologic examination, but without having changes in the work-up (lysosomal storage diseases, degenerative problems). These 2 categories may be considered neurologic cases, commonly diagnosed and treated by neurologists.

[c] Signs associated with age-related cognitive dysfunction are described by the acronym DISHAA: that is, disorientation, altered interactions, altered sleep-wake cycle, house-soiling, altered activity levels, anxiety.

brought significant progress in knowledge of this condition.[43] Inflammaging is characterized by the following 5 states[44]: low-grade, controlled, asymptomatic, chronic, and systemic. Normally, inflammatory responses fade away when proinflammatory factors in infection and tissue injuries are eliminated and then turn into a highly active and balanced state known as "resolving inflammation."[45] Conversely, the inflammation during inflammaging is in an uncontrolled and unbalanced state, named "nonresolving inflammation."[45] Such imbalance can be a major driving force for frailty and common age-related pathologies,[41] including the nervous and the musculoskeletal system.[33] It ultimately has negative impacts on metabolism, bone density, strength, exercise toler-ance, vascular system, cognitive function, and mood. Up to this date, inflammaging is considered a key factor in acceleration of the aging process and lifespan and, in humans, it is highly related to conditions including Alzheimer's disease,[46] Parkinson's disease, acute lateral sclerosis, multiple sclerosis, atherosclerosis, heart disease, age-related macular degeneration,[47] type II diabetes,[48] osteoporosis and insulin resis-tance,[49] cancer, and other diseases. Overall, inflammaging increases morbidity and mortality, seriously impairing the health and the quality of life of patients.[49] Although this has not been studied systematically yet, empirical observations in veterinary clinics and owners' reports suggest that this phenomenon also affects the quality of life and welfare of elderly dogs and cats.[36,50] It has also been suggested that chronic stress, through the effect on immunomodulation, might have a role on the onset of naturally occurring oncologic conditions in those species.[10]

PATHOPHYSIOLOGY OF INFLAMMAGING

As already anticipated, inflammaging implies elevated levels of circulating proinflam-matory cytokines,[51] including IL-6, IL-1β, IL-15, IL-18, TNF-α mRNA, and TNF-α pro-tein,[52] which, through different biochemical reactions and pathways,[53] induce the production of senescent cells. These cells must be effectively removed and replaced, otherwise their accumulation may contribute to the manifestations of aging. In turn, senescent cells secrete proinflammatory cytokines and other compounds,[54] devel-oping a senescence-associated secretory phenotype which contributes to the age-associated chronic low-grade inflammatory condition.

As mentioned earlier, chronic inflammation is a core-aging mechanism that appears to be relevant in the pathophysiology of tissues and organ systems, including brain tis-sue. There has been extensive investigation of age-associated neurodegenerative dis-ease in the dog. Chronic inflammation is involved in the loss of brain mass and function. Aberrant production of proinflammatory cytokines, including IL-1β, IL-6, and TNF-α, by microglia and astrocytes supports a neurotoxic milieu that contributes to neurodegeneration.[55,56] Signs of senescence have been detected in mammalian brains, highlighting their potential role in brain aging,[57] although information about the aged canine brain is still negligible. Conversely, some evidence of increased in-flammatory activity and gene expression patterns in aging canine brain tissue is available.[58]

Medicine is working toward the identification of suitable clinical markers which may help understand whether an organism's proinflammatory and anti-inflammatory status is in balance. Unfortunately, biological markers specific of the aging process have not yet been fully identified, which does not help in evaluating the degree of inflammaging. Based on the afore-mentioned underlying mechanisms, the most promising markers of inflammaging include immune cell markers (eg, CD8+ T cells, a decrease in CD4+ T cells and CD19+ B cells), serum cytokine markers (such as IL-1 and IL-10,[59] which have been identified in dogs and cats[36]), and microRNAs,[43] a class of molecules involved in the regulation of gene expression and biological pathways associated with inflammation, cellular senescence, and age-related diseases.[60]

THE CONCEPT OF ANTINFLAMMAGING

While inflammation could be beneficial to the organism by neutralizing an insult and restoring tissues early in life, it becomes detrimental in later years as inflammaging.[61] Inflammaging can be counter-acted by anti-inflammaging.[41] One of the endogenous counter-regulators recognized is cortisol.[62] However, besides being the main specific response and counterbalance to inflammaging, the activation of the HPA axis[63] becomes with chronic activation the cause of the decline of immunologic functions, leading from robustness to frailty.[64] Contrary to the altered inflammation markers level that signifies an earlier stage between cellular abnormalities and systems dysfunction, the frailty phenotype is an objectively measured indicator of advanced-stage aging that is characterized by organism-level dysfunction. Results from human observational studies and randomized controlled trials indicate that these objective measurements facilitate classification of older patients with chronic conditions into groups that vary in disease incidence, prognosis, and therapeutic response/toxicity.[65] In veterinary medicine, there has been given increasing attention to frailty in the assessment of aging dogs,[66–68] which is defined as a decline in an organism's physiologic reserves, resulting in increased vulnerability to stressors and a frailty index, which is directly related to survival and can be measured through scales[69] (a summary of frailty-related signs is presented in **Table 2**).[68]

To further complicate the picture, coexistence of immunosenescence and inflammaging[34] makes it difficult to establish whether the inflammation-related diseases are caused by one or the other process. Unfortunately, there is still need for integrated biological and clinical research before a causal relationship may be said to exist between inflammaging and diseases.[43]

While it is difficult to assess the degree of inflammaging in an individual, both human and veterinary medicine have focused on protective and preventative interventions. Several factors probably contribute to the increased inflammatory response in the elderly. Recent attention in geroscience has focused on alterations in cytokine receptor signaling,[73] the imbalance of redox factors,[74] changes in genotypes,[75] increased body fat,[76] and life-long antigenic exposure.[51] These are all likely candidates responsible for chronic immune system activation and inflammation associated to age, and acting against these factors would, therefore, help counter-act inflammaging. In humans, there is some evidence that antiaging interventions, such as exercise and dietary restriction, may mitigate inflammaging-related changes.[36,77] In the study of Alzheimer's disease, it has been observed that physical activity can improve neurogenesis and mitigate the age-related loss of brain mass both in the hippocampus and globally in the brain.[78] Similarly, veterinary medicine has started to recognize aging as a life-long process and healthy-aging as a goal that needs to be addressed early in life.[52] Aging research in veterinary medicine has brought some evidence that

Table 2
Frailty index proposed for dogs[23,70–72]

	Frailty
Domains	**Factors**
Physical condition (recorded by owner and veterinarian)	Body conditions score (BCS) Thigh girth deterioration (measure in cm) Unintentional weight loss (measure in Kg)
Physical activity	Customary activity (score form owner's observations) Gait speed(continuous duration in seconds)
Mobility	On leash/Off leash (continuous duration in seconds)
Strength	Climbing stairs (continuous duration in seconds)
Cognitive performance	Working memory (trails in cognitive tests) Learning behavior (score form owner's observations)
Mood and social relations	Anxiety/nervousness (score form owner's observations) Social avoidance (score form owner's observations)

environmental enrichments and physical activity might help preserve and ameliorate cognitive function in aging dogs,[79–81] while the effect of exercise on feline brain aging is still unexplored.[69]

INFLAMMATION AND BEHAVIOR FROM THE VETERINARY CLINICIAN'S PERSPECTIVE

Recently, several studies have suggested a causal link between ongoing inflammation and impaired mental health in humans.[6] Inflammation is considered a risk factor for depression and its correlation with behavior changes has been widely highlighted.[82] Dantzer and colleagues have reported that proinflammatory stimuli, such as LPS or IL-1β, increase activity in the tryptophan-metabolizing enzyme indoleamine 2,3-dioxygenase, resulting in lowered tryptophan availability and therefore decreased 5-HT synthesis.[6]

Psychological illness, including depression and anxiety disorders, and stress induce the same inflammation-related mechanisms and behavioral changes of sickness caused by diseases and infections[6] and might be responsible for the presence of an animal's SB.[5] For instance, SB has been shown to increase in cats with interstitial cystitis, for which a relationship to psychological stress has been well described.[83] Not only inflammatory and medical conditions in general have an important impact on the welfare of the animal, but they also have a role in the disruption of the human-animal bond and decisions such as relinquishment and euthanasia.[84–86]

Inflammation may also be linked to pain, by cyclooxygenase (COX) enzymes, mostly COX 2, which help synthesize prostaglandins found in elevated concentration at the inflammatory site.[87] In addition, there is evidence that cytokines (eg, IL-1β, TNF-α) are involved in the initiation as well as the maintenance of pain by directly activating nociceptive sensory neurons.[88] Pain-induced responses lead to several physiologic changes including a decreased serotonin activity in the brain,[87] that is also negatively influenced by the reduction of physical activity caused by pain.[89] Pain-induced alteration in motivation and emotional states results in a wide range of potential changes in behavior, that are the most commons sign of pain in itself[90] (**Fig. 4**, Video 1). Indeed, the modern approach to pain no longer focuses on measuring the intensity of pain but on subjective feelings[21,91,92] which, in non-human animals, should be based on the indirect evaluation through behavior changes and response to pain medication. The most common signs of pain are those related to a reduction of previously expressed behaviors and to the development of previously not expressed behaviors (See **Table 1**).[22]

A recent area of research explores the relationship between inflammation and aggressive behavior. Although there are relatively few small-scale studies so far, both peripheral cytokines and cytokines in the brain have been suggested to exert modulatory roles in aggressive behavior in non-human animals.[93] For example, activation of either the periaqueductal gray (PAG) or medial hypothalamus, which are known sites of localization of IL-1β, IL-2, and their receptors in the brain,[94,95] may functionally influence the aggressive response in cats.[96] In particular, the local administration of IL-1β and IL-2,[97] respectively, into the medial hypothalamus and PAG has been shown to induce aggressive behavior, causing cats to express behaviors such as hissing, pupillary dilatation, retraction of the ear, as well as increased blood pressure and heart rate in response to threat.[98] In dogs, a study on German shepherds presenting with aggressive behavior and no other clinical signs has indicated significantly higher serum levels of C-reactive protein and IL-6, when compared to matching dogs presenting with no aggressive behavior or other behavioral changes.[99] Additionally, there is increasing evidence of a relationship between inflammatory pathologies, such as

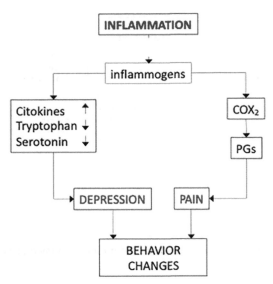

Fig. 4. The inflammation, depression, and pain cycle.

osteo-arthrosis and other osteo-muscular conditions, and behavior changes, including aggressive behavior.[21,23,100] It is not to be excluded that other behavior problems, like abnormal repetitive behavior, may also be caused or influenced by inflammation.[101] Further studies to examine the complex neural circuitry in which cytokines act to affect behaviors will be needed to understand the extent of these interactions. Meanwhile, it is advised that the clinician assesses for inflammatory and painful conditions in all animals presenting with a history of behavior problems.

Fundamentally, behavioral and medical diagnoses often coexist, as animal behavior reflects the individual physiologic state.[102] The traditional clinical approach to behavioral problems has been based on analyzing whether the behavioral changes were "purely behavioral" or secondary to physical conditions, excluded through comprehensive differential diagnoses. The potential influences of medical factors on behavior problems were viewed as diagnoses of exclusion.[103] More modern approaches consider behavior as an output of the whole behavior body system, which includes the central nervous system, but it is not limited to it. In other words, the display of specific behavior is one of the methods by which the individual seeks to establish equilibrium between internal factors, such as health, and the environment.[104] Any illness or treatment will have an effect on behavior, which should be kept into account, as behavioral and physical health are both components of an integrated system that should be managed and treated as a whole.[105] In parallel with human psychiatry and the multi-axis approach, veterinary clinicians are today encouraged to make a complete and exhaustive assessment of a case by collecting and organizing information about all the factors that, together, may contribute to behavioral and mental health problems in companion animals.[104] In veterinary behavioral medicine, efforts are made for referrals in different specialties in order to have a complete assessment of cases, to a more holistic collection of information regarding the management of the case, and to a synergetic vision regarding the therapy (Fig. 5). In addition, factors such as personality traits and social and physical environment have an influence on whether a particular individual will show a problem behavior[106] and even develop or display signs of illness.[10,50] In other words, it is essential to understand how behavioral

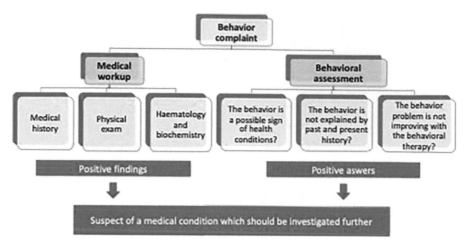

Fig. 5. Extended examinations and tests required during a behavioral assessment.

medicine and other specialties such as neurology, dermatology, gastroenterology, etc. are linked together to improve diagnosis and therapy process.[107–112]

SUMMARY

SB is evoked by proinflammatory cytokines released by macrophages, dendritic cells, and mast cells, which can trigger behavioral changes via the activation of sensory neurons or the secretion of immune signaling molecules from the microglia into the brain.[1–4] These pathways may be activated in response to infectious pathogens or stress,[8] particularly in the aged animals.[113] SB is therefore relevant in various contexts besides fighting infections. Behavioral changes include increased body temperature, sleep, loss of appetite as well as metabolism alterations causing weight loss. Sickness behavior and inflammation are possible factors to consider in the onset and maintenance of pain and should be viewed from a bio-psycho-social perspective.

CLINICS CARE POINTS

- Sickness behavior is a cytokine-mediated motivational adaptive response linked to infection and inflammation.
- Elderly animals present changes that are the result of the balance between inflammatory and anti-inflammatory activity in the body (senescence and inflammaging). There are no specific markers, therefore the behavior and the physical health of the animal need to be assessed.
- Overall, frailty should be assessed: physical condition (body condition score [BCS], muscular loss, weight loss), physical activity (decreased activity levels and gait speed), mobility on and off leash, strength, and cognitive changes (loss of memory, loss of learning), mood and social changes (anxiety, social avoidance).
- Frailty measures related to physical health should also be considered, including signs such as needing assistance standing up or eating, incontinence, sensory decline, osteo-muscular, metabolic, and dermatologic conditions.
- Physical and mental health are closely connected: behavioral and medical diagnoses often coexist.

- Veterinary clinicians should collect information about all the factors that may contribute to behavioral and mental health problems.
- Other factors such as personality traits and social and physical environment have an influence on whether a particular individual will show a problem behavior.

DISCLOSURE

The Authors have nothing to disclose.

SUPPLEMENTARY DATA

Supplementary data related to this article can be found online at https://doi.org/10.1016/j.cvsm.2023.08.006.

REFERENCES

1. Moieni M, Eisenberger NI. Effects of inflammation on social processes and implications for health: Effect of inflammation on social processes. Ann NY Acad Sci 2018;1428(1):5–13.
2. OConnor JC, Lawson MA, André C, et al. Lipopolysaccharide-induced depressive-like behavior is mediated by indoleamine 2,3-dioxygenase activation in mice. Mol Psychiatr 2009;14(5):511–22.
3. Dantzer R, Kelley KW. Twenty years of research on cytokine-induced sickness behavior. Brain Behav Immun 2007;21(2):153 60.
4. Kelley KW, Bluthé RM, Dantzer R, et al. Cytokine-induced sickness behavior. Brain Behav Immun 2003;17(1):112–8.
5. Hart BL. Biological basis of the behavior of sick animals. Neurosci Biobehav Rev 1988;12(2):123–37.
6. Dantzer R, O'Connor JC, Freund GG, et al. From inflammation to sickness and depression: when the immune system subjugates the brain. Nat Rev Neurosci 2008;9(1):46–56.
7. Kent S, Bluthe RM, Dantzer R, et al. Different receptor mechanisms mediate the pyrogenic and behavioral effects of interleukin 1. Proc Natl Acad Sci USA 1992;89(19):9117–20.
8. Miller AH, Maletic V, Raison CL. Inflammation and Its Discontents: The Role of Cytokines in the Pathophysiology of Major Depression. Biol Psychiatr 2009;65(9):732–41.
9. Ursin H, Eriksen HR. The cognitive activation theory of stress. Psychoneuroendocrinology 2004;29(5):567–92.
10. Cannas S, Berteselli GV, Piotti P, et al. Stress and Cancer in Dogs: Comparison Between a Population of Dogs Diagnosed with Cancer and a Control Population - A Pilot Study. Maced Vet Rev 2016;39(2):201–8.
11. Raison CL, Miller AH. When Not Enough Is Too Much: The Role of Insufficient Glucocorticoid Signaling in the Pathophysiology of Stress-Related Disorders. Aust J Pharm 2003;160(9):1554–65.
12. Ader Robert. Psychoneuroimmunology. 4th Edition. Academic Press; 2006.
13. Strouse TB. The relationship between cytokines and pain/depression: A review and current status. Curr Pain Headache Rep 2007;11(2):98–103.
14. Bluthé RM, Walter V, Parnet P, et al. Lipopolysaccharide induces sickness behaviour in rats by a vagal mediated mechanism. C R Acad Sci III 1994;317(6):499–503.

15. Watkins LR, Wiertelak EP, Goehler LE, et al. Neurocircuitry of illness-induced hyperalgesia. Brain Res 1994;639(2):283–99.
16. Romeo HE, Tio DL, Rahman SU, et al. The glossopharyngeal nerve as a novel pathway in immune-to-brain communication: relevance to neuroimmune surveillance of the oral cavity. J Neuroimmunol 2001;115(1–2):91–100.
17. Vitkovic L, Konsman JP, Bockaert J, et al. Cytokine signals propagate through the brain. Mol Psychiatr 2000;5(6):604–15.
18. Konsman JP, Vigues S, Mackerlova L, et al. Rat brain vascular distribution of interleukin-1 type-1 receptor immunoreactivity: Relationship to patterns of inducible cyclooxygenase expression by peripheral inflammatory stimuli. J Comp Neurol 2004;472(1):113–29.
19. Reyes TM, Sawchenko PE. Involvement of the arcuate nucleus of the hypothalamus in interleukin-1-induced anorexia. J Neurosci 2002;22(12):5091–9.
20. Ericsson A, Kovacs K, Sawchenko P. A functional anatomical analysis of central pathways subserving the effects of interleukin-1 on stress-related neuroendocrine neurons. J Neurosci 1994;14(2):897–913.
21. Piotti P, Albertini M, Lavesi E, et al. Physiotherapy Improves dogs' quality of life measured with the milan pet quality of life scale: is pain involved? Veterinary Sciences 2022;9(7):335.
22. Camps T, Amat M, Manteca X. A review of medical conditions and behavioral problems in dogs and cats. Animals 2019;9(12):1133.
23. Wrightson R, Albertini M, Pirrone F, et al. The Relationship between Signs of Medical Conditions and Cognitive Decline in Senior Dogs. Animals 2023; 13(13):2203.
24. Overall KL. Medical differentials with potential behavioral manifestations. Vet Clin Small Anim Pract 2003;33(2):213–29.
25. Bognár Z, Piotti P, Szabó D, et al. A novel behavioural approach to assess responsiveness to auditory and visual stimuli before cognitive testing in family dogs. Appl Anim Behav Sci 2020;228:105016.
26. Seibert LM, Landsberg GM. Diagnosis and management of patients presenting with behavior problems. Vet Clin Small Anim Pract 2008;38(5):937–50.
27. Foster ES, Carrillo JM, Patnaik AK. Clinical signs of tumors affecting the rostral cerebrum in 43 dogs. J Vet Intern Med 1988;2(2):71–4.
28. Shihab N, Bowen J, Volk HA. Behavioral changes in dogs associated with the development of idiopathic epilepsy. Epilepsy Behav 2011;21(2):160–7.
29. Packer RMA, McGreevy PD, Salvin HE, et al. Cognitive dysfunction in naturally occurring canine idiopathic epilepsy. PLoS One 2018;13(2):e0192182.
30. Fatjó J, Stub C, Manteca X. Four cases of aggression and hypothyroidism in dogs. Vet Rec 2002;151(18):547–8.
31. Stella JL, Lord LK, Buffington CAT. Sickness behaviors in response to unusual external events in healthy cats and cats with feline interstitial cystitis. JAVMA (J Am Vet Med Assoc) 2011;238(1):67–73.
32. Mushiake H. Neurophysiological perspective on allostasis and homeostasis: dynamic adaptation in viable systems. J Robot Mechatron 2022;34:710–7.
33. Franceschi C, Campisi J. Chronic Inflammation (Inflammaging) and Its Potential Contribution to Age-Associated Diseases. Journals of Gerontology Series A 2014;69(Suppl 1):S4–9.
34. Shaw AC, Goldstein DR, Montgomery RR. Age-dependent dysregulation of innate immunity. Nat Rev Immunol 2013;13(12):875–87.
35. Pawelec G, Adibzadeh M, Pohla H, et al. Immunosenescence: ageing of the immune system. Immunol Today 1995;16(9):420–2.

36. Day MJ. Ageing, Immunosenescence and Inflammageing in the Dog and Cat. J Comp Pathol 2010;142:S60–9.
37. Campbell D, Rawlings JM, Heaton PR, et al. Insulin-like growth factor-I (IGF-I) and its association with lymphocyte homeostasis in the ageing cat. Mech Ageing Dev 2004;125(7):497–505.
38. HogenEsch H, Thompson S, Dunham A, et al. Effect of age on immune parameters and the immune response of dogs to vaccines: a cross-sectional study. Vet Immunol Immunopathol 2004;97(1–2):77–85.
39. Horohov DW, Kydd JH, Hannant D. The effect of aging on T cell responses in the horse. Dev Comp Immunol 2002;26(1):121–8.
40. Pawelec G, Barnett Y, Forsey R, et al. T cells and aging january 2002 update. Front Biosci 2002;7(4):d1056–183.
41. Franceschi C, Capri M, Monti D, et al. Inflammaging and anti-inflammaging: A systemic perspective on aging and longevity emerged from studies in humans. Mech Ageing Dev 2007;128(1):92–105.
42. Franceschi C, Bonafè M, Valensin S, et al. Inflamm-aging: An Evolutionary Perspective on Immunosenescence. Ann N Y Acad Sci 2006;908(1):244–54.
43. Xia S, Zhang X, Zheng S, et al. An Update on Inflamm-Aging: Mechanisms, Prevention, and Treatment. Journal of Immunology Research 2016;2016:1–12.
44. Giunta S. Is inflammaging an auto[innate]immunity subclinical syndrome? Immun Ageing 2006;3(1):12.
45. Nathan C, Ding A. Nonresolving Inflammation. Cell 2010;140(6):871–82. https://doi.org/10.1016/j.cell.2010.02.029.
46. Giunta B, Fernandez F, Nikolic WV, et al. Inflammaging as a prodrome to Alzheimer's disease. J Neuroinflammation 2008;5(1):51.
47. Boren E, Gershwin ME. Inflamm-aging: autoimmunity, and the immune-risk phenotype. Autoimmun Rev 2004;3(5):401–6.
48. Franceschi C, Valensin S, Lescai F, et al. Neuroinflammation and the genetics of Alzheimer's disease: The search for a pro-inflammatory phenotype. Aging Clin Exp Res 2001;13(3):163–70.
49. Lencel P, Magne D. Inflammaging: The driving force in osteoporosis? Med Hypotheses 2011;76(3):317–21.
50. Piotti P, Karagiannis C, Satchell L, et al. Use of the Milan Pet Quality of Life Instrument (MPQL) to Measure Pets' Quality of Life during COVID-19. Animals 2021;11(5):1336.
51. De Martinis M, Franceschi C, Monti D, et al. Inflamm-ageing and lifelong antigenic load as major determinants of ageing rate and longevity. FEBS (Fed Eur Biochem Soc) Lett 2005;579(10):2035–9.
52. Adams AA, Breathnach CC, Katepalli MP, et al. Advanced age in horses affects divisional history of T cells and inflammatory cytokine production. Mech Ageing Dev 2008;129(11):656–64.
53. Sasaki M, Ikeda H, Sato Y, et al. Proinflammatory cytokine-induced cellular senescence of biliary epithelial cells is mediated via oxidative stress and activation of ATM pathway: A culture study. Free Radic Res 2008;42(7):625–32.
54. Freund A, Orjalo AV, Desprez PY, et al. Inflammatory networks during cellular senescence: causes and consequences. Trends Mol Med 2010;16(5):238–46.
55. Mattson MP, Arumugam TV. Hallmarks of brain aging: adaptive and pathological modification by metabolic states. Cell Metabol 2018;27(6):1176–99.
56. Yin F, Sancheti H, Patil I, et al. Energy metabolism and inflammation in brain aging and Alzheimer's disease. Free Radic Biol Med 2016;100:108–22.

57. Sikora E, Bielak-Zmijewska A, Dudkowska M, et al. Cellular Senescence in Brain Aging. Front Aging Neurosci 2021;13:646924. https://doi.org/10.3389/fnagi.2021.646924.
58. Head E. A canine model of human aging and Alzheimer's disease. Biochim Biophys Acta (BBA) - Mol Basis Dis 2013;1832(9):1384–9.
59. Minciullo PL, Catalano A, Mandraffino G, et al. Inflammaging and anti-inflammaging: the role of cytokines in extreme longevity. Arch Immunol Ther Exp 2016;64(2):111–26.
60. Olivieri F, Rippo MR, Monsurrò V, et al. MicroRNAs linking inflamm-aging, cellular senescence and cancer. Ageing Res Rev 2013;12(4):1056–68.
61. Miki C, Kusunoki M, Inoue Y, et al. Remodeling of the immunoinflammatory network system in elderly cancer patients: Implications of inflamm-aging and tumor-specific hyperinflammation. Surg Today 2008;38(10):873–8.
62. Dong J, Li J, Cui L, et al. Cortisol modulates inflammatory responses in LPS-stimulated RAW264.7 cells via the NF-κB and MAPK pathways. BMC Vet Res 2018;14(1):30.
63. Turnbull AV, Rivier CL. Regulation of the hypothalamic-pituitary-adrenal axis by cytokines: actions and mechanisms of action. Physiol Rev 1999;79(1):1–71.
64. Sergio G, Sergio G. Exploring the complex relations between inflammation and aging (inflamm-aging): anti-inflamm-aging remodelling of inflamm- aging, from robustness to frailty. Inflamm Res 2008;57(12):558–63.
65. Wu IC, Lin CC, Hsiung CA. Emerging roles of frailty and inflammaging in risk assessment of age-related chronic diseases in older adults: the intersection between aging biology and personalized medicine. BioMed 2015;5(1):1.
66. Hua J, Hoummady S, Muller C, et al. Assessment of frailty in aged dogs. AJVR (Am J Vet Res) 2016;77(12):1357–65.
67. Chen FL, Ullal TV, Graves JL, et al. Evaluating instruments for assessing health-span: a multi-center cross-sectional study on health-related quality of life (HRQL) and frailty in the companion dog. GeroScience 2023;13. https://doi.org/10.1007/s11357-023-00744-2.
68. Banzato T, Franzo G, Di Maggio R, et al. A Frailty Index based on clinical data to quantify mortality risk in dogs. Sci Rep 2019;9(1):16749.
69. Melvin RL, Ruple A, Pearson EB, et al. A review of frailty instruments in human medicine and proposal of a frailty instrument for dogs. Front Vet Sci 2023;10:1139308.
70. Mondino A, Khan M, Case B, et al. Activity patterns are associated with fractional lifespan, memory, and gait speed in aged dogs. Sci Rep 2023;13(1):2588.
71. Piotti P, Piseddu A, Aguzzoli E, et al. Two valid and reliable tests for monitoring age-related memory performance and neophobia differences in dogs. Sci Rep 2022;12(1):16175.
72. Tapp PD, Siwak CT, Estrada J, et al. Effects of age on measures of complex working memory span in the beagle dog (canis familiaris) using two versions of a spatial list learning paradigm. Learn Mem 2003;10(2):148–60.
73. Fulop T, Larbi A, Douziech N, et al. Cytokine receptor signalling and aging. Mech Ageing Dev 2006;127(6):526–37.
74. Chung HY, Sung B, Jung KJ, et al. The molecular inflammatory process in aging. Antioxidants Redox Signal 2006;8(3–4):572–81.
75. Grimble RF. Inflammatory response in the elderly. Curr Opin Clin Nutr Metab Care 2003;6(1):21–9.

76. Pedersen BK, Bruunsgaard H. Possible beneficial role of exercise in modulating low-grade inflammation in the elderly: Beneficial role of exercise in modulating low-grade inflammation. Scand J Med Sci Sports 2003;13(1):56–62.
77. Lawler DF, Larson BT, Ballam JM, et al. Diet restriction and ageing in the dog: major observations over two decades. Br J Nutr 2008;99(4):793–805.
78. Fabel K, Kempermann G. Physical Activity and the Regulation of Neurogenesis in the Adult and Aging Brain. Neuromol Med 2008;10(2):59–66.
79. Snigdha S, de Rivera C, Milgram NW, et al. Exercise enhances memory consolidation in the aging brain. Front Aging Neurosci 2014;6. https://doi.org/10.3389/fnagi.2014.00003.
80. Cotman CW, Berchtold NC. Physical activity and the maintenance of cognition: Learning from animal models. Alzheimer's Dementia 2007;3(2S). https://doi.org/10.1016/j.jalz.2007.01.013.
81. McKenzie BA. Comparative veterinary geroscience: mechanism of molecular, cellular, and tissue aging in humans, laboratory animal models, and companion dogs and cats. AJVR (Am J Vet Res) 2022;83(6). https://doi.org/10.2460/ajvr.22.02.0027.
82. Hughes MM, Carballedo A, McLoughlin DM, et al. Tryptophan depletion in depressed patients occurs independent of kynurenine pathway activation. Brain Behav Immun 2012;26(6):979–87.
83. Lai H, Gardner V, Vetter J, et al. Correlation between psychological stress levels and the severity of overactive bladder symptoms. BMC Urol 2015;15(1):14.
84. Duarte Cardoso S, Da Graça Pereira G, De Sousa L, et al. Factors behind the Relinquishment of Dogs and Cats by their Guardians In Portugal. J Appl Anim Welfare Sci 2022;1–12. https://doi.org/10.1080/10888705.2022.2087183. Published online June 13.
85. Pegram C, Gray C, Packer RMA, et al. Proportion and risk factors for death by euthanasia in dogs in the UK. Sci Rep 2021;11(1):9145.
86. Arome D, Onalike E, Sunday A, et al. Pain and inflammation: Management by conventional and herbal therapy. Indian J Pain 2014;28(1):5.
87. Chaouloff F. Effects of acute physical exercise on central serotonergic systems. Medicine &Science in Sports &amp Exercise 1997;29(1):58–62.
88. Özaktay AC, Kallakuri S, Takebayashi T, et al. Effects of interleukin-1 beta, interleukin-6, and tumor necrosis factor on sensitivity of dorsal root ganglion and peripheral receptive fields in rats. Eur Spine J 2006;15(10):1529–37.
89. Tsatsoulis A, Fountoulakis S. The Protective role of exercise on stress system dysregulation and comorbidities. Ann N Y Acad Sci 2006;1083(1):196–213.
90. Hellyer P, Rodan I, Brunt J, et al. AAHA/AAFP pain management guidelines for dogs and cats. J Feline Med Surg 2007;9(6):466–80.
91. Reid J, Scott EM, Calvo G, et al. Definitive Glasgow acute pain scale for cats: validation and intervention level. Vet Rec 2017;180(18):449.
92. Reid J, Wiseman-Orr L, Scott M. Shortening of an existing generic online health-related quality of life instrument for dogs: Measuring canine health-related quality of life. J Small Anim Pract 2018;59(6):334–42.
93. Takahashi A, Flanigan ME, McEwen BS, et al. Aggression, social stress, and the immune system in humans and animal models. Front Behav Neurosci 2018;12. https://doi.org/10.3389/fnbeh.2018.00056.
94. Hassanain M, Bhatt S, Zalcman S, et al. Potentiating role of interleukin-1β (IL-1β) and IL-1β type 1 receptors in the medial hypothalamus in defensive rage behavior in the cat. Brain Res 2005;1048(1–2):1–11.

95. Bhatt S, Zalcman S, Hassanain M, et al. Cytokine modulation of defensive rage behavior in the cat: Role of GABAa and interleukin-2 receptors in the medial hypothalamus. Neuroscience 2005;133(1):17–28.
96. Zalcman SS, Siegel A. The neurobiology of aggression and rage: Role of cytokines. Brain Behav Immun 2006;20(6):507–14.
97. Bhatt S, Siegel A. Potentiating role of interleukin 2 (IL-2) receptors in the midbrain periaqueductal gray (PAG) upon defensive rage behavior in the cat: Role of neurokinin NK1 receptors. Behav Brain Res 2006;167(2):251–60.
98. Siegel A, Roeling TAP, Gregg TR, et al. Neuropharmacology of brain-stimulation-evoked aggression. Neurosci Biobehav Rev 1999;23(3):359–89.
99. Re S, Zanoletti M, Emanuele E. Association of inflammatory markers elevation with aggressive behavior in domestic dogs. J Ethol 2009;27(1):31–3.
100. Barcelos AM, Mills DS, Zulch H. Clinical indicators of occult musculoskeletal pain in aggressive dogs. Vet Rec 2015;176(18):465.
101. Siracusa C, Provoost L, Lilly ML, et al. Compulsive self-licking and self-biting in dogs with paraesthesia: two cases. In: Denenberg S, editor. Proceedings of the 11th international veterinary behaviour meeting, 14-16th september 2017, samorin, Slovakia. 1st edition. CABI; 2017. p. 79–80. https://doi.org/10.1079/9781786394583.0079.
102. Herron ME. Advances in understanding and treatment of feline inappropriate elimination. Top Companion Anim Med 2010;25(4):195–202.
103. Overall KL. Natural models of human psychiatric conditions: assessment of mechanism and validity. Progress in neuro-psychopharmacology biological psychiatry 2000;24(727):776.
104. Fatjó J, Bowen J. Making the case for multi-axis assessment of behavioural problems. Animals 2020;10(3):383.
105. Uccheddu S. Management of specific fears and anxiety in the behavioural medicine of companion animals: punctual use of psychoactive medications. Dog Behavior 2019;5(2). https://doi.org/10.4454/db.v5i2.109.
106. Piotti P, Satchell LP, Lockhart TS. Impulsivity and behaviour problems in dogs: a reinforcement sensitivity theory perspective. Behav Process 2018;151:104–10.
107. Amadei E, Cantile C, Gazzano A, et al. The link between neurology and behavior in veterinary medicine: a review. Journal of Veterinary Behavior 2021;46:40–53.
108. Tynes VV, Sinn L. Abnormal repetitive behaviors in dogs and cats. Vet Clin Small Anim Pract 2014;44(3):543–64.
109. Mills DS, Demontigny-Bédard I, Gruen M, et al. Pain and problem behavior in cats and dogs. Animals 2020;10(2):318.
110. Bécuwe-Bonnet V, Bélanger MC, Frank D, et al. Gastrointestinal disorders in dogs with excessive licking of surfaces. Journal of Veterinary Behavior 2012;7(4):194–204.
111. Frank D. Recognizing behavioral signs of pain and disease. Vet Clin Small Anim Pract 2014;44(3):507–24.
112. Korte SM, Koolhaas JM, Wingfield JC, et al. The Darwinian concept of stress: benefits of allostasis and costs of allostatic load and the trade-offs in health and disease. Neurosci Biobehav Rev 2005;29(1):3–38.
113. Godbout JP, Chen J, Abraham J, et al. Exaggerated neuroinflammation and sickness behavior in aged mice after activation of the peripheral innate immune system. FASEB j 2005;19(10):1329–31.

Behavior Changes Associated with Metabolic Disease of Dogs and Cats

Lisa Radosta, DVM, DACVB

KEYWORDS

- Hypothyroidism • Aggression • Endocrine disease • Anxiety behavior

KEY POINTS

- Endocrine diseases in dogs and cats can, directly and indirectly, affect behavior patterns.
- Through operant conditioning, behavior changes associated with physical disease can progress to long-term behavior patterns which do not resolve with treatment of the primary endocrine disease.
- Emotional and physical processes in the body are inextricably linked and both can influence clinical signs which are historically characterized as behavioral.

INTRODUCTION

A healthy animal body can cope with a certain amount of change without entering a state of chronic stress and possible behavioral or physical disease. The amount of change that an individual can handle is referred to as "allostatic load." When the change exceeds the allostatic load, clinical signs of behavioral or physical disease can result (Sterling 2014). The allostatic load can be altered by medications (eg, phenobarbital, corticosteroids, benzodiazepines, antidepressants, tramadol, levetiracetam, gabapentin)[1–6]; gastrointestinal problems (eg, inflammatory bowel disease, intestinal neoplasia)[7,8]; dermatologic diseases (eg, atopy, food allergy, flea allergy dermatitis)[9]; orthopedic disease (eg, neoplasia, osteoarthritis),[10] metabolic disease (eg, hypothyroidism, hypoadrenocorticism, diabetes mellitus), and any disease that causes pain or discomfort. See **Table 1** for a list of clinical signs caused by metabolic diseases.

When a stressor is encountered, whether physical (eg, metabolic disease, acute injury, surgery, inflammatory disease, chronic disease) or emotional (eg, fear, anxiety, stress, conflict, and/or panic [FASCP]), the body launches a physiologic stress response. This response can be acute (ie, immediate) or chronic (eg, days, weeks, months). Acute stress will trigger an adaptive change, while chronic stress may be

Florida Veterinary Behavior Service, West Palm Beach, FL, USA
E-mail address: drlisaradosta@gmail.com

Vet Clin Small Anim 54 (2024) 17–28
https://doi.org/10.1016/j.cvsm.2023.08.004
0195-5616/24/© 2023 Elsevier Inc. All rights reserved.

Table 1 Behavioral clinical signs of endocrine disease		
Disorder	**Dogs**	**Cats**
Hypothyroidism	Aggression, coprophagia, poor focus and learning, fear of sounds, distress during separation, hyperactivity, difficulty training, mental dullness, lethargy, changes in mentation, disorientation, changes in interactions with family.	Lethargy, inappetence, decreased interactions with the environment.
Hyperthyroidism	Restlessness, anxiety, dysrexia, lethargy	Anxiety, restlessness, nighttime vocalization, increased appetite, hyperactivity, changes in litter box habits
Hypoadrenocorticism	Restlessness, increased anxiety, depression, changes in mentation, erratic behavior, disorientation, circling, aggression, lethargy	Behavioral periuria, perichezia, lethargy, depression, dysrexia, polyuria, polydipsia, changes in interactions with the pet parent, pica, increases in fear.
Hyperadrenocorticism	Panting, polyuria, polyphagia, lethargy	Lethargy, behavioral periuria, perichezia, urine spraying, aggression, polyphagia, polydipsia, polyuria, licking the vulva, vocalizing, rolling on the ground, head rubbing
Sex hormone–secreting adrenal tumors	Polyphagia, polydipsia, polyuria, panting	Hyperactivity, urine marking, estrus behavior (pacing, vocalizing, lordosis)
Diabetes mellitus	Polyuria, anxiety, polyphagia, polydipsia	Anxiety, irritability, aggression, altered sleep, changes in litter box habits, mental dullness, decreased activity, restlessness, increased sleep, confusion, difficulty jumping, reduced tolerance of handling.

maladaptive as it exceeds the allostatic load. Both acute and chronic stress result in behavior changes as the patient attempts to cope.

Behavior changes, including those resulting from changes in physiology due to metabolic disease, can be reinforced or punished intrinsically (eg, hormones, neurochemicals, alleviation of discomfort) or extrinsically (eg, environment, people, other animals). Through positive and negative consequences (ie, reinforcement, punishment), behavior changes associated with physical disease can progress to long-term behavior patterns. For example, a dog with polyuria and polydipsia due to hyperadrenocorticism may have urinary accidents in the home. Urination is intrinsically reinforced immediately when pressure on the bladder is alleviated. In this way, the dog may learn that urination in the home is reinforcing, which will in the end affect the consistency of elimination outside despite previous house-training. Despite the effective treatment of the hyperadrenocorticism, the learning cannot be undone; however, with appropriate behavior modification the urination in the house can be improved. The dog may need to be reminded of the previous house-training in order to eliminate the possibility of future accidents. In another example, a cat who vocalizes at night resulting from undiagnosed hyperthyroidism and is fed by the caregivers in order stop the meowing is reinforced for vocalizing and/or waking the caregivers up. When the hyperthyroidism is treated, the cat may feel healthy. However, he has learned that when he desires food, waking up the caregivers is the most effective way to satisfy that need.

In the past, veterinarians may have been encouraged to rule out physical problems before considering behavioral diagnoses or delay treatment for what was categorized as behavioral clinical signs while physical disease was ruled out. However, recent research supports the concept that emotional and physical processes in the body are inextricably linked and both can influence clinical signs that are historically characterized as behavioral.[10,11] In fact, "behavioral" clinical signs can be caused by diseases of any body system, with no real separation between the emotional and physical components, in spite of the fictitious distinction being often used for teaching purposes.

Therefore, clinicians must diagnose and treat all clinical signs, such as pain, fear, and distress, of the same condition immediately and simultaneously to improve the health and welfare of a patient. The early recognition of behavioral clinical signs and the associated reinforcement and punishment of resulting behaviors allow the veterinary health care team to educate the caregivers immediately and prevent negative progression of behavior patterns. Additionally, treatment with diet, supplements, medications, probiotics, pheromone analogues, environmental changes, and behavior modification can immediately alleviate stress and potentially reduce the progression of the negative behavior while diagnostics are being performed and treatment is initiated for the physical disease.

For any of the endocrine diseases discussed later, it is possible for patients to present with only behavioral changes. This emphasizes the importance of a complete diagnostic workup on all pets presenting with behavior problems, even if the caregivers feel strongly that the problem is not health-related.[12] A complete workup includes a physical examination, complete blood count, serum chemistry, thyroid analysis (free thyroxine measured by equilibrium dialysis [fT4 (ED)] in dogs and total thyroxine [TT4] in cats), urinalysis, fecal examination antigen, and fecal float.[13,14] Additional diagnostics should be at the veterinarian's discretion and may include ultrasound, radiographs, blood pressure measurement, and/or urinary culture.

If the clinical signs at presentation are consistent with FASCP, treatment with psychotropic medications, supplements, probiotics, pheromone analogues, and/or diets should be instituted. Avoid the use of medications that may alter testing (**Table 2**). Instruct clients to avoid interactions or situations which stimulate the FASCP-related behavior patterns. Recommend changes in the environment and behavior of the caregivers to reduce reinforcement and punishment of behavior patterns.

For example, if a dog shows aggression when pushed or pulled, recommend that the caregivers use food or toys to lure the dog from that spot to the desired area instead of physically handling the dog. If the dog is aggressive on walks, recommend

Table 2
Medications and ingredients which may affect testing for common endocrine disease

Effect	Medication/Ingredient
Hypoglycemia	SSRIs, L-theanine
Hyperglycemia	TCAs, benzodiazepines, glucocorticoids
Altered cortisol/ACTH	Clonidine, trazodone, dexmedetomidine
Altered thyroid	Glucocorticoids, TCA, SSRI

Abbreviations: ACTH, adrenocorticotropic hormone; SSRI, selective serotonin reuptake inhibitors; TCA, tricyclic antidepressant.

that they refrain from walking the dog at peak times or entirely if they have a yard in which the dog can exercise. For cats who vocalize overnight, recommend that the caregivers ignore the cat at those times and utilize an automatic feeder set to open prior to when the cat wakes the caregivers up. For cats who have changes in litter box habits, recommend that the caregivers offer the ideal number of boxes for the household, ideal size boxes with the cat's preferred shape and side height, and about 3 inches of litter depth, placed in the cat's core area. While working with a positive reinforcement training professional cannot change metabolic changes in the body, it can help the caregivers to understand environmental changes and adopt alternative strategies for living with their pet and so should be recommended.

Disorders of the Thyroid Gland

Proposed mechanisms for thyroid-related behavior changes and influences on behavior disorders include a lowered threshold for aggression due to primary clinical signs (eg, changes in appetite, energy level), impaired transmission of serotonin at the postsynaptic $5-HT_{2A}$ receptors in the cerebral cortex,[15] regulation of noradrenergic function,[16] alterations in monoamine (ie, dopamine, epinephrine, serotonin) synthesis, turnover, and release,[17] and increased metabolism of serotonin in the cerebrospinal fluid.[18,19]

Several medications which are commonly used to treat behavior problems can affect serum thyroid levels. Clomipramine (Clomicalm) at a dose of 3 mg/kg PO q12, has been shown to reduce serum thyroxine (T4), fT4 (ED), and triiodothyronine (T3) in dogs after 28 days of use and decreases continued through 112 days (end of study). In the aforementioned study, there was no effect on thyrotropin-releasing hormone or thyroid-stimulating hormone (TSH).[20] Proposed mechanisms include the binding of iodine by clomipramine, decreasing iodine availability in the thyroid gland, and irreversible inhibition of the synthesis of thyroid peroxidase which oxidizes iodide ions used in the production of T4 and T3.[21] Selective serotonin reuptake inhibitors (SSRIs) can reduce serum T4, fT4, and T3 in humans; however, results are inconsistent.[22,23] Avoid the use of tricyclic antidepressants (eg, clomipramine, imipramine, amitriptyline) and potentially SSRIs (eg, fluoxetine, sertraline, paroxetine) until thyroid status is known.

Hypothyroidism
Hypothyroidism is a multisystemic disorder with the potential for dermatologic, cardiac, neurologic, metabolic, gastrointestinal, hematologic, and ocular clinical signs.[24] Well-recognized behavioral clinical signs in dogs include mental dullness, lethargy, changes in mentation, disorientation, and altered social interactions.[15] Anecdotally, hypothyroidism in dogs has been linked to noise and storm phobia, separation-related disorders,

hyperactivity, poor focus and learning, compulsive behaviors, training disorders, copro-phagia, and aggression.[25–28] In fact, aggression may be the only presenting complaint in some cases.[29]

While hypothyroidism is the most common endocrine disease in pet dogs, its prev-alence is only 0.2% in the population.[30,31] Because of the low prevalence in the gen-eral population, finding an aggressive dog who is also hypothyroid may be as difficult as finding a needle in a haystack. Additionally, aggression is a common presentation in dogs with normal thyroid concentrations. In a study measuring TT4, fT4, total triio-dothyronine (TT3), free triiodothyronine (fT3), thyroglobulin autoantibodies (TgAA), TSH, triiodothyronine autoantibodies, and thyroxine autoantibodies (T4AA) in[31] aggressive and nonaggressive dogs, aggressive dogs had higher concentrations of T4AA when compared to non-aggressive dogs; however, T4AA values were still within normal range.[32] In a second study comparing TT4 and TSH in 39 aggressive and nonaggressive dogs, TT4 was higher in aggressive dogs but was not outside the normal range.[33]

In a case report, a hypothyroid (low T4, increased TSH) dog diagnosed with aggres-sion was treated with levothyroxine for 1 month at which time, owner-directed aggres-sion was decreased; however, territorial aggression was not.[17] In a case series of 4 dogs who were presented for aggression to familiar and unfamiliar people and also had thyroid values consistent with hypothyroidism, all dogs responded to treatment with supplementation and management recommendations, but none resolved completely.[20] In cases of hypothyroid dogs presenting with aggression, some clini-cians recommend treatment for 1 month before reassessment.[34,35] Aggression has been associated with increased TgAA concentrations, along with normal TT4 and TSH concentrations in dogs.[26]

Inappropriate or unnecessary supplementation of thyroid hormone may lead to tachycardia, irritability, aggression, nervousness, and weight loss in dogs. In addition, because thyroid hormone is functionally linked to brain dopamine and serotonergic systems, L-thyroxine supplementation, even in euthyroid patients, may affect the same systems involved in canine aggression disorders; therefore, improvement with thyroid supplementation does not confirm that the cause is thyroid-related. However, in a study examining the effect of T4 supplementation on behavior change and serum levels of prolactin and serotonin in hypothyroid[36] dogs, the only behavior change seen was increased activity and there were no changes in serum serotonin or prolactin levels.[37] In a double-blinded, placebo-controlled study examining the effect of thyroid supplementation on dogs who directed aggression at family members and had fT4 in or below the lower 20th percentile of the normal range; TT4, TT3, or fT3 in or below the lower 30th percentile of the normal range; or the presence of TgAA, no difference was found between the supplemented and placebo groups in the level of aggression.[38] At this time, evidence supporting the safety and efficacy of supplementation with levo-thyroxine in euthyroid dogs is lacking. For that reason, supplementation without testing supportive of hypothyroidism is not recommended.[5]

Hypothyroidism in cats is rare. In fact, it is the least common endocrine disorder in cats. Most commonly, it occurs in kittens and in cats following radioiodine treatment; however, adult-onset hypothyroidism has been reported.[39] Behavioral clinical signs include lethargy, inappetence, and lack of interest in the environment.[30,40–42]

Hyperthyroidism

Hyperthyroidism is rare in dogs; however behavior changes such as restlessness, anx-iety, dysrexia, and lethargy have been noted in dogs with thyroid cancers (eg, thyroid carcinoma) leading to clinical hyperthyroidism and resolution after thyroidectomy.[43,44]

Hyperthyroidism is the most common endocrine disease in cats.[45] Behavioral clinical signs are common and include anxiety, restlessness, nighttime vocalization, increased appetite, hyperactivity, and changes in litter box habits.[46] Because hyperthyroidism is more common in cats over 10 years of age, complicating factors, including cognitive dysfunction, may be present. Cats over 11 years of age may display increased aggression, marking, behavioral periuria, vocalization, restlessness, changes in interactions and sociability, and aggression as a normal part of aging or due to cognitive dysfunction complicating the clinician's ability to distinguish the etiology of behavioral clinical signs.[47]

Disorders of the Adrenal Gland

Changes in the secretion of sex hormones, mineralocorticoids, or glucocorticoids due to impaired adrenal gland function can result from excessive secretion of adrenocorticotropic hormone (ACTH) by the pituitary gland most likely due to a pituitary tumor; excessive secretion of cortisol by the adrenal gland (adrenal tumor), iatrogenic medication administration (eg, glucocorticoids, ketoconazole), and excessive sex hormone (androgens, estrogen) secretion (adrenal tumor).[48,49]

Administration of exogenous glucocorticoids in dogs has been associated with increases in startle response, fear, vigilance, avoidance of people, barking, and aggression and decreases in recovery from stressful events, exploratory behavior, and play.[1-3] Glucocorticoids have been shown to alter post-TSH values (endogenous), lower serum TT4 (endogenous and exogenous), and lower fT4 (exogenous) measurements potentially through inhibition of TSH secretion in the pituitary gland, changes in thyroid binding, and/or metabolism.[4-6]

Along the hypothalamic-pituitary-adrenal axis, there are alpha-1 and alpha-2 adrenergic receptors and as such its production of hormones can be affected by medications that modulate binding at those receptors. For example, in humans, trazodone can decrease plasma cortisol levels when compared to placebo.[50,51] The literature is conflicting regarding clonidine's effect on ACTH and cortisol levels. In 1 study in humans, clonidine decreased cortisol and ACTH concentrations in adults and in a subsequent study, it had no effect.[52,53] In a study in children, clonidine reduced plasma ACTH and cortisol.[54] Dexmedetomidine is commonly used for sedation in dogs prior to procedures. The transmucosal preparation (Sileo) has been used off-label as a pre-visit pharmaceutical to reduce stress during procedures and veterinary visits.[55] Studies in dogs appear to demonstrate that at higher doses or with prolonged use of injectable dexmedetomidine given intravenously, basal cortisol levels can decrease and the response to ACTH stimulation can be blunted.[56,57] Because of the potential for alterations in cortisol and ACTH secretion, clinicians should consider avoiding trazodone,[58] dexmedetomidine,[56,57,59] and clonidine[52] in patients for whom impaired adrenal function is suspected until testing is complete. Evidence is lacking at this time as to the effect, if any, of a transmucosal preparation of dexmedetomidine on cortisol and ACTH.

Hypoadrenocorticism

Hypoadrenocorticism (Addison's disease) can result from the destruction of the adrenal cortices (primary) or a decrease in ACTH secretion from the pituitary gland (secondary). Patients can be deficient in mineralocorticoids and glucocorticoids (typical) or only glucocorticoids (atypical). It is more common in dogs than cats. Aside from the clinical signs directly resulting from changes in adrenal hormone levels, the presence of a tumor may exert its own behavioral clinical signs such as restlessness, increased anxiety, depression, changes in mentation, erratic behavior, disorientation, circling, and aggression.[60,61]

The most common behavioral clinical sign of hypoadrenocorticism in dogs is lethargy although some dogs with atypical hypoadrenocorticism exhibit polydipsia. The behavioral clinical signs associated with hypoadrenocorticism in cats include behavioral periuria, perichezia, lethargy, depression, dysrexia, polyuria, polydipsia, changes in interactions, pica, and increases in fear.[62,63,64]

Hyperadrenocorticism (Cushing's disease)
Typically, clinical signs result from excessive secretion of cortisol from the adrenal cortex; however, clinical signs can result from oversecretion of aldosterone, testosterone, androstenodione, progesterone, and estrodiol.[3,65–67]

Behavioral clinical signs in dogs include panting, polyuria, polyphagia, and lethargy.[68] Hyperadrenocorticism is rare in cats; however, it has been reported.[3] Behavioral clinical signs in cats include lethargy, behavioral periuria, perichezia, urine spraying, aggression, polyphagia, polydipsia, polyuria, licking the vulva, vocalizing, rolling on the ground, and head rubbing.[3,37,69,70] About 80% of cases in cats have concurrent diabetes mellitus.[71]

Sex hormone–secreting adrenal tumors
Behavior changes such as aggression (eg, people, other cats), hyperactivity, urine marking, and estrus behavior (pacing, vocalizing, lordosis) have been reported in cats with sex hormone–secreting tumors such as an adrenocortical carcinoma.[40] In dogs, behavioral clinical signs may be similar to typical hyperadrenocorticism and include polyuria, polydipsia, panting, and polyphagia.[52]

Disorders of the Pancreas

Diabetes mellitus
Behavioral clinical signs in dogs include polyuria, anxiety, polyphagia, and polydipsia.[72,73] Clinical signs of diabetes mellitus in cats include anxiety, irritability, aggression, altered sleep, changes in litter box habits, mental dullness, decreased activity, restlessness, increased sleep, and confusion.[37] Diabetic neuropathy is more common in cats than dogs. Cats with diabetes may have difficulty jumping and an aversion to being petted or handled due to discomfort resulting from diabetic neuropathy.

L-theanine, a common ingredient in antianxiety supplements, has several effects on the endocrine system. In rats, L-theanine has been shown to have insulin-like actions, increasing glucose tolerance, and lowering blood glucose.[74] In humans, SSRIs such as fluoxetine and sertraline can have a hypoglycemic effect, normalize glucose homeostasis, and increase insulin sensitivity.[75] Tricyclic antidepressants (imipramine, clomipramine) can cause a hyperglycemic effect.[67] Benzodiazepines such as diazepam may induce hyperglycemia in diabetic rats; however, it may reduce hyperglycemia related to stress in nondiabetic mice.[76,77] More research is needed to determine if this effect is reliably present in dogs.

SUMMARY

Like many physical disorders, clinical signs associated with metabolic diseases affecting thyroid, adrenal, and pancreatic function are reflective of nonspecific changes in behavior. Additionally, patients who have underlying disorders of FASCP may be under treatment with medications that alter basal thyroid, glucose, and cortisol levels. Through reinforcement and punishment of behaviors associated with clinical signs caused by organic or iatrogenic endocrine disease, behaviors can be perpetuated and become persistent behavior patterns. Screening all patients presenting with a primary behavior complaint or those with behavioral clinical signs for endocrine diseases is essential. Alleviating stress immediately while completing a physical and diagnostic workup or treating metabolic disease alleviates suffering and may stave off the adoption of behavior patterns in a more permanent way.

CLINICS CARE POINTS

- Screening all patients presenting with a primary behavior complaint or those with behavioral clinical signs for endocrine diseases is essential.
- Treat behavioral clinical signs immediately with medications, supplements, pheromone analogues, probiotics, and/or diet, with consideration given to the medications and ingredients which may alter testing.
- Make recommendations for environmental and behavioral changes immediately.

DISCLOSURE

Dr L. Radosta currently serves on advisory boards for Purina, Zoundz, and Ellevet.

REFERENCES

1. Elkholly DA, Brodbelt DC, Church DB, et al. Side Effects to Systemic Glucocorticoid Therapy in Dogs Under Primary Veterinary Care in the UK. Front Vet Sci 2020 Aug 14;7:515.
2. Notari L, Burman O, Mills D. Behavioural changes in dogs treated with corticosteroids. Physiol Behav 2015;151:609–16.
3. Notari L, Mills D. Possible behavioral effects of exogenous corticosteroids on dog behavior: A preliminary investigation. J. Vet. Behav 2011;6:321–7.
4. Peterson ME, Ferguson DC, Kintzer PP, et al. Effects of spontaneous hyperadrenocorticism on serum thyroid hormone concentra- tions in the dog. Am J Vet Res 1984;45:2034–8.
5. Torres SM, McKeever PJ, Johnston SD. Effect of oral administration of prednisolone on thyroid function in dogs. Am J Vet Res 1991;52:416–21.
6. Daminet S, Paradis M, Refsal KR, et al. Short-term influence of prednisone and phenobarbital on thyroid function in euthyroid dogs. Can Vet J 1999;40:411.
7. Bécuwe-Bonnet V, Bélanger MC, Frank D, et al. Gastrointestinal disorders in dogs with excessive licking of surfaces. Journal of Veterinary Behavior 2012;7(4):194–204.
8. Frank D, Bélanger MC, Bécuwe-Bonnet V, et al. Prospective medical evaluation of 7 dogs presented with fly biting. Can Vet J 2012;53:1279.
9. Harvey ND, Craigon PJ, Shaw SC, et al. Behavioural Differences in Dogs with Atopic Dermatitis Suggest Stress Could Be a Significant Problem Associated with Chronic Pruritus. Animals 2019;9:813.
10. Mills DS, Demontigny-Bedard I, Gruen M, et al. Pain and problem behavior in cats and dogs. Animals 2020;10:318.
11. Dinwoodie IR, Zottola V, Dodman N. An investigation into the effectiveness of various professionals and behavior modification programs, with or without medication, for the treatment of canine aggression. J Vet Behav 2021;43:46–53.
12. Boag AK, Neiger R, Church DB. Trilostane treatment of bilateral adrenal enlargement and excessive sex steroid hormone production in a cat. J Small Anim Pract 2004;45:263–6.

13. Ferguson DC. Testing for hypothyroidism in dogs. VCNA: Small Animal Practice 2007;37:647–69.
14. Camps T, Amat M, Mateca X. A review of medical conditions and behavioral problems in dogs and cats. Animals 2019;9:1–17.
15. Henley WN, Valdic F. Hypothyroid-induced changes in autonomic control have a central serotonergic component. Am J Physiol 1997;272:894–903.
16. Whybrow PC, Prange AJ Jr. A hypotheses of thyroid-catecholamine-eceptor interaction. Arch Gen Psychiatr 1981;38:106–13.
17. Hassan WA, Rahman TA, Aly MS, et al. Alterations in monoamines level in discrete brain regions and other peripheral tissues in young and adult male rates during experimental hyperthyroidism. Int J Dev Neurosci 2013;31:311–8.
18. Henley WN, Chen S, Klettner C, et al. Hypothyroidism increases serotonin turnover and sympathetic activity in the adult rat. Can J Physiol Pharmacol 1991; 69:205–10.
19. Bauer M, Heinz A, Whybrow PC. Thyroid hormones, serotonin and mood: of synergy and significance in the adult brain. Mol Psychiatr 2002;7:140–56.
20. Gulikers KP, Panciera DL. Evaluation of the effects of clomipramine on canine thyroid function tests. J Vet Intern Med 2003;17:44–9.
21. Rousseau A, Comby F, Buxeraud J, et al. Spectroscopic analysis of charge transfer complex formation and peroxidase inhibition with tricyclic antidepressant drugs: potential anti-thyroid action. Biol Pharm Bull 1996;19:726–8.
22. Caye A, Pilz LK, Maia AL, et al. The impact of selective serotonin reuptake inhibitors on the thyroid function among patients with major depressive disorder: a systematic review and meta analysis. Eur Neuropsychopharmacol 2020,33: 139–45.
23. Gitlin M, Altshuler LL, Frye MA, et al. Peripheral thyroid hormones and response to selective serotonin reuptake inhibitors. J Psychiatr Neurosci 2004 Sep 1;29(5): 383–6.
24. Nelson RW, Couto CG. Small animal internal medicine - E-book (small animal medicine). Kindle Edition. St Louis, MO: Elsevier Health Sciences; 2014. p. 2104.
25. Aronson LP, Dodds WJ. The effect of hypothyroid function on canine behavior. In: Current research in veterinary behavioral medicine. West Lafayette: Purdue University Press; 2005. p. 131–8.
26. Fatjo J, Amat M, Manteca X. Animal behavior case of the month. J Am Vet Med Assoc 2003;223:623–6.
27. Beaver BV, Haug LI. Canine behaviors associated with hypothyroidism. J Am Anim Hosp Assoc 2003;39:431–4.
28. Barlow TA, Casey RA, Bradshaw JWS, et al. An investigation of the relationship between thyroid status and behavior in dogs. St Louis, MO: Scientific Proceedings of the British Small Animal Veterinary Association Congress; 2003. p. 614.
29. Fatjo J, Stub C, Manteca X. Four cases of aggression and hypothyroidism in dogs. Vet Rec 2002;151:547–8.
30. Panciera DL. Hypothyroidism in dogs: 66 cases (1987-1992). J Am Vet Med Assoc 1994;204:761–7.
31. Kour H, Chhabra S, Randhawa CS. Prevalence of hypothyroidism in dogs. Pharma Innov J 2020;9:70–2.
32. Radosta LA, Shofer FS, Reisner IR. Comparison of thyroid analytes in dogs aggressive to familiar people and in non-aggressive dogs. Vet 2012;192:472–5.
33. Carter G, Scott-Moncrieff JC, Luescher AU, et al. Serum total thyroxine and thyroid stimulating hormone concentrations in dogs with behavior problems. J Vet Behav 2009;4:230–6.

26   Radosta

34. Beaver BV. Canine social behavior. In: Beaver BV, editor. Canine behavior: a guide for veterinarians. Philadelphia: WB Saunders Co; 1999. p. 152–81.
35. Dodman NH, Mertens PA, Aronson LP. Animal behavior case of the month. J Am Vet Med Assoc 1995;207:1168–71.
36. Graham PA, Lundquist RB, Refsal KR, et al. Reported clinical signs in 8317 cases of canine hypothyroidism and 2647 cases of subclinical thyroiditis529. Birmingham, UK: Proceedings of BSAVA; 2004.
37. Hrovat A, De Keuster T, Kooistra HS, et al. Behavior in dogs with spontaneous hypothyroidism during treatment with levothyroxine. J Vet Intern Med 2019;33:64–71.
38. Dodman NH, Aronson L, Cottam N, et al. The effect of thyroid replacement in dogs with suboptimal thyroid function on owner-directed aggression: A randomized, double-blind, placebo-controlled clinical trial. J Vet Behav 2013;8:225–30.
39. Rand J, Levine J, Best S, et al. Spontaneous adult-onset hypothyroidism in a cat. J Vet Intern Med 1993;7:272–6.
40. Greco DS. Diagnosis of Congenital and Adult-Onset Hypothyroidism in Cats. Clin Tech Small Anim Pract 2006;21:40–4.
41. Peterson ME. Primary goitrous hypothyroidism in a young adult domestic longhair cat: diagnosis and treatment monitoring. Journal of Feline Medicine and Surgery Open Reports 2015;1(2). 2055116915615153.
42. Galgano M, Spalla I, Callegari C, et al. Primary hypothyroidism and thyroid goiter in an adult cat. J Vet Intern Med 2014;28:682–6.
43. Tullio C, Uccheddu S. Symptomatic Hyperthiroidism associated with Carcinoma in a Dog. Dog behavior 2021;7.
44. Scharf VF, Oblak ML, Hoffman K, et al. Clinical features and outcome of functional thyroid tumours in 70 dogs. J Sm An Pract 2020;61:504–11.
45. Peterson ME. Hyperthyroidism and cats: What's causing this epidemic of thyroid disease and can we prevent it? J Fel Med and Surg 2012;14:804–18.
46. Bellows J, Center S, Daristotle L, et al. Evaluating aging in cats: How to determine what is healthy and what is disease. J Fel Med Surg 2016;18:551–70.
47. Sordo L, Breheny C, Halls V, et al. Prevalence of disease and age-related behavioural changes in cats: past and present. Vet Sciences 2020;7:85.
48. Sullivant AM, Lathan P. Ketoconazole-induced transient hypoadrenocorticism in a dog. Can Vet J 2020;61:407.
49. Sumner JP, Hulsebosch SE, Dudley RM, et al. Sex-hormone producing adrenal tumors causing behavioral changes as the sole clinical sign in 3 cats. Can Vet J 2019;60:305.
50. Settimo L, Taylor D. Evaluating the dose-dependent mechanism of action of trazodone by estimation of occupancies for different brain neurotransmitter targets. J Psychopharmacol 2018;32:96–104.
51. Monteleone P. Effects of trazodone on plasma cortisol in normal subjects. A study with drug plasma levels. Neuropsychopharmacology 1991;5:61–4.
52. Lanes R, Herrera A, Palacios A, et al. Decreased secretion of cortisol and ACTH after oral clonidine administration in normal adults. Metabolism 1983;32:568–70.
53. Kim MH, Hahn TH. The effect of clonidine pretreatment on the perioperative proinflammatory cytokines, cortisol, and ACTH responses in patients undergoing total abdominal hysterectomy. Anesth Analg 2000;90:1441–4.
54. Muñóz-Hoyos A, Fernández-García JM, Molina-Carballo A, et al. Effect of clonidine on plasma ACTH, cortisol and melatonin in children. J Pineal Res 2000;29:48–53.

55. Hauser H, Campbell S, Korpivaara M, et al. In-hospital administration of dexme-detomidine oromucosal gel for stress reduction in dogs during veterinary visits: a randomized, double-blinded, placebo-controlled study. Journal of veterinary behavior 2020;39:77–85.

56. Maze M, Virtanen R, Daunt D, et al. Effects of dexmedetomidine, a novel imid-azole sedative-anesthetic agent, on adrenal steroidogenesis: in vivo and in vitro studies. Anesth Analg 1991;73:204–8.

57. Guan W, Feng X, Zhang L, et al. Evaluation of post-operative anti-stress response of dexmedetomidine in dogs. J Northeast Agric Univ (English Edition) 2018;25: 27–32.

58. Morris EM, Kitts-Morgan SE, Spangler DM, et al. The impact of feeding cannabi-diol (CBD) containing treats on canine response to a noise-induced fear response test. Front Vet Sci 2020;7:569565.

59. Bisht DS, Jadon NS, Kandpal M, et al. Clinicophysiological and haematobio-chemical effects of dexmedetomidine-etomidate-sevoflurane anaesthesia in dogs. Indian J Vet Surg 2016;37:77–81.

60. Barnhart KF, Edwards JF, Storts RW. Symptomatic granular cell tumor involving the pituitary gland in a dog: a case report and review of the literature. Vet Path 2001;38:332–6.

61. Nixon S. Seizures and anxiety with a case of hypoadrenocorticism in a dog. Sci-ence Week 2013;27.

62. Hock CE. Atypical hypoadrenocorticism in a Birman cat. Can Vet J 2011;52: 893–6.

63. Giudice E, Macrì F, Crinò C, et al. Hypoadrenocorticism in a young dwarf cat-case report. Vet Arh 2016;86:591–600.

64. Peterson ME, Greco DS, Orth DN. Primary hypoadrenocorticism in ten cats. J Vet Intern Med 1989;3:55–8.

65. Boord M, Griffin C. Progesterone secreting adrenal mass in a cat with clinical signs of hyperadrenocorticism. J Am Vet Med Assoc 1999;214:666–9.

66. Rossmeisl JH, Scott-Moncrieff JCR, Seims j, et al. Hyperadrenocorticism and hy-perprogesteronemia in a cat with adrenocortical adenocarcinoma. JAAHA 2000; 36:512–7.

67. Syme HM, Scott-Moncrieff JC, Treadwell NG, et al. Hyperadrenocorticism asso-ciated with excessive sex hormone production by an adrenocortical tumor in two dogs. J Am Vet Med Assoc 2001;219:1725–8.

68. Peterson ME. Diagnosis of hyperadrenocorticism in dogs. Clin Tech Sm An Pract 2007;22:2–11.

69. Millard RP, Pickens EH, Wells KL. Excessive production of sex hormones with an adrenocortical tumor. J Am Vet Med Assoc 2009;234:505–8.

70. Meler EN, Scott-Mongrief JC, Peter AT, et al. Cyclic estrous-like behavior in a spayed cat associated with excessive sex-hormone production by an adrenocor-tical carcinoma. J Feline Med Surg 2011;13:473–8.

71. Nelson RW, Couto CG. Small animal internal medicine - E-book (small animal medicine). Kindle Edition. St Louis, MO: Elsevier Health Sciences; 2014. p. 2395.

72. Catchpole B, Ristic JM, Fleeman LM, et al. Canine diabetes mellitus: can old dogs teach us new tricks? Diabetologia 2005;48:1948–56.

73. Lokes-Krupka TP, Tsvilichovsky MI, Karasenko AU. Features of correction of a pathological condition of small animals at the diabetes mellitus with obesity. Sci-entific Messenger of LNU of Veterinary Medicine and Biotechnologies. Series: Vet Sci 2021;23:50–4.

74. Saeed M, Naveed M, Arif M, et al. Green tea (Camellia sinensis) and l-theanine: Medicinal values and beneficial applications in humans—A comprehensive review. Biomed Pharmacother 2017;95:1260–75.
75. McIntyre RS, Soczynska JK, Konarski JZ, et al. The effect of antidepressants on glucose homeostasis and insulin sensitivity: synthesis and mechanisms. Expet Opin Drug Saf 2006;5:157–68.
76. Salice VS, Valenza FV, Pizzocri MP, et al. Benzodiazepines induce hyperglycemia in rats by affecting peripheral disposal of glucose. Crit Care 2013;17:1–200.
77. Surwit RS, McCubbin JA, Kuhn CM, et al. Alprazolam reduces stress hyperglycemia in ob/ob mice. Psychosom Med 1986;48:278–82.

Separation-related Problems and Their Interaction with Physical Disease

Hagar Hauser, DVM, DACVB

KEYWORDS

- Dog • Behavioral health • Physical health • Separation anxiety
- Separation-related problems

KEY POINTS

- The condition of separation-related problems (SRP) is common in owned dogs and should be identified by clinicians.
- Differential diagnoses of physical disease for the clinical signs of SRP should be considered in each case.
- Appropriate diagnostics should be performed to rule out physical disease that may present as or exacerbate SRP.

 Video content accompanies this article at http://www.vetsmall.theclinics.com

INTRODUCTION
Terminology

The term "separation anxiety" has most often been used to describe dogs' undesirable behaviors that occur in absence of their owners. Anxiety is an emotion of apprehension to an anticipated danger or threat. However, when dogs exhibit undesirable behaviors during an owner's absence, they do not always show signs of anxiety.[1] Newer research suggests the use of alternative terminology because there are other potential motivations causing the observed behaviors, such as frustration and panic associated with the loss of an attachment figure.[2,3] Other terms used to describe the condition include separation-related problems (SRPs); separation-related behavior; separation-related distress; and separation-related disorders.[2] To consider all the potential components, the author will be using the term SRPs throughout the article.

Prevalence

SRP is one of the most common behavioral disorders in dogs with approximately 17% to 29% of dogs reported to have signs consistent with SRP.[4–8] It represents 20% to

Metropolitan Veterinary Associates, 2626 Van Buren Avenue, Norristown, PA 19403, USA
E-mail address: hhauser@metro-vet.com

Vet Clin Small Anim 54 (2024) 29–42
https://doi.org/10.1016/j.cvsm.2023.08.003
vetsmall.theclinics.com
0195-5616/24/© 2023 Elsevier Inc. All rights reserved.

40% of the caseload at behavior specialty clinics in North America.[9] This condition can affect the quality of life of the pet and the owner as well as place a burden on the human–animal bond.[4] With its high prevalence, there are two medications that are approved and labeled by the Food and Drug Administration to treat "separation anxiety" in dogs: Clomicalm (or the generic clomipramine hydrochloride) and Reconcile.[10–13]

Clinical Signs

In the literature, SRP in dogs is described as specific behaviors exhibited when dogs are alone, perceived to be alone, and/or when they cannot access their owner.[1,6,14,15] The most common owner complaints of dogs with SRP include house soiling, destruction, excessive vocalization, and increased repetitive motor activity in the owner's absence.[11,13,14,16,17] Video observation of dogs with SRP shows that they often vocalize and become destructive immediately after the owner's departure but signs may not occur until 10 to 30 minutes later.[14,18] If the dog is destructive, they often target exit points and they can cause severe property damage in an attempt to access their owners or escape the environment, as seen in **Fig. 1**.[4] However, dogs may go undiagnosed if they exhibit signs that do not leave evidence such as pacing, panting, and whining.[4] Other less frequently noted signs of SRP may include tachycardia, tachypnea, trembling, anorexia, vomiting, diarrhea, and decreased activity.[9,16] They may also exhibit excessive excitement or anxiety on the owner's return.[16]

PHYSICAL DISEASE AND SEPARATION-RELATED PROBLEM

Behavioral conditions in dogs are often considered diagnoses of exclusion after medical causes are ruled out. However, physical illnesses can exacerbate behavioral conditions as well as cause a relapse, regression, or recurrence of a behavioral condition

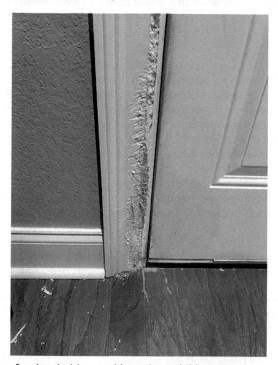

Fig. 1. Destruction of a threshold caused by a dog exhibiting SRP.

and vice versa, which will be shown in the case studies later in this article. Changes in behavior are often the first sign of illness and owners may be more likely to notice behavioral changes than physical ones. Therefore, it is important for every clinician evaluating a patient presenting with SRP to first consider and rule out the medical differential diagnoses. Often, physical illness can be ruled as unlikely in the presence of a consistent trigger, such as the owner's departure, but should still be considered. We review some physical pathologies that should be considered as possible differential diagnoses and comorbidities when observing behavior changes commonly associated with SRP. See **Table 1** for a complete list of medical differential diagnoses for canine SRP.

Destructive Behavior

Destructive behavior by a dog exhibiting SRP may include digging, scratching, or chewing. Seizures and hepatic encephalopathy should be considered.[9] Owners may not be able to distinguish destruction from pica, so it is important for the clinician to differentiate between them. Pica, ingestion of inanimate objects, is more likely to be a sign of a gastrointestinal disorder rather than behavioral.[19] If the dog is getting into the trash or stealing objects, causes of polyphagia should be considered. Medical conditions that result in polyphagia including systemic disease (eg, diabetes mellitus, hyperadrenocorticism, hepatic disease), thalamic lesions, and pets on calorie restriction for weight loss.[20,21]

Medications that cause polyphagia include corticosteroids, diuretics, and benzodiazepines. Corticosteroids can cause additional signs consistent with SRP including inappropriate elimination, panting, and an increase in anxiety.[20] Other medication classes that can result in increased agitation and secondary destructive behavior include antihistamines (cyproheptadine), selective serotonin reuptake inhibitors, tricyclic antidepressants, barbiturates (phenobarbital), and Janus kinase inhibitors (oclacitinib).[19,22]

Inappropriate Elimination

Physical conditions to consider in dogs exhibiting inappropriate elimination include those that result in increased volume or frequency of urine or stool, increased discomfort during elimination, decreased control of sphincters (incontinence), and diseases affecting cortical homeostasis **(Fig. 2)**.[20] The medical history collection should include information regarding water consumption, diet, pica-like behaviors, volume and frequency of elimination, signs of pain during elimination, mobility or sensory concerns, changes in appearance of feces or urine, and a description of the act of elimination.[23]

Impaired cognitive function may lead to disorientation and loss of learned behaviors, including house training.[23] Conditions that affect mobility, such as arthritis or neuromuscular disorders, and sensory decline can alter elimination habits as they have difficulty accessing or navigating their elimination areas.[23] Medical conditions that increase anxiety or androgens (eg, interstitial cell tumors) could result in an escalation in marking behavior.[23] See **Table 2** for a summary of medical causes of fecal and urinary house soiling in dogs.

Medications that can result in inappropriate elimination include those that relax the urethral sphincter (prazosin), stimulate appetite and/or result in polyphagia (benzodiazepines), cause polyuria and polydipsia (corticosteroids, phenobarbital), increase urine or fecal volume (diuretics), and cause diarrhea (chemotherapeutic agents).[23]

Repetitive Motor Activity

Common repetitive behaviors that dogs with SRP may exhibit include pacing and circling, as seen in Video 1. Medical differential diagnoses for increased motor activity

Table 1
Differential diagnoses of physical disease for clinical signs of canine separation-related problem

Clinical Sign of SRP	Differential Diagnoses-Related to Physical Disease
Destructive behavior	Gastrointestinal (pica) Metabolic/endocrine (hepatic encephalopathy, hepatic dysfunction or failure, diabetes mellitus, hyperadrenocorticism) Neoplasm (thalamic lesions causing polyphagia, pica, and so forth) Infectious (rabies) Dog on calorie restricted diet for weight loss Partial (focal) seizures
Inappropriate urination	Developmental (ectopic ureter, portosystemic shunting) Acquired (urolithiasis, polyp) Metabolic/endocrine (diabetes mellitus, renal insufficiency or failure, hypercalcemia, hyperadrenocorticism, primary polydipsia) Neurogenic (lesions in the brain, upper motor neuron disease, lower motor neuron disease) Inflammatory (cystitis, vaginitis, prostatitis) Infectious (pyelonephritis, pyometra) Hormonal disease (testicular neoplasm)
Inappropriate defecation	Developmental (hydrocephalus) Acquired (tumor, prostatic disease, hernia) Metabolic/endocrine (hyperadrenocorticism) Neurogenic (lesions in the brain, upper motor neuron disease, lower motor neuron disease) Inflammatory (enteritis, colitis) Infectious (parasitemia) Diet (high fiber)
Repetitive motor activity	Degenerative (meningoencephalitis, cauda equina syndrome) Metabolic/endocrine (hypocalcemia, hypomagnesemia) Neoplastic (lesions in the frontal lobe, internal capsule, caudate nuclei) Sensory deficits (blindness) Infectious (rabies) Hepatic encephalopathy Toxicity
Inactivity	Developmental (portosystemic shunting, lysosomal storage disease) Metabolic/endocrine (hepatic encephalopathy, hepatic dysfunction or failure, hypothyroidism, hyperkalemia, hyperadrenocorticism) Neoplastic (thalamic, subthalamic, midbrain, frontal lobe, intracranial) Toxicity (heavy metal, medications) Traumatic (cerebral injury)
Panting, hypersalivation	Thermal regulation (hyperthermia, fever) Respiratory disease Cardiovascular disease Metabolic/endocrine disease (hyperadrenocorticism) Hypertension Pain Toxicity (marijuana)

(continued on next page)

Table 1 (continued)	
Clinical Sign of SRP	**Differential Diagnoses-Related to Physical Disease**
Self-directed behaviors	Degenerative (meningoencephalitis, cauda equina syndrome) Metabolic/endocrine (hypocalcemia, hypomagnesemia, hepatocutaneous syndrome, hepatic encephalopathy) Neoplastic (lesions in the brain) Pain (neuropathy, neuritis, postoperative incision) Dermatologic (hypersensitivity reaction, food allergy, parasites, acral lick dermatitis, symmetric lupoid onychodystrophy) Infectious (bacterial, fungal, parasitic) Immune-mediated Foreign body
Anorexia	Gastrointestinal (nausea) Metabolic/endocrine (hypothyroidism) Neoplasm (GI lymphoma) Immune-mediated diseases Pain
Excessive vocalization	Hepatic encephalopathy Pain (neurologic, orthopedic, musculoskeletal, visceral) Cognitive dysfunction

Data from Refs.[6,9,19–21]

or ritualistic behaviors include degenerative causes (meningoencephalitis, cauda equina syndrome), endocrine or metabolic causes (hypocalcemia, hypomagnesemia), neurologic causes (lesions in the frontal lobe, central neurologic disease), sensory deficits (blindness), infectious causes (rabies), and toxic causes (tetanus, botulism).[9,21]

Medications that have the potential to increase activity via a paradoxic effect include behavior-modifying medications (benzodiazepines, selective serotonin reuptake inhibitors, tricyclic antidepressants), antihistamines, corticosteroids, phenylpropanolamine, phenobarbital, and oclacitinib.[20,22]

Inactivity

In contrast with repetitive behavior, some dogs exhibiting SRP will experience inactivity, such as lying by the exit door during the owner's absence. Medical differential diagnoses for inactivity, sometimes referred to as depression or listlessness, include developmental causes (portosystemic shunting, lysosomal storage disease), endocrine or metabolic causes (hepatic encephalopathy, hepatic failure, hypothyroidism, hyperadrenocorticism), neoplastic causes (thalamic, subthalamic, midbrain, or frontal

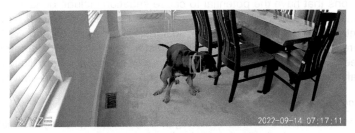

Fig. 2. A dog defecating while home alone secondary to SRP.

Table 2
Medical differential diagnoses for canine fecal and urinary house soiling

Medical Causes of Fecal House Soiling	Examples	Medical Causes of Urinary House Soiling	Examples
Increased fecal volume	Maldigestion, malabsorption, high-fiber diets	Increased volume of urine (polyuria)	Renal, hepatic, hypercalcemia, pyometra, hyperadrenocorticism, diabetes mellitus or insipidus
Increased voiding frequency	Colitis, diarrhea	Increased voiding frequency	Urinary tract infection (UTI), cystic calculi, bladder neoplasm
Reduced control (incontinence)	Compromised neurologic function (impairments of a peripheral nerve, the spine, sphincter)	Reduced control (incontinence)	Compromised neurologic function (impairments of a peripheral nerve, the spine, sphincter)
Painful defecation	Arthritis, anal sacculitis, colitis	Painful urination (pollakiuria)	Arthritis, UTI, cystic calculi, prostatitis
Cranial disease	Neoplasm, encephalitis	Cranial disease	Neoplasm, encephalitis
Sensory decline	Blindness	Sensory decline	Blindness
Canine cognitive dysfunction syndrome	Disorientation, loss of learned behaviors	Canine cognitive dysfunction syndrome	Disorientation, loss of learned behaviors
Altered mobility	Arthritis, neuromuscular	Altered mobility	Arthritis, neuromuscular
Medications altering stool consistency	Chemotherapeutics	Medications altering urine frequency or volume	Corticosteroids
		Marking	Increased anxiety, hormonal (androgen-producing tumors)

Adapted from Ref.[23]; with permission. The original table was published in Behavior Problems of the Dog & Cat, 3rd Ed., G. Landsberg, W. Hunthausen, L. Ackerman, Pg 274, Copyright Elsevier (2013).

lobe lesions), toxic causes (heavy metal, medication overdoses), and traumatic causes (cerebral injury).[21]

Medications that have the potential to cause sedation include behavior-modifying medications (benzodiazepines, selective serotonin reuptake inhibitors, tricyclic antidepressants, and others), antihistamines, analgesics, and many others.[20,22] In a study on dogs presenting to a specialty clinic with a history of corticosteroid treatment for at least 1 week, they found that those patients were significantly more likely to be in a negative affective state and significantly less likely to present a high-activity level.[24]

Panting and Hypersalivation

Panting can be associated with thermal regulation, fever, respiratory disease, cardiovascular disease, metabolic disease, endocrine disease, hypertension, toxin exposure, and pain.[9,19,25,26] Hypersalivation may be secondary to an increase in panting or primarily due to dental disease, gastrointestinal disease, neurologic disease, toxin exposure, and pain.[19] Any medication that increases anxiety and agitation can increase the frequency of secondary panting. Panting is also a side effect of various medications, including corticosteroids.[20]

Self-Directed Behaviors

Dogs with SRP may exhibit behaviors that are targeted at themselves including excessive licking or chewing of their body. Medical differential diagnoses for self-directed or self-injurious behaviors include conditions causing pain or pruritus (hypersensitivity reactions, neuropathies, symmetric lupoid onychodystrophy, postoperative incision), infectious causes (bacterial, fungal, parasitic), endocrinopathies, neoplasia, immune-mediated diseases, and dermatologic disorders associated with systemic disease (hepatocutaneous syndrome).[20] According to Sherman, specific medical diagnoses to consider include neuritis, dermatitis, foreign body, parasites, acral lick dermatitis, and hepatic encephalopathy.[9] **Fig. 3** provide an example of acral lick dermatitis. In a study on psychogenic alopecia study in cats, 76% of cases had a medical etiology with a combination of adverse food reaction and atopy being the most common.[27]

Miscellaneous Behaviors

Dogs with SRP can exhibit nonspecific signs of anxiety, including anorexia and excessive vocalization. Anorexia can be caused by many medical conditions, therefore, a thorough history collection is recommended to narrow down the list of medical differential diagnoses. Excessive vocalization can be caused by primary neurologic disease, hepatic encephalopathy, and conditions resulting in pain or discomfort.[6,9] Anorexia is a common side effect of medications, including behavior-modifying agents (selective serotonin reuptake inhibitors). Medications causing an increase in agitation can secondarily cause excessive vocalization due to anxiety.

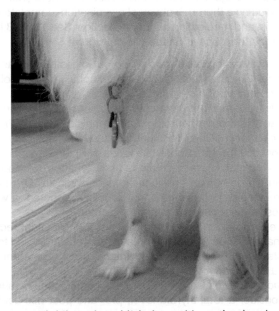

Fig. 3. Dog presenting with bilateral acral lick dermatitis on the dorsal aspect of the carpi.

AGE OF PRESENTATION AND DIFFERENTIAL DIAGNOSES
Patients Under 1 Year of Age

In puppies, some medical differential diagnoses for SRP are more likely than in an adult patient. Puppies that are destructive when home alone should be assessed for congenital defects, such as portosystemic shunting, and proper caloric intake as they grow. If they are eliminating in the home, the clinician should screen for gastrointestinal parasites and congenital conditions, such as ectopic ureter. The clinician should also inquire about whether their expected increased frequencies for urination and defecation are being considered. Behavioral differential diagnoses that should be considered in younger patients include boredom, incomplete house training, and normal separation distress in puppies less than 6 months of age.[28]

Senior Patients

In patients of an older age, medical conditions causing signs of SRP should be considered, especially if the SRP did not start until their older age. Older patients are more likely to have multiple medical conditions (eg, deafness, blindness, arthritis) that may present as SRP. They are also more susceptible to senile changes that reduce their ability to cope with separation from attachment figures and changes to their environment.[28] In older patients, age-related physical ailments, including degenerative joint disease, are likely to exacerbate behavior problems.[29] Older patients should also be screened for cognitive dysfunction syndrome as this condition has clinical signs that overlap with SRP including increased anxiety, elimination in the home due to disorientation or loss of learned behaviors, repetitive motor activity, and increased attachment to the owner.

DIFFERENTIAL DIAGNOSES: PHYSICAL DISEASE

The veterinary clinician must rule out differential diagnoses of physical disease for each SRP sign (**Fig. 4**). Dogs presenting with anxiety disorders should undergo baseline diagnostics including a thorough physical examination, complete blood cell count, chemistry, urinalysis, and medication history collection. See **Table 3** for a summary of diagnostic tests to perform based on the clinical sign of SRP.

- *Destructive behavior to obtain food*: Rule out digestive disease or pica with a gastrointestinal (GI) panel testing for levels of cobalamin and folate, fecal examination, and collection of a diet history.
- *Other destructive behaviors* (scratching, digging): Consider infectious disease testing and an MRI if other neurologic abnormalities are identified.
- *Inappropriate urination*: Consider a urine culture and sensitivity, abdominal ultrasound, cystoscopy, pre- and post-bile acids, MRI for a neoplastic lesion, examination for a scrotal mass in males, and gonadotropin hormone-releasing hormone (GnRH) or human chorionic gonadotropin (hCG) response tests for testosterone in males.[20] If diabetes insipidus is suspected, a water deprivation or desmopressin response test may be indicated.[23]
- *Inappropriate defecation*: Consider a diet history collection, rectal examination, fecal examination, GI panel testing for levels of cobalamin and folate, pancreatic function tests, novel protein diet trial, antacid or GI protectant trial, abdominal ultrasound, ± colonoscopy.[20,23]
- *Repetitive motor activity*: Consider toxin testing, infectious testing, and an MRI.
- *Inactivity*: Consider a total thyroid level, pre- and post-bile acids, toxin testing, and an MRI.

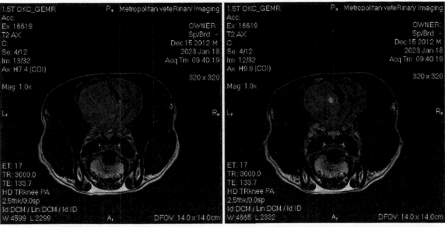

Fig. 4. Axial T2 (*left*) and T1 post-contrast images of a 10-year-old mixed breed dog that was presented to a veterinary neurologist for behavioral changes (increased anxiety when home alone, pacing, inappropriate elimination in the home). MRI conclusions: Extensive plaque-like extra-axial contrast enhancing mass in the left forebrain with expansile tracking in the falx cerebri/longitudinal fissure, marked left forebrain edema, and resultant severe mass effect that results in rightward subfalcine and caudal transtentorial herniation. There is coning and nearly foraminal herniation of the cerebellum though the cerebellar tissue does not extend through the foramen magnum at the time of imaging. Primary differentials include lymphoma, histiocytic sarcoma, granular cell tumor, or less likely an atypical meningioma. Although considered much less likely without a history of travel to a known endemic region, fungal granulomatous disease cannot be excluded. (Images provided by Melissa Logan, PhD, DVM, DACVIM [Neurology]).

- *Panting and hypersalivation*: Consider total thyroid level, temperature reading, blood pressure, 4DX or titers for tick-borne diseases, thoracic radiographs, echocardiogram, and toxin testing.
- *Self-directed behavior*: Dermatologic diseases should be ruled out with cytology of skin lesions, hair pluck, skin scrape, food trial, and intradermal skin testing. An analgesic medication trial can rule out pain-related causes of self-injurious behavior.

In combination with other clinical signs, the clinician should be able to narrow down the diagnostic list to determine potential causes of anorexia and excessive vocalization.

BRIEF OVERVIEW OF FELINE SEPARATION-RELATED PROBLEM

SRP can be observed in cats as well. There is limited research on SRP in cats, but early retrospective studies were performed by veterinary behaviorist Dr Stefanie Schwartz. In those studies, the most common signs of SRP in cats included inappropriate urination, inappropriate defecation, excessive vocalization, destructive behavior, and psychogenic grooming.[30] When cats inappropriately urinated while home alone, 75% urinated on their owner's bed.[30] Some sex differences were noted as inappropriate defecation was significantly higher in neutered females than neutered males, psychogenic grooming was only identified in females, and destructive behavior was only observed in neutered males.[30] Risk factors for SRP in cats were often

Table 3
Diagnostics to rule out medical causes of canine separation-related problem

Clinical Signs of SRP	Diagnostics to Rule out Causes of Physical Disease (In Addition to a Physical Examination, Complete Blood Cell Count (CBC), Chemistry, Urinalysis)
Destructive behavior	GI panel (cobalamin/folate), fecal examination, diet history collection, infectious testing, MRI
Inappropriate urination	Urine culture and sensitivity, abdominal ultrasound, cystoscopy, pre- and post-bile acids, MRI, GnRH or hCG response tests, water deprivation or desmopressin response test if diabetes insipidus is suspected
Inappropriate defecation	Diet history collection, rectal examination, fecal examination, GI panel (cobalamin/folate), pancreatic function tests, novel protein diet trial, antacid or GI protectant trial, abdominal ultrasound, ± colonoscopy
Repetitive motor activity	Toxin testing, infectious testing, MRI
Inactivity	Total thyroid level, pre- and post-bile acids, MRI, toxin testing
Panting, hypersalivation	Total thyroid level, temperature reading, blood pressure, 4DX or titers for tick-borne diseases, thoracic radiograph, echocardiogram, toxin testing
Self-directed behaviors	Dermatologic tests (cytology of skin lesions, hair pluck, skin scrape, food trial, intradermal skin testing), analgesic trial, MRI, infectious testing
Anorexia, excessive vocalization	All tests may be considered but narrow down based on other clinical signs

dependent on the owner's lifestyle, such as having an owner who worked long hours, changes in the owner's work schedule, frequent travel by the owner, and an increase in time the owner spent with family or friends.[28,30,31] In addition, cats were more at risk for SRP when there was death or removal of a housemate from the home, when the cats had a history of shelter adoption after 3 months of age, in cats that followed their owners around the home, neutered cats, and cats owned by a single individual.[28] In another study on behavioral associations with breed coat type and eye color in cats, SRP was seen in cats lacking the dominant allele for a full-colored or traditional coat pattern, including lilac coat-colored, Siamese, Burmese, and Tonkinese cats.[32]

In a more recent study, approximately 13% of cat owners surveyed reported that their cat met at least one of the behavioral criteria used to define SRP and of those, 90% reported that their cat displayed two or more behaviors indicative of SRP.[33] In that study, the most commonly reported SRP behaviors were destructive behavior (66%), excessive vocalization (63%), inappropriate urination (60%), and depression–apathy (53%).[33] Lower frequency behaviors included aggression (37%), agitation–anxiety (37%), and inappropriate defecation (23%).[33]

A representative case study of a cat with SRP is included below.

CASE STUDIES
Canine

S, an approximately 9-year-old male neutered German Wirehaired Pointer mix weighing 19.5 kg, was presented to the author for a 2-year history of pacing, barking, whining, panting, and destructive behavior when home alone. When S was adopted by his owner, B, around 3-years-old, he exhibited barking when B was absent, especially when he was crated. B discontinued use of the crate and began to gate S into the kitchen where he relaxed during owner absences.

When S was 7-years-old, he began to exhibit ataxia and was diagnosed by a veterinary neurologist via MRI with a left spinal arachnoid diverticulum at T11–T12, T11–12 fusion (suspected to be congenital), right L7–S1 disc protrusion, and intervertebral foramen stenosis. His owner noticed that he began to show signs of pain and was prescribed prednisolone and gabapentin which addressed his signs of discomfort. S also began to attend physical therapy which improved his ataxia and mobility.

About 2 months after S's neurologic evaluation, he began to whine and bark when separated from his owner by the gate, when she was home, mostly overnight. When home alone, he began to jump over the gate and became destructive (eg, chewing on objects). Nine months before behavioral evaluation, the primary care veterinarian prescribed fluoxetine 0.5 to 2 mg/kg by mouth every 24 hours with minimal improvement observed by his owner.

After behavioral evaluation by the author, S was diagnosed with SRP. He was prescribed clonidine 0.01 to 0.03 mg/kg by mouth 1 hour before departures, weaned off the fluoxetine due to lack of effect, and started to receive melatonin 2 to 3 mg before bedtime to address whining when separated from his owner at night. The owner was instructed to implement behavior modification including relaxation exercises and graduated departures to achieve improvement in his clinical signs.

This is an example of a dog that was predisposed to SRP but had improved with straightforward management when first adopted. However, once he was diagnosed with physical disease causing pain and mobility changes, his SRP returned and increased with severity, requiring more intensive treatment.

Feline

H, a 3-year-old male neutered domestic shorthair weighing 3.6 kg, was presented to the author for a 5-month history of vomiting when home alone. H vomited bile and undigested food if his owner, E, was absent for at least 10 hours (none if < 10 hours, 50% chance if 10–12 hours, 100% chance if overnight). E was away overnight about once per month and when E was going out of town, a pet sitter came to the home once per day to observe H. E began to leave the television on and placed a blanket on the couch that H enjoyed spending time on. Another behavior that began 5 months before presentation was H's vocalization if a door was closed between him and E when she was home, so E did not close doors between them. Before presentation for behavior evaluation, H was started on Zylkene (alpha casozepine) 75 mg by mouth once every 24 hours per the recommendation of a veterinary internist. E reported that there was minimal improvement in vomiting during absences while on the supplement for more than 4 weeks. E also attempted FELIWAY Classic diffusers in the kitchen and living room for a few months with no significant improvement.

Two years before presentation to the author for a behavior consultation, H was experiencing chronic mucoid vomiting. The vomitus at that time had a different appearance from the vomitus found after E's absences. H had an extensive workup performed with his primary care veterinarian followed by two internal medicine specialists which included abdominal radiographs with a barium series, abdominal ultrasound, thoracic radiographs, and exploratory laparotomy and biopsy. Histopathology revealed mild lymphocytes enteritis, nodal small cell lymphoproliferation, and gastric *Helicobacter pylori*. H was treated with prednisolone, Leukeran for suspected lymphoma, and enrofloxacin. The Leukeran and prednisolone were discontinued, and H was started on cisapride 2 mg by mouth once every 12 hours with a commercial diet of duck and peas. At that time, he was diagnosed with food allergies and the mucoid vomiting stopped with the diet change. In addition to the vomiting, H began to exhibit constipation that resolved on the diet change and with the addition of mineral oil.

After behavioral consultation, H was diagnosed with SRP and prescribed buspirone 0.7 mg/kg by mouth once every 12 hours for 1 week, then increased to 1.4 mg/kg by mouth once every 12 hours in combination with behavior modification and environmental management. Video recording was recommended to investigate for other signs of SRP. After 6 months of treatment, E reported that H's vomiting secondary to SRP improved on buspirone as he only vomited if E was absent for at least 3 days including overnights. H's food allergies continued to be well-controlled on his diet.

This case is an example of how a clinical sign of SRP, vomiting, must be differentiated from a primary cause of physical disease. This is an uncommon presentation of SRP in a cat but with the cat's history of food allergies, he was more likely to exhibit gastrointestinal upset as a clinical sign of an anxiety-based condition.

SUMMARY

SRP is a common behavioral diagnosis in companion dogs and there are numerous physical diseases that have clinical signs overlapping with SRP. In addition, physical conditions can exacerbate signs of SRP and cause regression in its treatment, so the clinician should be aware of the relationship. It is important for clinicians to appropriately screen for SRP, diagnose it, and provide appropriate treatments.

CLINICS CARE POINTS

- Separation-related problem (SRP) is defined as a dog exhibiting specific behaviors when they are alone, perceived to be alone, and/or when they cannot access their owner.
- The most common owner complaints of dogs with SRP include house soiling, destruction, excessive vocalization, and increased repetitive motor activity in the owner's absence. Other clinical signs include pacing, panting, whining, tachycardia, tachypnea, trembling, anorexia, vomiting, diarrhea, and decreased activity.
- If a dog is getting into the trash or stealing objects when they are home alone, differential diagnoses of physical disease should be considered for pica and polyphagia.
- Physical conditions to consider in dogs exhibiting inappropriate elimination include those that result in increased volume or frequency of urine or stool, increased discomfort during elimination, decreased control of sphincters (incontinence), and diseases affecting cortical homeostasis.
- Differential diagnoses of physical disease for increased motor activity or ritualistic behaviors include degenerative causes, endocrine or metabolic causes, neurologic causes, sensory deficits, nutritional causes, infectious causes, and toxic causes.
- Differential diagnoses of physical disease for inactivity, often referred to as depression or listlessness, include developmental causes, endocrine or metabolic causes, neoplastic causes, toxic causes, and traumatic causes.
- Panting can be associated with thermal regulation, fever, respiratory disease, cardiovascular disease, metabolic disease, endocrine disease, hypertension, toxin exposure, and pain. Hypersalivation may be secondary to an increase in panting or primarily due to dental disease, gastrointestinal disease, neurologic disease, toxin exposure, and pain.
- Differential diagnoses of physical disease for self-directed behaviors include conditions causing pain or pruritus, infectious causes, endocrinopathies, neoplasia, immune-mediated diseases, and dermatologic disorders associated with systemic disease.

- Anorexia can be caused by many physical conditions, so a thorough history collection is recommended to narrow down the list of medical differential diagnoses.
- Excessive vocalization can be caused by primary neurologic disease, hepatic encephalopathy, and conditions resulting in pain or discomfort.
- Dogs presenting with anxiety should undergo baseline diagnostics including a thorough physical examination, complete blood cell count, chemistry, urinalysis, and medication history collection. Additional diagnostics should be considered based on the clinical signs being observed.

DISCLOSURE

The author has no commercial or financial conflicts of interest or funding sources to disclose.

SUPPLEMENTARY DATA

Supplementary data related to this article can be found online at https://doi.org/10.1016/j.cvsm.2023.08.003.

REFERENCES

1. Landsberg GM, Hunthausen W, Ackerman L. Fears phobias, and anxiety disorders. In: of the dog and cat. 3rd edition. New York: Saunders Limited; 2013. p. 181-210.
2. Ogata NN. Separation anxiety in dogs: what progress has been made in our understanding of the most common behavioral problems in dogs? J Vet Behav 2016;16(C):28–35.
3. de Assis LS, Matos R, Pike TW, et al. Developing diagnostic frameworks in veterinary behavioral medicine: Disambiguating separation related problems in dogs. Front Vet Sci 2020;6:499.
4. Ballantyne KC. Separation, Confinement, or Noises: What is Scaring That Dog? Vet Clin North Am Small Anim Pract 2018;48:367–86.
5. Tiira K, Sulkama S, Lohi H. Prevalence, comorbidity, and behavioral variation in canine anxiety. J Vet Behav 2016;16(C):36–44.
6. Sherman BL, Mills DS. Canine anxieties and phobias: an update on separation anxiety and noise aversions. Vet Clin North Am Small Anim Pract 2008;38(5):1081–106.
7. Bradshaw JWS, McPherson JA, Casey RA, et al. Aetiology of separation-related behaviour in domestic dogs. Vet Rec 2002;151(2):43–6.
8. Bamberger M, Houpt KA. Signalment factors, comorbidity, and trends in behavior diagnoses in dogs: 1,644 cases (1991-2001). J Am Vet Med Assoc 2006;229(10):1592–601.
9. Sherman BL. Separation Anxiety in Dogs. Compendium 2008;1:27–42.
10. Seksel K, Lindeman MJ. Use of clomipramine in treatment of obsessive-compulsive disorder, separation anxiety and noise phobia in dogs: a preliminary, clinical study. Aus Vet J 2001;79:252–6.
11. King JN, Sherman BL, Overall KL, et al. Treatment of separation anxiety in dogs with clomipramine: results from a prospective, randomized, double-blind, placebo-controlled, parallel-group, multicenter clinical trial. Appl Anim Behav Sci 2000;67(4):255–75.
12. Landsberg GM, Melese P, Sherman BL, et al. Effectiveness of fluoxetine chewable tablets in the treatment of canine separation anxiety. J Vet Behav 2008;3(1):12–9.

13. Sherman BL, Landsberg GM, Reisner IR, et al. Effects of reconcile (fluoxetine) chewable tablets plus behavior management for canine separation anxiety. Vet Therapeut 2007;8(1):18–31.
14. Palestrini C, Minero M, Cannas S, et al. Video analysis of dogs with separation-related behaviors. Appl Anim Behav Sci 2010;124(1–2):61–7.
15. Overall K. Abnormal canine behaviors and behavioral pathologies not primarily involving pathologic aggression. In: Manual of clinical behavioral medicine for dogs and cats. Elsevier Health Sciences; 2013. p. 231–311.
16. Flannigan G, Dodman NH. Risk factors and behaviors associated with separation anxiety in dogs. J Am Vet Med Assoc 2001;219(4):460–6.
17. Storengen LM, Boge SCK, Strøm SJ, et al. A descriptive study of 215 dogs diagnosed with separation anxiety. Appl Anim Behav Sci 2014;159:82–9.
18. Blackwell EJ, Casey RA, Bradshaw JWS. Efficacy of written behavioral advice for separation-related behavior problems in dogs newly adopted from a rehoming center. J Vet Behav 2016;12:13–9.
19. Frank D. Recognizing behavioral signs of pain and disease. Vet Clin North Am Small Anim Pract 2014;44(3):507–24.
20. Landsberg GM, Hunthausen W, Ackerman L. Is it behavioral, or is it medical?. In: Landsberg GM, Hunthausen W, Ackerman L, editors. Behavior problems of the dog and cat. 3rd edition. New York: Saunders Limited; 2013. p. 75–94.
21. Overall KL. Medical differentials with potential behavioral manifestations. Vet Clin North Am Small Anim Pract 2003;33:213–29.
22. Siracusa C. Treatments affecting dog behaviour: something to be aware of. Vet Rec 2016;179:460–1.
23.. Landsberg GM, Hunthausen W, Ackerman L. Canine housesoiling. In: Landsberg GM, Hunthausen W, Ackerman L, editors. Behavior problems of the dog and cat. 3rd edition. New York: Saunders Limited; 2013. p. 269–79.
24. Notari L, Burman O, Mills DS. Is there a link between treatments with exogenous corticosteroids and dog behaviour problems? Vet Rec 2016;179:462.
25. Melian C, Pérez-Alenza MD, Peterson M. Hyperadrenocorticism in dogs. In: Ettinger SJ, Feldman EC, editors. Textbook of veterinary internal medicine. Diseases of the dog and cat. 7th edition. St Louis (MO): Saunders Elsevier; 2010. p. 1816–40.
26. Forney S. Dyspnea and tachypnea. In: Ettinger SJ, Feldman EC, editors. Textbook of veterinary internal medicine. Diseases of the dog and cat. 7th edition. St Louis (MO): Saunders Elsevier; 2010. p. 253–5.
27. Waisglass SE, Landsberg GM, Yager JA, et al. Underlying medical conditions in cats with presumptive psychogenic alopecia. J Am Vet Med Assoc 2006;228(11):1705–9.
28. Schwartz S. Separation anxiety syndrome in dogs and cats. J Am Vet Med Assoc 2003;222:1526–32.
29. Chapman BL, Voith VL. Behavioral problems in old dogs: 26 cases (1984-1987). J Am Vet Med Assoc 1990;196:944–6.
30. Schwartz S. Separation anxiety syndrome in cats: 136 cases (1991-2000). J Am Vet Med Assoc 2002;220:1028–33.
31. Patronek GJ, Glickman LT, Beck AM, et al. Risk factors for relinquishment of cats to an animal shelter. J Am Vet Med Assoc 1996;209:582–8.
32. Wilhelmy J, Serpell J, Brown D, et al. Behavioral associations with breed, coat type, and eye color in single-breed cats. J Vet Behav 2016;13:80–7.
33. de Souza MD, Oliveira PMB, Machado JC, et al. Identification of separation-related problems in domestic cats: A questionnaire survey. PLoS One 2020;15(4):e0230999.

The Relationship Between Aggression and Physical Disease in Dogs

Marta Amat, DVM, PhD, DipECAWBM*, Susana Le Brech, DVM, MSc, PhD, Xavier Manteca, DVM, PhD, DipECAWBM

KEYWORDS

- Canine aggression • Physical disease • Pain • Neurologic problems
- Endocrine disease • Dermatologic problems • Microbiome • Diagnostic protocol

KEY POINTS

- Aggression is a very common behavioral problem in dogs and has a negative influence on dogs' welfare.
- Physical disease can influence the development of aggression problems in dogs.
- A physical examination with the necessary diagnostic tests should be done when addressing aggression problems in dogs.

INTRODUCTION

Aggression problems are very common in dogs[1–4] and have a negative influence on dogs' welfare, as most of them are linked to the experience of stress[5] and aggression is one of the main reasons for relinquishment and euthanasia of healthy dogs.[6–8] Moreover, aggression seems to be associated with a negative cognitive bias and a related negative emotional state.[9] Besides their effect on dogs' welfare, aggression problems pose a risk to public health.[10,11]

Some forms of aggression can be part of dogs' normal behavioral repertoire despite being problem behaviors. Some examples of "normal" aggression are intermale aggression, resource-related aggression, and maternal aggression.[12] Moreover, ontogenetic factors could have an effect on the development of aggression problems. For instance, an inappropriate socialization could facilitate the appearance of fear-related aggression because it happens when puppies do not have appropriate contact with people and/or other animals.[13,14] Similarly, an inappropriate management, including

The authors are fully employed by the Autonomous University of Barcelona and have no economic interest that could interfere with their role as authors of this article.
School of Veterinary Medicine, Universitat Autònoma de Barcelona, Cerdanyola del Vallés 08193, Spain
* Corresponding author.
E-mail address: marta.amat@uab.es

vetsmall.theclinics.com

inadequate punishment or inconsistent handling could cause fear-related or/and frustration-related aggression.[15] Finally, medical conditions can have a significant effect on the development of aggression problems, by either eliciting the aggressive behavior or worsening an already existing problem, because it often happens because of dogs being in pain.[16,17]

The objectives of this article are to (1) review from a practical standpoint the most important medical conditions that could trigger or worsen aggressive behavior in dogs and (2) to suggest a diagnostic protocol for aggressive dogs. We have also included a discussion on the link between aggressive behavior and changes in the microbiome. Indeed, although such changes are not necessarily associated to a disease, there is increasing evidence suggesting that many health-related issues can modify behavior by altering the microbiome.

PAIN AND AGGRESSION

Pain is a psychophysical phenomenon in which the physical perception (nociception) is elaborated by the central nervous system (CNS) to generate the pain experience and response. Therefore, the main sign of pain is a change in behavior. According to a study published by Beaver (1983), pain-related aggression accounts for 2% to 3% of the behavior caseload.[18] However, much more recent research carried out in several referral behavior centers indicates that pain is involved in a much higher percentage of cases.[19]

Pain can modify both the frequency or the intensity of a certain behavior (eg, dogs in pain play less) or it can trigger the appearance of a new behavior (eg, dogs can start showing tail chasing because of pain). The same happens with aggression, as pain can worsen an existing aggression problem, or it can trigger aggression in a nonaggressive dog. In fact, in a study carried out with dogs that had a painful condition and were aggressive toward family members, the authors identified 2 groups of dogs: dogs that showed aggression because they had pain and which reacted with impulsivity when being manipulated and dogs that showed a worsening of aggression due to pain and exhibited aggression in the same contexts in which they reacted aggressively before being in pain, although with higher intensity.[20]

In another study, dogs with musculoskeletal pain tended to show aggression when they were approached while lying down, directing a soft bite mainly toward the victim' legs.[21] Moreover, a study carried out with military dogs concluded that the appearance of aggression was one of the most frequent behavior problems in individuals with multilevel lumbosacral stenosis.[22]

Pain can have a negative effect on aggression through several mechanisms. First, aggression can be a defensive reaction to avoid a particular handling that the dog anticipates as potentially painful.[23] Second, the stress response associated with pain reduces serotonin activity[24]; and third, pain can decrease physical activity, which further reduces serotonin activity in the CNS.[25] A reduction in serotonin activity in the CNS has been linked to aggressive behavior in dogs.[26]

ENDOCRINE DISEASES AND AGGRESSION

Hypothyroidism is a common disease in dogs and its relationship with aggressive behavior has been the focus of many investigations. The relationship between aggression and hypothyroidism seems to be related to the effect of this condition on the serotonergic system. Thyroid hormones seem to have an effect on the concentration of serotonin in blood and in different brain regions, and they also modulate serotonin turnover in the brain.[27,28] The importance of the serotonergic system in dogs with aggression has been established in several publications[29–31] and may explain, at least in part, the relationship between hypothyroidism and certain behavior problems.

According to some publications, the aggression showed by hypothyroid dogs can appear in the absence of other symptoms of hypothyroidism.[32] For instance, an article reported 4 cases of dogs presenting hypothyroidism and aggression as its only symptom, and aggression was reduced after supplementation with thyroid hormones.[33]

It should be kept in mind, however, that thyroid hormones do not have a predictable effect on aggressive behavior. For example, in a cross-sectional study conducted to examine the association between aggression toward family members and serum thyroid hormone concentrations, no differences were found between aggressive and nonaggressive dogs.[34] Hrovat and colleagues (2019)[35] evaluated behavioral changes and serum serotonin concentrations in clinically hypothyroid dogs after levothyroxine supplementation for a period of 6 months and only found changes in activity level but not in aggressive behavior and serotonin concentrations. It should be considered, however, that the latter study had some limitations, including a small sample size and a lack of control group. Finally, Dodman and colleagues (2013) studied the effect of thyroid hormone supplementation in dogs with values of thyroid hormones at the low end of the normal range (borderline) that showed aggression toward family members, and did not find a clear beneficial effect of such supplementation.[36] This study suggests that thyroid hormone supplementation in euthyroid patients (low total T4 but free T4 and thyroid stimulating hormone [TSH] within normal values) is not recommended, even when there is a behavioral problem, because the behavior problem and the thyroid disturbance are unlikely to be related.

In humans, *hyperadrenocorticism* (or Cushing disease, CS) has been associated with a wide range of psychiatric disorders, including depression, anxiety, and panic disorders,[37] and with alterations in cognitive function.[38] Dogs with CS show behavioral and cognitive changes more frequently than dogs of the same age not affected by CS.[39] Regarding aggressive behavior, however, there are no studies showing a direct relationship between aggression and CS. However, it has been reported that exogenous glucocorticoids can cause aggressive behavior in dogs.[40–42] For instance, dogs under corticosteroid treatment were reported by their owners to be significantly more aggressive in the presence of food and more prone to reacting aggressively when disturbed than control dogs.[41] In a more recent study, aggression was also found to be a possible side effect of systemic glucocorticoid therapy in dogs.[43]

NEUROLOGIC PROBLEMS AND AGGRESSION

Many neurologic problems can cause behavior changes such as aggression,[16,17,44] especially when the limbic system is affected[45] (**Box 1**).

The incidence of *brain tumors* in dogs is around 3.0%. Some breeds such as the Boxer, Doberman Pinscher, Golden Retriever, or Scottish Terrier have a higher-than-average risk of developing intracranial tumors.[46] The clinical signs of intracranial tumors depend on their location and size. In dogs, seizures and behavioral changes (ie, irritability, hiding, decreased activity, repetitive behaviors, and so forth) are frequent signs.[47,48] In fact, seizures are one of the most frequent clinical signs when there is a neurologic lesion.[49] Sometimes, if the tumor is in one of the silent areas of the CNS (frontal and prefrontal cortex), behavioral changes could be the only sign.[44] In a study done with 43 dogs with rostral brain tumors, 5 of them showed only behavioral changes and the rest either had seizures and behavioral changes or had only seizures.[47]

Idiopathic epilepsy (IE) is the most common problem diagnosed in dogs with seizures[49] and often manifests with behavioral changes just as it occurs in people.[50]

Box 1
Most common neurologic diseases that could cause aggressive behavior[16,17]

Neurovascular diseases

Inflammatory and infectious diseases (eg, meningitis and encephalitis)

Brain trauma

Congenital anomalies (eg, lissencephaly and hydrocephalus)

Metabolic disease (eg, portosystemic shunt)

Toxic diseases (eg, lead toxicosis)

Neoplasia (eg, in the pituitary gland, hypothalamus, frontal lobe, pyriform lobe, temporal lobe, and in the spinal cord)

Neurodegenerative diseases

Several studies have observed this association, and between 38% and 71% of dogs with IE show behavioral changes such as defensive aggression.[51,52]

Some hepatic diseases that affect the CNS, such as *portosystemic shunt*, can cause *hepatic encephalopathy* (HE). In this condition, various toxins, including ammonia, are not metabolized and eliminated by the liver and their accumulation affects the CNS.[53] This pathology is more frequent in purebred dogs such as the Maltese, Bichon Frise, Shih Tzu, Miniature Schnauzer, Australian Cattle Dog, Border Collie, Jack Russell Terrier, and Irish Wolfhound. The most common signs are seizures, head pressing, and ataxia but other behavioral changes such as anxiety, fear-related behaviors, and aggression are also common.[44,53,54] In fact, in one study on dogs with HE, 29% of them showed altered behaviors.[55] Signs could be intermittent and can be worse after meals.[53]

Other neurologic problems that can cause aggression are inflammatory and infectious diseases caused by viruses, such as distemper and rabies.[16] Rabies is a fatal encephalitis caused by lyssaviruses. Transmission of rabies is through the bite of a rabid animal, which introduces the virus present in its saliva into the bite wound. Major clinical signs in dogs are behavior changes such as aggression, excessive barking, excessive salivation, and neurologic signs such as paralysis or mastication muscle paralysis.[56]

In addition, although it is not very common, developmental disorders such as hydrocephalus could cause aggression. Hydrocephalus results from the accumulation of an excessive amount of cerebrospinal fluid in the brain,[57] and it could be congenital or acquired. Congenital hydrocephalus is the most common brain malformation in dogs and small brachycephalic breeds are predisposed.[58] Besides unspecific signs, several behavior changes including aggression have been reported in dogs with hydrocephalus. In addition, hydrocephalic dogs can have difficulties to cope with stressful events, cognitive impairment, and learning difficulties as well as other behavior problems such as fearfulness.[57] Acquired hydrocephalus does not cause skull malformation and can develop at any age, causing the same signs than congenital hydrocephalus.[57]

Furthermore, there are several substances that can be toxic to dogs.[16,17] For example, ingestion of lead-containing materials can cause gastrointestinal (GI) and neurologic symptoms.[59] Additionally, dogs may display behavioral changes such as lethargy, hysteria, vocalizations, or aggressive behaviors.[60,61] This problem is more common in puppies and young dogs because they tend to explore more than adult dogs. Furthermore, puppies are more sensitive to the effects of lead because their blood–brain barrier is more permeable to it than that of adult dogs.[62] Other substances, such as certain recreational drugs, can also cause aggressive behavior in dogs. Finally, it has been described that amphetamines and methamphetamines, as well as some types of mushrooms, can cause aggressive behavior.[63]

DERMATOLOGIC DISEASES AND AGGRESSION

There are several studies on the association between dermatologic problems and quality of life (QOL) and behavior of dogs.[64–67] Most of them include dogs with *atopic dermatitis* (AD), a chronic disease that causes pruritus. Almost all of them agree that there is an inverse correlation between QOL and pruritus. Furthermore, an association was observed between pruritus due to AD and behavioral problems. Specifically, dogs that had a moderate-to-severe level of pruritus showed significantly more problems related to anxiety and fear, as well as increased aggressiveness and excitability than healthy dogs in the control group.[67] Regarding aggression problems, dogs with AD were more likely to show owner-directed aggression, familiar-dog aggression, and stranger-directed aggression. Interestingly, people with AD show chronic sympathetic overactivation, as well as an excessive sympathetic response to itching sensation,[68] and the same could happen in dogs.[67]

MICROBIOME AND AGGRESSION

The link between the CNS and the GI system has been well established and it is commonly referred to as the "brain-gut-axis."[69] It is widely acknowledged that the relationship between brain and gut is bidirectional, and one of the mechanisms whereby the digestive tract can affect brain and behavior is through the microbiome, which produces a variety of neurotransmitters and precursors, including tryptophan, serotonin, GABA, dopamine, acetylcholine, and noradrenaline (**Table 1**).[70,71] All these molecules have the potential to modify behavior, and, for example, several studies have shown the relationship between low levels of serotonin and aggressive behaviors.[29,72–74]

It has been showed that changes in the microbiome can have an effect on the behavior of laboratory rodents.[76] Research on this particular topic is far less advanced in dogs but it has been reported that the microbiome of aggressive dogs is different

Table 1	
Some neurotransmitters produced by the gut microbiome[75]	
Microorganism	**Neurotransmitter**
Lactobacillus spp	GABA
Bifidobacterium spp	GABA
Escherichia spp	Noradrenaline
Bacillus spp	Noradrenaline
Saccharomyces spp	Noradrenaline
Candida spp	Serotonin
Streptococcus spp	Serotonin
Escherichia spp	Serotonin
Enterococcus spp	Serotonin
Bacillus	Dopamine
Lactobacillus spp	Acetylcholine

Table 2
Main information that should be included in the anamnesis

Dog Data	Age, Environment during Early Development, Age of Adoption, Breed, Neutering Status
Environment and family members	Housing, outdoor access, profile of family members
Owner complaint/s	Description of the aggressive episodes (beginning, target, posture, context, previous treatments)
Handling	Use of punishment, type of punishment, handling, routines (meals and type of food, play, walks, other activities, time left alone, and so forth)
Social behavior	Toward other dogs, unknown people, and family members
Elimination behavior	Description, onset
Phobias	Description, onset
Repetitive behaviors	Description, onset
Medical history	

from that of nonaggressive dogs.[69,77] Moreover, one study seems to indicate that changes in the microbiome lead to changes in behavior in dogs, although this study did not look at aggressive behavior.[78]

As the microbiome can change because of medical conditions,[71] the links between the microbiome and brain function and behavior could be one of the mechanisms whereby physical disease can result in behavioral changes. Clearly, this is an area that deserves further studies.

DIAGNOSTIC PROTOCOL: PRACTICAL APPROACH

We suggest that the diagnostic protocol when dealing with aggressive dogs should include, first of all, an interview with the owner aimed at obtaining all the relevant information about the dog and the owner complain (**Table 2** and **Fig. 1**). Sometimes,

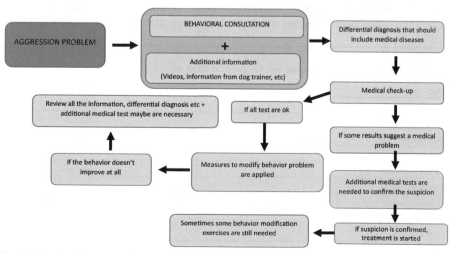

Fig. 1. Diagnostic protocol. Steps to follow within the diagnostic protocol when dealing with an aggressive dog.

some additional information will be needed, such as video recordings of the dog's behavior. In addition and based on the possible effect of many diseases on the development of aggression, a medical check-up should be done. This check-up should include a thorough physical examination to rule out painful conditions, a neurologic examination, a complete blood count, and biochemistry including T4 and TSH.

If some parameters are altered, additional test should be performed. For instance, if a neurologic problem is suspected, an imaging test such as an MRI might be needed, whereas if a portosystemic shunt is considered, a more specific biochemistry panel including bile acids and/or an abdominal ultrasound scan should be done.

In summary, as we have seen throughout the article, many medical conditions, including physical disease and psychophysical problems such as pain can cause or contribute to aggressive behavior in dogs. Therefore, a complete medical checkup is needed to make a proper diagnosis of such problems.

CLINICS CARE POINTS

- Pain can cause or worsen an aggression problem.
- Aggression can be the only symptom in some dogs with hypothyroidism.
- Dogs treated with corticosteroids can show aggressive behavior.
- Aggressive behavior can be a symptom of several neurologic problems. IE and portosystemic shunt, both very common, are some examples.
- Dogs with pruritus are more likely to show behavior problems including aggression.
- Changes in the microbiome could facilitate the appearance of aggressive behavior.
- The diagnostic protocol should consider the physical diseases that can change the dog's behavior.

REFERENCES

1. Bamberger M, Houpt KA. Signalment factors, comorbidity and trends in behaviour diagnosis in dogs: 1,644 cases (1991–2001). J Am Vet Med Assoc 2006; 229:1591–8.
2. Fatjó J, Amat M, Mariotti VM, et al. Analysis of 1040 cases of canine aggression in a referral practice in Spain. J Vet Behav Clin Appl Res 2007;2:158–65.
3. Col R, Day C, Phillips CJC. An epidemiological analysis of dog behavior problems presented to an Australian behavior clinic, with associated risk factors. J Vet Behav 2016;15:1–11.
4. Lord M, Loftus BA, Blackwell EB, et al. Risk factors for human-directed aggression in a referral level clinical population. Vet Rec 2017;181:44.
5. Kruk MR, Halász J, Meelis W, et al. Fast positive feedback between the adrenocortical stress response and a brain mechanism involved in aggressive behavior. Behav Neurosci 2004;118(5):1062–70.
6. Salman MD, New JG Jr, Scarlett JM, et al. Human and animal factors related to relinquishment of dogs and cats in 12 selected animal shelters in the United States. J Appl Anim Welfare Sci 1998;1(3):207–26.
7. De Keuster T, Lamoureux J, Kahn A. Epidemiology of dog bites: a Belgian experience of canine behaviour and public health concerns. Vet J 2006;172(3):482–7.
8. Pike A. Managing Canine Aggression in the Home. Vet Clin North Am Small Anim Pract 2018;48(3):387–402.

9. Barnard S, Wells DL, Milligan ADS, et al. Personality traits affecting judgement bias task performance in dogs (Canis familiaris). Sci Rep 2018;8(1):6660.
10. Westgarth C, Brooke M, Christley RM. How many people have been bitten by dogs? A cross-sectional survey of prevalence, incidence and factors associated with dog bites in a UK community. J Epidemiol Community Health 2018;72(4): 331–6.
11. Ramgopal S, Brungo LB, Bykowski MR, et al. Dog bites in a U.S. county: age, body part and breed in paediatric dog bites. Acta Paediatr 2018;107(5):893–9.
12. Luescher AU, Reisner IR. Canine aggression toward familiar people: a new look at an old problem. Vet Clin North Am Small Anim Pract 2008;38(5):1107–vii.
13. Appleby DL, Bradshaw JWS, Casey RA. Relationship between aggressive and avoidance behaviour by dogs and their experience in the first six months of life. Vet Rec 2002;150:434–8.
14. Arai S, Ohtani N, Ohta M. Importance of bringing dogs in contact with children during their socialization period for better behavior. J Vet Med Sci 2011;73(6): 747–52.
15. Casey RA, Loftus B, Bolster C, et al. Human directed aggression in domestic dogs (Canis familiaris): Occurrence in different contexts and risk factors. Appl Anim Behav Sci 2014;152:52–63.
16. Reisner I. The pathophysiologic basis of behavior problems. Vet Clin North Am Small Anim Pract 1991;21(2):207–24.
17. Overall KL. Medical differentials with potential behavioral manifestations. Vet Clin North Am Small Anim Pract 2003;33(2):213–29.
18. Beaver BV. Clinical classification of canine aggression. Appl Anim Ethol 1983; 10:35.
19. Mills DS, Demontigny-Bédard I, Gruen M, et al. Pain and Problem Behavior in Cats and Dogs. Animals (Basel) 2020;10(2):318.
20. Camps T, Amat M, Mariotti VM, et al. Pain-related aggression in dogs: 12 clinical cases. J Vet Behav 2012;7:99–102.
21. Barcelos AM, Mills DS, Zulch H. Clinical indicators of occult musculoskeletal pain in aggressive dogs. Vet Rec 2015;176(18):465.
22. Dodd T, Jones J, Holásková I, et al. Behavioral problems may be associated with multilevel lumbosacral stenosis in military working dogs. J Vet Behav 2020; 35:8–13.
23. Rutherford KMD. Assessing pain in animals. Anim Welf 2002;11:31–53.
24. Mellor DJ, Cook CJ, Stafford KJ. Quantifying some responses to pain as a stressor. In: Moberg GP, Mench JA, editors. The biology of animal stress. Basic principles and implications for animal welfare. 2002. Wallingford, UK: CAB International; 2000. p. 171–98.
25. Chaouloff F. Effects of acute physical exercise on central serotonergic systems. Med Sci Sports Exerc 1997;29(1):58–62.
26. Tsatsoulis A, Fountoulakis S. The protective role of exercise on stress system dysregulation and comorbidities. Ann N Y Acad Sci 2006;1083:196–213.
27. Reisner IR, Mann JJ, Stanley M, et al. Comparison of cerebrospinal fluid monoamine metabolite levels in dominant-aggressive and non-aggressive dogs. Brain Res 1996;714(1–2):57–64.
28. Bauer M, Heinz A, Whybrow PC. Thyroid hormones, serotonin and mood: of synergy and significance in the adult brain. Mol Psychiatr 2002;7(2):140–56.
29. Bauer M, London ED, Silverman DH, et al. Thyroid, brain and mood modulation in affective disorder: insights from molecular research and functional brain imaging. Pharmacopsychiatry 2003;36(Suppl 3):S215–21.

30. Cakiroğlu D, Meral Y, Sancak AA, et al. Relationship between the serum concentrations of serotonin and lipids and aggression in dogs. Vet Rec 2007;161(2): 59–61.

31. Rosado B, García-Belenguer S, Palacio J, et al. Serotonin transporter activity in platelets and canine aggression. Vet J 2010;186(1):104–5.

32. Beaver BV, Haug LI. Canine behaviors associated with hypothyroidism. J Am Anim Hosp Assoc 2003;39(5):431–4.

33. Fatjó J, Stub C, Manteca X. Four cases of aggression and hypothyroidism in dogs. Vet Rec 2002;151(18):547–8.

34. Radosta LA, Shofer FS, Reisner IR. Comparison of thyroid analytes in dogs aggressive to familiar people and in non-aggressive dogs. Vet J 2012;192(3): 472–5.

35. Hrovat A, De Keuster T, Kooistra HS, et al. Behavior in dogs with spontaneous hypothyroidism during treatment with levothyroxine. J Vet Intern Med 2019;33: 64–71.

36. Dodman NH, Aronson L, Cottam N, et al. The effect of thyroid replacement in dogs with suboptimal thyroid function on owner-directed aggression: A randomized, double-blind, placebo-controlled clinical trial. J Vet Behav 2013;8:225–30.

37. Conner SH, Solomon SS. Psychiatric Manifestations of Endocrine Disorders. J Hum Endocrinol 2017;1:007.

38. Forget H, Lacroix A, Bourdeau I, et al. Long-term cognitive effects of glucocorticoid excess in Cushing's syndrome. Psychoneuroendocrinology 2016;65:26–33.

39. Castilhos da Silva C, Cavalcante I, Carvalho de Carvalho G, et al. Cognitive dysfunction severity evaluation in dogs with naturally-occurring Cushing's syndrome: A matched case-control study. J Vet Behav 2021;46:74–8.

40. Notari L, Burman O, Mills D. Behavioural changes in dogs treated with corticosteroids. Physiol Behav 2015;1(151):609–16.

41. Notari L, Burman O, Mills D. Is there a link between treatments with exogenous corticosteroids and dog behaviour problems? Vet Rec 2016;179(18):462.

42. Notari L, Kirton R, Mills DS. Psycho-Behavioural Changes in Dogs Treated with Corticosteroids: A Clinical Behaviour Perspective. Animals (Basel) 2022; 12(5):592.

43. Elkholly DA, Brodbelt DC, Church DB, et al. Side Effects to Systemic Glucocorticoid Therapy in Dogs Under Primary Veterinary Care in the UK. Front Vet Sci 2020;7:515.

44. Camps T, Amat M, Manteca X. A Review of Medical Conditions and Behavioral Problems in Dogs and Cats. Animals (Basel) 2019;9(12):1133.

45. Amadei E, Cantile C, Gazzano A, et al. The link between neurology and behavior in veterinary medicine: A review. J Vet Behav 2021;46:40–53.

46. Snyder JM, Shofer FS, Van Winkle TJ, et al. Canine intracranial primary neoplasia: 173 cases (1986-2003). J Vet Intern Med 2006;20(3):669–75.

47. Foster ES, Carrillo JM, Patnaik AK. Clinical signs of tumors affecting the rostral cerebrum in 43 dogs. J Vet Intern Med 1988;2(2):71–4.

48. PJJ Mandigers, Van Nes JJ, Voorhout G. Intracranial tumors: a diagnostic challenge. Vet Q 1994;16(sup1):62.

49. Podell M, Fenner WR, Powers JD. Seizure classification in dogs from a nonreferral-based population. J Am Vet Med Assoc 1995;206(11):1721–8.

50. Levitin H, Hague DW, Ballantyne KC, et al. Behavioral Changes in Dogs With Idiopathic Epilepsy Compared to Other Medical Populations. Front Vet Sci 2019; 6:396.

51. Watson F, Packer RMA, Rusbridge C, et al. Behavioural changes in dogs with idiopathic epilepsy. Vet Rec 2020;186(3):93.
52. Shihab N, Bowen J, Volk HA. Behavioral changes in dogs associated with the development of idiopathic epilepsy. Epilepsy Behav 2011;21(2):160–7.
53. Konstantinidis AO, Patsikas MN, Papazoglou LG, et al. Congenital Portosystemic Shunts in Dogs and Cats: Classification, Pathophysiology, Clinical Presentation and Diagnosis. Vet Sci 2023;10(2):160.
54. Tivers M, Lipscomb V. Congenital portosystemic shunts in cats: investigation, diagnosis and stabilisation. J Feline Med Surg 2011;13(3):173–84.
55. Lidbury JA, Cook AK, Steiner JM. Hepatic encephalopathy in dogs and cats. J Vet Emerg Crit Care 2016;26(4):471–87.
56. Thiptara A, Atwill ER, Kongkaew W, et al. Epidemiologic trends of rabies in domestic animals in southern Thailand, 1994-2008. Am J Trop Med Hyg 2011; 85(1):138–45.
57. Thomas WB. Hydrocephalus in dogs and cats. Vet Clin North Am Small Anim Pract 2010;40(1):143–59.
58. Schmidt M, Ondreka N. Hydrocephalus in Animals. Pediatric Hydrocephalus 2019;53–95.
59. Bates N. Lead toxicosis in cats and dogs. Companion Animal 2018;23(12): 674–82.
60. Koh TS. Diagnosis of lead poisoning in dogs. Aust Vet J 1985;62(11):392–4.
61. Pokras MA, Kneeland MR. Lead poisoning: using transdisciplinary approaches to solve an ancient problem. EcoHealth 2008;5(3):379–85.
62. Toyomaki H, Yabe J, Nakayama SMM, et al. Factors associated with lead (Pb) exposure on dogs around a Pb mining area, Kabwe, Zambia. Chemosphere 2020;247:125884.
63. Oster E, Čudina N, Pavasović H, et al. Intoxication of dogs and cats with common stimulating, hallucinogenic and dissociative recreational drugs. Vet Anim Sci 2023;19:100288.
64. Favrot C, Linek M, Mueller R, et al, International Task Force on Canine. Atopic Dermatitis. Development of a questionnaire to assess the impact of atopic dermatitis on health-related quality of life of affected dogs and their owners. Vet Dermatol 2010;21(1):63–9 [published correction appears in Vet Dermatol 2010 Oct;21(5):544].
65. Linek M, Favrot C. Impact of canine atopic dermatitis on the health-related quality of life of affected dogs and quality of life of their owners. Vet Dermatol 2010;21(5): 456–62.
66. Klinck MP, Shofer FS, Reisner IR. Association of pruritus with anxiety or aggression in dogs. J Am Vet Med Assoc 2008;233(7):1105–11.
67. McAuliffe LR, Koch CS, Serpell J, et al. Associations Between Atopic Dermatitis and Anxiety, Aggression, and Fear-Based Behaviors in Dogs. J Am Anim Hosp Assoc 2022;58(4):161–7.
68. Tran BW, Papoiu AD, Russoniello CV, et al. Effect of itch, scratching and mental stress on autonomic nervous system function in atopic dermatitis. Acta Derm Venereol 2010;90(4):354–61.
69. Mondo E, Barone M, Soverini M, et al. Gut microbiome structure and adrenocortical activity in dogs with aggressive and phobic behavioral disorders. Heliyon 2020;6(1):e03311.
70. Cryan JF, O'Mahony SM. The microbiome-gut-brain axis: from bowel to behavior. Neuro Gastroenterol Motil 2011;23(3):187–92.

71. Dinan TG, Cryan JF. The Microbiome-Gut-Brain Axis in Health and Disease. Gastroenterol Clin N Am 2017;46(1):77–89.
72. Peremans K, Audenaert K, Coopman F, et al. Estimates of regional cerebral blood flow and 5-HT2A receptor density in impulsive, aggressive dogs with 99mTc-ECD and 123I-5-I-R91150. Eur J Nucl Med Mol Imag 2003;30(11):1538–46.
73. Coccaro EF, Fanning JR, Phan KL, et al. Serotonin and impulsive aggression. CNS Spectr 2015;20(3):295–302.
74. O'Mahony SM, Clarke G, Borre YE, et al. Serotonin, tryptophan metabolism and the brain-gut-microbiome axis. Behav Brain Res 2015;277:32–48.
75. Lyte M. Microbial Endocrinology and the Microbiota-Gut-Brain Axis. In: Lyte M, Cryan J, editors. Microbial endocrinology: the microbiota-gut-brain Axis in health and disease. Advances in experimental medicine and biology, 817. New York: Springer; 2014. https://doi.org/10.1007/978-1-4939-0897-4_1.
76. Kelly JR, Borre Y, O' Brien C, et al. Transferring the blues: Depression-associated gut microbiota induces neurobehavioural changes in the rat. J Psychiatr Res 2016;82:109–18.
77. Kirchoff NS, Udell MAR, Sharpton TJ. The gut microbiome correlates with conspecific aggression in a small population of rescued dogs *(Canis familiaris)*. PeerJ 2019;7:e6103.
78. McGowan RTS, Barnett HR, Czarnecki-Maulden G, et al. Tapping into those 'gut feelings': Impact of BL999 (Bifidobacterium longum) on anxiety in dogs. ACVB Veterinary Behavior Symposium; July 12, 2018; Denver, Colorado.

Behavior Problems Associated with Pain and Paresthesia

Daniel S. Mills, BVSc, PhD, CBiol, FRSB, FHEA, CCAB, Dip ECAWBM (BM), FRCVS, RCVS[a],*, Fergus M. Coutts, BVM&S, MSc, MRCVS[b], Kevin J. McPeake, BVMS, PGDip(CABC), PhD, AFHEA, CCAB, DipECAWBM(BM), MRCVS[c]

KEYWORDS

- Adjunctive behavior • Discomfort • Dysesthesia • Pain • Paresthesia
- Problem behavior

KEY POINTS

- Many forms of discomfort are implicated in problem behavior.
- Discomfort is commonly implicated in problem behavior.
- There are many nontraditionally recognized behaviors that can aid assessment of pain.
- Failure to make expected progress with a rational treatment plan often indicates discomfort.
- Behavioral comorbidities are a common feature of pain-related problem behaviors.

INTRODUCTION: PAIN, PARESTHESIA, AND DYSESTHESIA IN VETERINARY PRACTICE

The International Association for the Study of Pain (IASP) defines pain, as *"An aversive sensory and emotional experience typically caused by, or resembling that caused by, actual or potential tissue injury."*[1] Importantly, this definition and the accompanying notes highlight the following:

- Pain is usually an adaptive response, even though it may impact on the functioning of an individual.
- Pain and nociception are not the same.
- Pain is always a subjective experience influenced by biological, psychological, and social factors.

[a] Animal Behaviour Cognition and Welfare Group, Department of Life Sciences, University of Lincoln, Lincoln, UK; [b] Pain Management and Rehabilitation Centre, Broadleys Veterinary Hospital, Craigleith Road, Stirling FK7 7LE, UK; [c] The Royal (Dick) School of Veterinary Studies, Easter Bush Campus, Midlothian EH25 9RG, UK
* Corresponding author.
E-mail address: dmills@lincoln.ac.uk

Vet Clin Small Anim 54 (2024) 55–69
https://doi.org/10.1016/j.cvsm.2023.08.007
0195-5616/24/© 2023 Elsevier Inc. All rights reserved.
vetsmall.theclinics.com

- An individual's expression of pain (which does not need to be verbal) should be accepted and respected (and while the IASP refer to people in this regard, we would suggest the same standard should be applied to nonhuman animals).

By contrast, paresthesia is considered as an abnormal prickling, tingling, or burning sensation typically felt in the skin of the limbs[2]; the term "dysesthesia" may also be used to refer to abnormal painful sensations arising from innocuous cutaneous stimulation which are also often felt as a burning sensation that outlasts the stimulus.[3] Paresthesia may occur when the nerve supply to a region is compromised, for example, by compression or entrapment (such as from local inflammation) or as a result of direct damage (such as from herpes viral infection); it can also be seen in humans as a consequence of the hyperventilation associated with panic attacks or when the circulation to a region is compromised in a way that results in poor local nerve functioning, for example, when animals have been out in the snow for a while.[4] Although paresthesia can be chronic, the transient nature of many poses a diagnostic challenge when dealing with nonverbal individuals. Nonetheless, given their general biological basis, it is fair to say that paresthesia is probably far more common than is widely recognized in veterinary medicine, especially when there are signs of vertebral compression without signs of overt pain. The same probably applies to dysesthesia. Both phenomena can be expected to cause fear/anxiety as patients may experience spontaneous abnormal sensations during movement. For the purposes of this article, the authors refer to pain and/or paresthesia and/or dysesthesia as sources of discomfort.

CASE VIGNETTE: CHANGE IN CUTANEOUS SENSATION AND SELF-MUTILATION IN A DOG

A 6.5-year-old Labrador was presented with a history of having been hit by a car 8 months earlier. Advanced imaging showed multiple fractures of vertebral transverse processes, cervical cord contusion, and damage to the left brachial plexus. He was presented to a pain management clinic with marked left forelimb lameness and a "lick granuloma" over the medial aspect of the left carpus (**Fig. 1**). There was an absence of pin-prick sensation in and around this lesion, and consistent with neuropathy, there was presumed to be dysesthesia/pain in an area of hypoesthesia. He was also found to be hypothyroid. Treatment of neuropathic pain and thyroid supplementation decreased the licking without further behavior modification and the lesion healed (**Fig. 2**).

CLASSIFICATION OF DISCOMFORT AND ITS IMPLICATIONS

There are several systems used to describe and classify discomfort:

Temporal: Acute or chronic: Although this involves an arbitrary time-based distinction, it has some clinical utility, contrasting acute pain, for example, from a surgical setting, with chronic pain which is associated with conditions where pain lasts more than 3 months.[5] Nonetheless, there are challenges to the biological validity of this distinction.[6] This classification poorly describes the transition from the mechanisms behind inflammatory pain, which is mostly acute, to the changes in processing associated with neuropathic pain, often characterized by longer term tissue damage with central and peripheral sensitization.

Adaptive or maladaptive: As defined by Woolf "adaptive pain contributes to survival by protecting the organism from injury or promoting healing when injury has occurred. Maladaptive pain, in contrast, is an expression of the pathologic operation of the nervous system; it is pain as disease."[7] However, this assumption about malfunction giving rise to maladaptiveness may not be sound.[8]

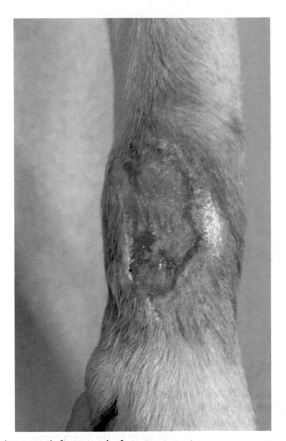

Fig. 1. Lick granuloma on left carpus before treatment.

Organ system affected: Although this description can help communicate the localization of discomfort, it can also lead to a belief that there is a specific "recipe" based on the locality of the pain. Conditions affecting certain organs may frequently recruit specific pain mechanisms, but effective management relies on understanding and recognition of the more fundamental pain mechanisms involved, regardless of the organ or tissue system affected.

Pathogenesis: Understanding the neurobiology involved in the discomfort being presented allows treatment with drugs to target specific mechanisms (peripheral sensitization, neuropathic pain, central sensitization, nociplastic pain). This provides the most valid basis for management.

Successful management of discomfort is optimized when using a multimodal approach, where pain mechanisms become therapeutic targets and approached with pharmacologic and non-pharmacologic treatment. The discussion of multimodal treatment is beyond the scope of this article, and the principles are well described in the World Small Animal Veterinary Association (WSAVA) Global Pain Council Guidelines[9] and related texts.[10,11]

PAIN AND DISCOMFORT: A BIOBEHAVIORAL PERSPECTIVE

The "biobehavioral model" of pain[12] recognizes, as noted above, that neurobiological mechanisms and behavioral contributors interact. Discomfort is not just a sensory

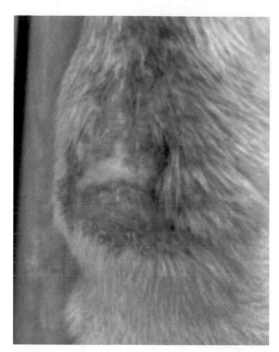

Fig. 2. Left carpus following treatment.

phenomenon but has a bidirectional relationship with both the emotional (affective) state and cognition of the patient, which will impact on their behavior. Protective strategies can be expected lead to an increased risk of anxiety and aggressive behavior,[4] but in other cases, the changes in behavior may be much more subtle. For example, joint hypermobility is a chronically uncomfortable condition for people[13] and in dogs is a risk factor for canine hip dysplasia,[14] which has recently been found to be associated with potentially problematic emotional arousal in dogs.[15] Some changes may also occur as a result of the increased cognitive load associated with discomfort, which can lower pain thresholds and the overall capacity of the sufferer to cope with environmental stressors.[16] The individual may then exhibit not only increased sensitivity to mildly noxious stimuli (eg, noise)[17] but also ordinarily innocuous stimuli, such as handling and touch, may also be perceived as potentially painful (a form of allodynia)[17] and thus threatening. This may manifest as an alteration in the way in which an individual animal interacts with others[18] and their environment[19] as they seek to avoid or change the nature of their responses to avoid discomfort. Indeed, in the case of animals under human care, the bidirectional relationship may extend to include the behavior of the carer, because the carer's behavior may affect both the perception of discomfort by the animal and their concerns about discomfort clearly affect their own mental well-being and behavior.[19,20] Accordingly, we must recognize that the relationships that exist between discomfort and behavior can be highly complex. It must also be acknowledged that although many potential relationships between discomfort and behavior are suggested, it is difficult to present definitive evidence of these. However, given the guidance of IASP[1] to accept and respect expressions of pain, which can be nonverbal, we should be open to at least provisionally accepting these relationships with discomfort, until it can be shown otherwise. Accordingly, veterinarians should be open to the implementation of management strategies for discomfort in cases of problem behavior; accepting that the relationship may not be an obvious one and that there is enormous variability between individuals.

This biobehavioral model also establishes a basis for identifying discomfort and assessing the pain burden an animal is experiencing.

- Nociceptors in the peripheral nervous system transduce injury to generate electrical activity in afferent sensory nerves.
- The release of inflammatory mediators in injured tissue lowers the threshold of nociceptors, causing a "nociceptive barrage."
- This barrage leads to central sensitization in the dorsal horn, where sensory signals are amplified and distorted before projection to the brain.
- The brain's perception of pain is altered by psychological influences, for example, reduced by distraction[21] or enhanced by anticipation.[22]

Further discussion of pain mechanisms is beyond the scope of this article, but further details can be found elsewhere, for example, Bell.[23]

RELATIONSHIP BETWEEN DISCOMFORT AND PROBLEM BEHAVIOR

There are several ways in which discomfort can contribute significantly to the presentation of problem behavior.

1. *Discomfort can be the overt or covert cause of the problem*: All veterinarians will be familiar with the painful animal that protects itself through aggressive behavior. However, the relationship between pain and aggressive behavior is often much more subtle than this, especially when the discomfort has had an insidious onset, as is often the case with chronic osteoarthritis or enteritis.
2. *Discomfort can exacerbate the signs or create a particular profile for a given problem behavior*: Associations between aggressive behavior and chronic musculoskeletal pain have been described in several case series,[18,24] which indicate certain features of the aggressive behavior that might be suggestive of pain involvement. These include greater impulsivity, greater generalization (extension of contexts in which the behavior occurs), bites to the extremities more than other regions, and "attacks" that are more easily broken up. In general, discomfort can be expected to produce some or all of the following general changes that might moderate the problem in various ways depending on its primary cause:
   a. Animals can be expected to be more anxious and/or avoidant as they seek to avoid exacerbating their discomfort. This anxieties may be more severe, that is, intense or extreme in their response, or triggered more readily (in response to otherwise innocuous stimuli that might be predictive of something leading to increased discomfort) than expected.[18,24] In non-anxiety/fear-related conditions, the individual may appear more withdrawn or less willing to engage in certain activities, such as going out for a walk or walking down steps to go into the garden.
   b. The increased and prolonged psychological and potentially physiologic load caused by an ongoing medical issue leading to discomfort will reduce the individual's resilience.[25] This might make the individual more irritable but also prone to other minor ailments. For example, in the case of atopy, a potential bidirectional relationship between the condition and the ability of the individual to cope has been shown.[26]
   c. Individuals may appear clingier/attention seeking as social support can reduce the perception of pain or threat of pain.[27] This higher level of interaction can lead to the conditioning and reinforcement of a range of problem behaviors, as

seems to have occurred during the COVID pandemic, during the lockdown period.[28] Preexisting signs of separation-related problems may be a particular risk factor for the development of a range of other problems in this regard. Perhaps somewhat paradoxically, despite these changes, the individual might avoid physical contact, and perhaps become more aggressive, as they seek to avoid handling which presumably exacerbates their discomfort.

d. The problem behavior might be accompanied by other changes in behavior (see **Box 1**). These include an increase in behaviors such as yawning, sniffing, body-shaking, stretching, and many bizarre behaviors such as air-snapping, surface

---

Box 1
Some common signals and cues to discomfort

The following are signs of discomfort that might be noticed in association with a behavior problem:

Increased blinking, lip-licking, nose-licking, yawning, air-sniffing and hesitant paw-lifting are widely used when individuals feel uncomfortable. These signals, except for slow blinking, are less common in cats.

A *change in the look* of a dog. Owners may struggle to identify what has changed in their dog's face, but both a softening of the eyes when approached (appeasement gesture) and a harder stare (expression of pain) with exposure of the white of the eye (whale eye) may occur with discomfort.

A tendency to *turn the head or body away* from a familiar individual when they approach, ultimately leading to the individual walking away (perhaps unexpectedly from the owner' perspective) can be a gentle way for an animal to signal that they do not want to engage or be touched. In many cases, the animal may walk away very slowly, not because it is physically uncomfortable but in order not to increase the excitement of the situation. Sudden changes in social exchanges can result in rapid escalation of threat.

Animals may *freeze* out of discomfort or as a sign of tolerance to the proximity of another. This often occurs as a normal behavioral response when a smaller dog meets a larger one, but if this there is a change in the frequency with which this response occurs, or a larger dog starts to do this type of response to a smaller dog when it previously did not, then this might indicate the animal is uncomfortable.

Air-licking and licking of surfaces have been associated with gastrointestinal discomfort, for example, due to Giardia or inflammatory bowel disease.

Play is typically reduced when animals are uncomfortable; but play bows in dogs and lateral lying in front of an individual in cats and dogs are often used to defuse a tense situation. So, potentially this behavior might be seen to increase in conspecifics with whom the uncomfortable individual shares a home, as they respond to the increased irritability of the uncomfortable housemate.

Coat changes, including increased dandruff and premature greying, may be signs of chronic stress. This may relate to chronic discomfort and so should be noted as part of the clinical examination. Changes to the nature of the coat, for example, curling of the hair over a muscle group, might also occur if there has been damage to the underlying tissue with consequent disruption to the blood supply and nutrition of hair follicles.

Increased scratching and grooming of a specific area may occur as a result of sensory disturbance related to paresthesia; ear scratching in the absence of overt ear disease may reflect head pain or discomfort in the upper neck.

A *general change in personality or fluctuating mood.* Many animals in discomfort are described as having a "Jekyll and Hyde" personality, moody, or unpredictable. Other more consistent changes are increased irritability/grumpiness and a reduction in play. Any of these changes, especially if they have developed over time, are highly suggestive of discomfort.

licking, and sudden postural freezing which may all be signs of mild discomfort.[4] Animals may also become more destructive, perhaps as a form of displaced/redirected aggressive behavior associated with the discomfort.[29] There may also be a decrease in potentially uncomfortable behaviors like going upstairs (in the case of cats, this might be manifest in reduced use of an upstairs litter box with or without a concomitant house soiling issue developing as a result) or going for a walk. In some cases, animal's will adapt by adopting strange postures or ways of doing routine behaviors, such as frequently appearing to be about to lie down and then stopping, before finally dropping very suddenly; lying or sitting in an unusual way; an unusual gait or way of defecating (perhaps squatting for a short while and then moving or walking on before trying again). In the case of cats with sore hips, they might adopt a standing posture to eliminate, which might be mistaken for spray marking. In some cases, the cat will continue to use the litter box, but in others, an association between eliminating and location may develop, so the animal develops a wandering pattern of house soiling (this might then be a primary behavioral complaint). Another general change might be restlessness as the animal may not be comfortable to lie still for a prolonged period. This can be manifested as the primary problem being accompanied by a separation-related problem; in other instances, the separation-related problem might be the primary complaint and other problems secondary. Thus, superficially unrelated behavioral comorbidities featuring separation-related problems or attention seeking should be given particular clinical attention.

e. Increased possessiveness, which may manifest as a shift in resting area to a more comfortable area (eg, sleeping on the sofa rather than their pet bed) and protectiveness of resources such as food, may also arise when an individual is in a state of discomfort. Resources in fact may become more valuable due to an increased need for certain resources such as comfortable resting places as well as a perceived increased personal cost (due to the pain involved) in reacquiring them if lost. Aggressive displays may be directed toward the human family or other animals in the home. Once again, owner reinforcement may play a substantial role in how this issue is finally manifested by the time the primary problem is presented, and it might not escalate to a primary problem but be considered an annoying feature of the pet's character. Accordingly, the potential for this change should be enquired about in all types of behavioral problem and, when such changes are noted as a behavioral comorbidity (as with apparent attachment-related issues described above), then careful clinical examination for a source of discomfort is warranted.

There are many potential adaptive mechanisms underpinning these types of observation, even if there is not definitive evidence. As already mentioned, animals in pain will feel more at risk and so will express higher levels of anxiety. Individuals in pain are also at greater risk of frustration as they are unable to access the resources they want or perceive certain resources as more valuable as the cost of access increases with the degree of pain associated with gaining it. Increased frustration will also increase the likelihood of displacement behaviors occurring if there is not an acceptable solution, and these might be the origin of the collection of signs commonly described as "calming signals"[30] (see **Box 1** on "Some common signals and cues to pain"). The occurrence of such behaviors may serve to increase endorphin release and thus alleviate some of the discomfort. Engaging in a social interaction with an owner, and as such attention-seeking behaviors[31] might have a similar effect (see case vignette below).

Enquiring about these changes can be illuminating and will certainly increase a clinician's awareness of the potential importance of discomfort in a range of behavioral complaints. This highlights the importance of close veterinary oversight of these cases. This oversight should extend to the treatment period as well, as the significance of discomfort and its effective management might only become apparent at this time in some incidences as discussed in the next section.

3. *Discomfort might reduce or completely block successful treatment of a behavior problem:* Although it is probably true to say that it is possible to train an animal to not show overt signs of pain, it is probably not true to say that this means that the animal ceases to feel pain. In some instances, training may mask the signs of discomfort, and its involvement or significance may only become apparent after behavior modification has begun. If the treatment plan is appropriate and well implemented then the animal should respond. A slower than expected or plateauing response to behavior modification exercises is, in our experience, much less often associated with poor owner compliance than it might be widely believed. More often, the issue relates to pain limiting the animal's ability to proceed. Consider, for example, a plan that involves an animal lying for a prolonged period, but the animal cannot lie comfortably. In this case, as the plan proceeds to increase the time required for the animal to remain lying, the chance of failure due to discomfort increases. Likewise, techniques depending on desensitization may be limited if the animal is already struggling to cope with discomfort. Accordingly, such limitation in progress can not only call for a reassessment of the case behaviorally but also medically.

CASE VIGNETTE: SLEEP DISTURBANCE AND ATTENTION-SEEKING ASSOCIATED WITH HIP DYSPLASIA

A 9-month-old, intact, male Labrador was referred to a pain management clinic with hip dysplasia. A murmur was discovered and the cardiologist reported an atrial septal defect, tricuspid valve dysplasia, and pulmonic valve stenosis. He had become clingy and did not sleep well at night, moving around and when awake seek out the owner for comfort. After treatment for the dysplasia, he was found to sleep through the night without specific behavioral intervention; it was noted that he did have some unusual sleep postures (**Fig. 3**), which might reflect his medical issues.

Identification of Discomfort

Inferences about whether an animal is in discomfort are drawn by owners and clinicians from their observations of the animal's behavior, and in the case of problem behavior, this often involves the assessment of low-grade persistent or intermittent discomfort. Individuals may inhibit or suppress signs of discomfort in certain contexts,[32] and so signs might not be obvious within the context and time of a standard veterinary consultation Thus, careful observation of the patient over a sustained period is essential. In a simple case, this may involve observing lameness to identify pain in a limb or identifying obvious effects on an animal's ability to move through its environment, for example, climbing stairs, enjoying walks, and rising with ease from a lying position. However, in more complex cases, the effect of pain on an animal's behavior may be less obvious, especially where there are subtle changes in gait rather than lameness. In some of these cases, owners are aware something is wrong, but may be unable to describe what. Video footage that can be viewed in slow motion is often helpful in these instances, with advice on how to capture this freely available online.[33] In this

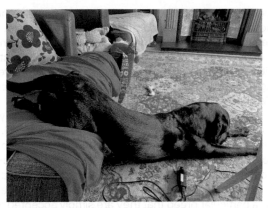

Fig. 3. Unusual sleep posture of dog with hip dysplasia.

instance, a range of parameters should be assessed. For example, animals with bilateral elbow osteoarthritis may have a short stride and elbow abduction, but not show the weight transference associated with a limp. In these cases, the animal may be presented with the owners reporting less obvious changes in behavior, such as those described in the **Box 1** above "Some common signals and cues to discomfort." Of course, none of these are pathognomonic for pain but may signify "yellow flags" for clinicians and should prompt closer examination such as the use of the "Dog pain screen" provided at the end of this article. All of the available evidence should then be carefully triangulated to make an assessment of the likelihood of the occurrence of discomfort and an on-the-spot risk assessment made, which includes the consequences of a failure to recognize discomfort before the next steps are decided.

PERSISTENT MYTHS ABOUT PAIN

Major barriers to clinicians identifying a source of discomfort for a problem behavior are.

- A failure to acknowledge or recognize that a range of conditions are actually painful or cause discomfort
- A belief that the problem is just "behavioral", and thus, a failure to undertake a systematic clinical examination with a view to thoroughly testing the idea "how might these signs be related to discomfort?"

However, there are also several myths that persist around pain in animals, which can affect both an owner's ability to seek help for a potentially painful problem in a timely way and a veterinarian's decision to intervene. These myths include:

- Behavior is distinct from disease and so behavior problems do not require veterinary assessment. Not only is this counter to the biobehavioral model of pain but also such a belief seems to deny the self-evident truth that the reason why most medical cases are presented to a veterinarian is because of a change in behavior, ranging from the lameness of the dog to the development of diarrhea (which is behavior of the gut). At a practical level, this can lead to a partial (eg, performing a cursory physical assessment) or complete failure to undertake a medical examination of a case presented for problem behavior.
- The absence of specific behavioral signs means that pain cannot be present. Examples include the lack of yelping when a painful area is palpated or used. In

other instances, signs of pain like lameness might be mild and so their significance as a potential source of discomfort could be dismissed. This is especially common when the relationship with other behavioral signs is not recognized.

- The absence of obvious or any physical evidence from diagnostic imaging. Many painful conditions, for example, muscular pain will not be revealed using traditional imaging techniques, but even when mild lesions are identified, these are sometimes deemed to be insignificant.

- The belief that certain conditions are not painful, unless they require surgical intervention. Common examples include a range of orthopedic problems such as luxating patellae (see case vignette below) or angular limb deformities; eye problems such as keratoconjunctivitis sicca; skin problems such as otitis externa and atopic dermatitis; and gastrointestinal problems such as acute and chronic inflammatory bowel disease. Indeed, in some instances, certain conditions are so common in a particular breed that they are simply accepted as being "normal" for that breed, without any consideration given to the discomfort they cause.

- Willingness to engage in certain activities like play or extended walks means that the animal cannot be in pain. This is most evident in dogs who are highly motivated to engage in particular activities, for example, chasing squirrels in the park or playing fetch with their ball on walks, which will induce the caregivers to think that "it can't be pain as he still runs around like a puppy at times." Although we may see a reduction in engagement exercise and play in some animals with pain,[34] many continue to engage in these activities in spite of being in pain.

- Related to the previous point, there is sometimes a perceptual blind spot to accepting that abnormalities in young animals can be painful. Some seem unwilling to accept that a young animal can be afflicted with a chronically painful condition such as osteoarthritis.

- The belief that pain is inevitable and just needs to be accepted. This is not uncommon when the state of older animals is considered. In these cases, the lack of intervention may sometimes be justified by an erroneous calculation of the benefits versus risks of analgesic intervention. Although painful conditions especially arising from degenerative conditions such as osteoarthritis are common, awareness must be raised on the early identification of pain and appropriate management to maintain the welfare of these patients.

- A short or single course of analgesia did not make obvious differences, so the condition cannot be painful or no amount of analgesia will work. In this case, there is often a failure to appreciate the heterogeneity of the mechanisms involved or the need for a multimodal approach.[9–11]

CASE VIGNETTE: LUXATING PATELLA AND AGGRESSION IN A DOG

A 2-year-old, male neutered, Chihuahua-cross was referred to a veterinary behaviorist for problems involving vocalizing when separated, barking and lunging at dogs on walks, and sudden and unpredictable episodes of growling, snarling, snapping, and biting toward his owners, usually when resting on their lap. He would still regularly jump on their lap, seemed to seek out physical contact and attention regularly, and weeks could pass without any aggressive behaviors occurring in this context. There were no other environmental triggers identified for these episodes, and physical causes were suspected and explored. The dog was identified as having a pelvic limb lameness where his owners had also seen him "skipping" (pulling one hind leg up abruptly) regularly when walking and running. A grade 2 unilateral luxating patella was identified. A behavior modification program was developed, and this included an analgesia trial in the short term. This led to an improvement in the severity of the signs, but not a resolution likely due to continued patellar luxation. Corrective surgery was performed and after recovery, the lameness was resolved, and no further episodes of aggressive behavior occurred even once pain relief was withdrawn.

REFLECTIONS FROM SPECIALIST CLINICAL PRACTICE

In preparation of this article, the authors each reviewed the last 100 dog cases seen in their referral clinics. DSM and KJM each run a behavior referral clinic; FMC runs a pain management referral clinic. We offer the following additional insights for reflection on the relationship between pain and behavior.

1. Of those 100 cases referred to each of the authors' behavior clinics, DSM found 76% had suspected physical problems (75% causing pain/discomfort); KJM found 58% had suspected physical problems (53% causing pain/discomfort); for FMC, running a pain management clinic, 100% had painful conditions as expected.
2. The perception of the case as behavioral or painful seems to strongly influence the level of clinical attention given to the assessment of the case before referral. If the problem is thought by the referring veterinarian to be behavioral rather than pain-related, there is high probability that relevant physical (usually relating to discomfort) issues will not be identified by them. Relevant physical problems (even if their significance was not identified) were missed by the referring veterinarian in more than half of the behavior cases referred. This most often included gait abnormalities, signs of chronic enteropathy, and bizarre oral behaviors. Among the behavioral cases, it was also noted that even when a veterinarian had identified a physical issue, other physical problems often went unrecognized.
3. Whether or not the animal is perceived to be in pain is strongly associated with the emphasis given in the presenting complaint. For example, the emotional sensitivity of the patient was emphasized in around three-quarters or more of behavior cases presented, but in less than half of those referred for pain management. By contrast functional issues, such as the ability to undertake normal activities like going for a walk or groom the dog was emphasized in more than 90% of pain referrals but less than 50% of behavior referrals.
4. Clinical comorbidities (ie, conditions not contributing to the primary cause of pain), and multiple comorbidities, are common in the cases seen and often have a direct bearing on treatment plans, for example, affecting drug choices (non-steroidal anti-inflammatory drug [NSAID] precluded in dogs with gastrointestinal disease or impaired renal function), treating hypothyroidism, or seeking additional advice from cardiology or neurology services. Among the most common comorbidities seen are, being overweight (which obviously exacerbates musculoskeletal discomfort), dermatologic issues, gastrointestinal issues, heart disease, and endocrine disorders.
5. In both types of referral, owners are generally very quick to recognize and accept the relevance and relationship between discomfort and the behavioral issues they face.
6. Chronic osteoarthritis is commonly implicated in both types of referral and this often affects more than one site. Spinal tenderness was not uncommon, even when there was no pathologic finding on radiography or advanced imaging. Long-standing postural and gait change can lead to myofascial discomfort, evident from sensitivity around the shoulder and lumbar musculature.
7. Successful management of pain is optimized when using a multimodal approach, where pain mechanisms become therapeutic targets and approached with

pharmacologic and non-pharmacological treatment. Behavioral intervention may be required to address established avoidance responses.

CONCLUDING COMMENTS

Veterinarians should routinely consider and reflect on how discomfort might affect the presentation of a problem behavior, appreciating that this does not require overt manifestation of pain and that discomfort may be transient or intermittent. In line with the principle of erring in favor of an animal's well-being, we should not completely discount the potential role that pain/discomfort plays in any problem behavior case, even if the link seems unlikely or is not yet documented in published literature. Trial analgesia may not be sufficient to definitively confirm a focus of discomfort. However, it will safeguard the welfare of the patient, illustrate compassion for the patient, and may negate the need for a behavior modification program that the owner may struggle to undertake. For these reasons, it is our recommendation that it is often better to treat suspected discomfort first rather than consider its significance only after diagnostic assessment reveals clear physical evidence of pathology (which may not be possible) or when the animal does not respond to behavior therapy.

CLINICS CARE POINTS

- Pain and paresthesia are commonly implicated in problem behavior through a range of direct and indirect effects.

- Veterinarians should always consider discomfort in any case presenting with a problem behavior.

- Veterinarians should maintain oversight of problem behavior cases if referred to a non-veterinary behaviorist, as the relevance of discomfort may become apparent at any stage of the diagnostic or treatment process.

DOG PAIN SCREEN (MILLS REPRODUCED WITH PERMISSION)

Client questionnaire to be used for cases of problem behavior in conjunction with a clinical examination.

Main behavior problem of concern:

Other problem behaviors:

General

- Have you struggled to teach your dog certain actions?
  - If so which ones?
- Would you say your dog is moody, has a changeable temperament or Jekyll and Hyde type personality?
- Would you describe your dog as clingy or occasionally clingy for no apparent reason?
- When your dog is scared does she/he tend to seek you out or take off and be alone?
- Does your dog wake you at night?
- Does your dog seem scared sometimes for no apparent reason?

Adjunctive Behaviors

- Does your dog show any of the following behaviors?
  - Arching her/his neck and fixing position while looking up (Stargazing),

- o Snapping jaws for no apparent reason (Fly snapping, jaw snapping),
- o Excessive licking of surfaces or "air licking"
- o Excessive licking or grooming of any region of the body or limbs
- o Frequent licking of others
- o An appetite for non-food related items (eg, plaster, wood, plastic, but not including plants or feces) (Pica)
- o A strong appetite for green plants for example, grass or leaves
- o Any abnormalities of gait or load bearing (including tending to prop itself up)
- o Unusual sitting or lying postures (frog-sitting or lying with the legs sticking straight out behind) or always lying with one hip down
- o Hesitant or unusual elimination behavior, including vocalizing while eliminating (urine of feces)
- o Sudden skin flinches
- o Yelping for no apparent reason
- o Excessive sniffing behavior or sniffing for no apparent reason
- o Excessive yawning
- o Frequent stretching and body shaking
- o Moaning

Movement and Activity

- Is your dog reluctant to move sometimes?
- Does your dog avoid being touched sometimes or in relation to particular body regions?
- Does your dog avoid walking on very warm or cold surfaces?
- Does your dog occasionally refuse to continue on a walk or go into a part of the home?
- If you work or do specific physical activities with your dog, would you say your dog tends to underperform or that its performance has dropped off?
  - o Does your dog seem to be "one-sided" in any aspect of behavior or work?
  - o Does your dog take time to get going?
  - o Does your dog have poor stamina for no apparent reason?
  - o Are there certain activities your dog avoids doing or seems to enjoy less without good reason?

DISCLOSURE

D.S. Mills and F.M. Coutts have both received funding from Boehringer Ingelheim for veterinary education activities related to pain in dogs.

REFERENCES

1. Available at: https://www.iasp-pain.org/resources/terminology/#pain. Accessed September 18, 2023.
2. Available at: https://www.ninds.nih.gov/health-information/disorders/paresthesia. Accessed September 18, 2023.
3. Available at: https://www.ncbi.nlm.nih.gov/medgen/97901. Accessed September 18, 2023.
4. Mills DS, Demontigny-Bédard I, Gruen M, et al. Pain and problem behavior in cats and dogs. Animals 2020;10(2):318.
5. Voscopoulos C, Lema M. When does acute pain become chronic? Br J Anaesth 2010;105(suppl_1):i69–85.

6. Finnerup NB, Nikolajsen L, Rice AS. Transition from acute to chronic pain: a misleading concept? Pain 2022;163(9):e985–8.
7. Woolf CJ. Pain: moving from symptom control toward mechanism-specific pharmacologic management. Ann Intern Med 2004;140(6):441–51.
8. Mills DS. Medical paradigms for the study of problem behaviour: a critical review. Appl Anim Behav Sci 2003;81(3):265–77.
9. World Small Animal Veterinary Association. Global Pain Council Guidelines. Available at: https://onlinelibrary.wiley.com/doi/10.1111/jsap.13566 Accessed 18th January 2023.
10. Self I., BSAVA guide to pain management in small animal practice, 2019, British Small Animal Veterinary Association. Gloucester, UK.
11. Pye C, Bruniges N, Peffers M, et al. Advances in the pharmaceutical treatment options for canine osteoarthritis. J Small Anim Pract 2022;63(10):721–38.
12. Flor H, Turk DC. Chapter 4: Psychobiological mechanisms in chronic pain. In: Chronic pain: an integrated biobehavioral approach. Philadelphia, USA: Lippincott Williams & Wilkins; 2015. p. 89–135.
13. Kumar B, Lenert P. Joint hypermobility syndrome: recognizing a commonly overlooked cause of chronic pain. Am J Med 2017;130(6):640–7.
14. Lust G, Williams AJ, Burton-Wurster N, et al. Joint laxity and its association with hip dysplasia in Labrador retrievers. Am J Vet Res 1993;54(12):1990–9.
15. Bowen J, Fatjó J, Serpell JA, et al. First evidence for an association between joint hypermobility and excitability in a non-human species, the domestic dog. Sci Rep 2019;9(1):8629.
16. Rooney NJ, Clark CC, Casey RA. Minimizing fear and anxiety in working dogs: A review. J Vet Behav 2016;16:53–64.
17. Merola I, Mills DS. Behavioural signs of pain in cats: an expert consensus. PLoS One 2016;11(2):e0150040.
18. Barcelos AM, Mills DS, Zulch H. Clinical indicators of occult musculoskeletal pain in aggressive dogs. Vet Rec 2015;176(18):465.
19. Lopes Fagundes AL, Hewison L, McPeake KJ, et al. Noise sensitivities in dogs: an exploration of signs in dogs with and without musculoskeletal pain using qualitative content analysis. Front Vet Sci 2018;5:17.
20. Barcelos AM, Kargas N, Maltby J, et al. Theoretical foundations to the impact of dog-related activities on human hedonic well-being, life satisfaction and eudaimonic well-being. Int J Environ Res Publ Health 2021;18(23):12382.
21. Frankenstein UN, Richter W, McIntyre MC, et al. Distraction modulates anterior cingulate gyrus activations during the cold pressor test. Neuroimage 2001; 14(4):827–36.
22. Ploghaus A, Tracey I, Gati JS, et al. Dissociating pain from its anticipation in the human brain. Science 1999;284(5422):1979–81.
23. Bell A. The neurobiology of acute pain. Vet J 2018;237:55–62.
24. Camps T, Amat M, Mariotti VM, et al. Pain-related aggression in dogs: 12 clinical cases. Journal of Veterinary Behavior 2012;7(2):99–102.
25. Mackay EL, Zulch H, Mills DS. Trait-Level Resilience in Pet Dogs—Development of the Lincoln Canine Adaptability Resilience Scale (L-CARS). Animals 2023; 13(5):859.
26. Harvey ND, Craigon PJ, Shaw SC, et al. Behavioural differences in dogs with atopic dermatitis suggest stress could be a significant problem associated with chronic pruritus. Animals 2019;9(10):813.
27. Coan JA, Schaefer HS, Davidson RJ. Lending a hand: Social regulation of the neural response to threat. Psychol Sci 2006;17(12):1032–9.

28. Sherwell EG, Panteli E, Krulik T, et al. Changes in Dog Behaviour Associated with the COVID-19 Lockdown, Pre-Existing Separation-Related Problems and Alterations in Owner Behaviour. Veterinary Sciences 2023;10(3):195.

29. Beaver BV. Aggressive behavior problems. Vet Clin N Am Equine Pract 1986;2(3): 635–44.

30. Rugaas T. *On talking terms with dogs: calming signals*, 2006. Carlsborg, WA, USA.

31. Mills DS, Beral A, Lawson S. Attention seeking behaviour in dogs: what owners love and loathe. J Vet Behav Clin Appl Res 2010;5(1):60.

32. Crombez G, Eccleston C. To express or suppress may be function of others' distress. Behav Brain Sci 2002;25(4):457–8.

33. Obtaining gait footage of your dog public version: Available at: https://www.youtube.com/watch?v=OFlraJLWZ3M&ab_channel=WhatMakesYouClick%3F.

34. Rowland T, Pike TW, Reaney-Wood S, et al. Using network analysis to detect associations between suspected painful health conditions and behaviour in dogs. Vet J 2023;293:105954.

Repetitive Behaviors in Dogs

Jonathan Bowen, BVetMed, MRCVS, Dip (AS)CABC[a],
Jaume Fatjó, DVM, PhD, Dipl.ECAWBM-BM[b],*

KEYWORDS

- Compulsive-disorder • Stereotypy • Dog • Behavior • Anxiety • Compulsiveness

KEY POINTS

- Dysfunctional repetitive behaviors indicate a state of poor welfare and/or health issues.
- The early detection of such behaviors can be challenging; they often go unnoticed due to more prominent behavioral problems, such as aggression, or are perceived as harmless or even amusing.
- A clinical assessment should include an accurate description of the problem behavior, information on related temperament traits, a medical examination, a description of the environment, and an assessment of the impact of the problem on the quality of life of both the animal and the family.
- Behavior modification strategies should include environmental enrichment and training the animal in alternative, functional behaviors.
- Adjunctive pharmacological treatment is usually required, with fluoxetine being the first-line drug for the treatment of dysfunctional repetitive disorders in dogs.

INTRODUCTION

The consideration of repetitive behaviors in companion animals started in the early1990s with the articles by Luescher and colleagues, in the present journal,[1] and by Rapoport and colleagues.[2] Luescher and colleagues suggested parallels between some stereotypies in companion animals and obsessive-compulsive disorders (OCD) in people.[1] This assumption was based on the observation that repetitive disorders show some degree of face, predictive, and construct validities with human OCD: Some repetitive behaviors in dogs resemble OCD (face validity), they can be treated with the same drugs (predictive validity), and they share some biological mechanisms with them (construct validity). In support of this, that article cited a just-in-press case report on the successful treatment of a canine patient diagnosed with acral-lick dermatitis (ALD) with clomipramine.[3] The following year, Rapoport and colleagues went on to propose ALD as an animal model of human OCD.[2]

a Queen Mother Hospital for Small Animals, Royal Veterinary College, Hawkshead Lane, North Mymms, Hertfordshire, UK; b Autonomous University of Barcelona and Institut Hospital del Mar d'Investigacions Mèdiques, Barcelona, Spain
* Corresponding author.
E-mail address: jaume.fatjo@uab.es

Vet Clin Small Anim 54 (2024) 71–85
https://doi.org/10.1016/j.cvsm.2023.09.003
0195-5616/24/© 2023 Elsevier Inc. All rights reserved.
vetsmall.theclinics.com

The list of repetitive behaviors that Luescher and colleagues produced[1] has remained influential in the identification of these behaviors throughout the 3 decades since it was published. The repetitive behaviors that we see in the clinic are generally derived from species-typical behaviors, including locomotion (eg, circling), predation (eg, tail-chasing), and grooming (eg, ALD) and eating/sucking (eg, pica and flank-sucking) (**Table 1**). According to Mason, the 3 main types of "source behavior" are escape attempts, surrogates for natural behavior patterns, and a third category of heterogeneous forms that probably reflect underlying dysfunction.[4]

From the very beginning, there have been issues around the terminology and definitions relating to repetitive behavior. Historically, the term "stereotypy" seems to be associated with the welfare literature in production, zoo, and laboratory species,

Table 1 Repetitive behaviors in dogs	
	Breed Predisposition Identified
General	
Spinning	English Bull Terrier Staffordshire Bull terrier
Chasing lights and/or shadows	Border Collie
Pacing and fence running	
Freezing	English Bull Terrier
Snapping at air	
Involving self-trauma, self-mutilation, self-directed	
Tail-chasing (can be combined with tail-mutilation)	German Shepherd Belgian Shepherd Australian Cattle Dog Anatolian Shepherd Dog Bull Terrier Shiba Inu
Tail-mutilation, tail-chewing (can be combined with tail-chasing)	
Face and neck scratching	
Acral lick dermatitis	Large breeds Labrador Retriever German Shepherd Great Dane Saint Bernard
Compulsive licking or chewing	
Claw biting	
Self-nursing	
Flank-sucking	Doberman Pinscher
Checking rear	Miniature Schnauzer
Ingestive	
Pica	
Sucking	
Polyphagia	
Psychogenic polydipsia	

Based on the original list proposed by Luescher et al[1] and subsequently modified by other authors. It includes information about known breed predispositions from Gough et al.[5]

whereas "compulsive disorder" is more associated with domestic pets. Attempts to settle on a single universally accepted term have faltered.

Behaviors in dogs such as tail-chasing or ALD are just phenotypic descriptions or behavioral syndromes that could be linked to several nonbehavioral underlying factors. In humans, repetitive behaviors are not only a symptom of OCDs; they can also be a symptom of Tourette's syndrome and autism spectrum disorders among other conditions. As a result, it may be best using etiologically agnostic terms, such as dysfunctional repetitive behaviors.

This problem of finding a satisfactory, universal terminology for repetitive behaviors in animals reflects the rather greater issues faced by research on human OCDs and psychiatric disorders in general.

Current research in human psychiatry has shifted from an approach focused on discrete diagnostic categories, such as OCD, to transdiagnostic traits, such as compulsivity, impulsivity, or anxiety.[6] These offer a more mechanistic understanding of problems that helps to better identify genetic and environmental factors, as well as new diagnostic and treatment approaches.

PREVALENCE

Repetitive behaviors in dogs are apparently far less prevalent than other behavior problems such as aggression, separation-related disorders, social fears, and noise-reactivity.[7-10] For instance, in a study of the demographics of behavior problems in a convenience sample of 4114 dogs, 16% of participants reported that their dogs showed a repetitive behavior problem at some point in their lives.[11] However, there is also evidence that they may be substantially unrecognized.[10,12]

There is a high level of comorbidity with other behavior problems, including noise sensitivity, anxiety and fear, house-soiling, excessive barking, and destructiveness[11] but particularly aggression, separation-related problems, and hyperactivity/impulsivity.[7]

However, often the client's list of presenting behavioral complaints does not include repetitive behavior. Perhaps, this is because repetitive behaviors are overshadowed by the influence of other problems such as aggression or separation anxiety on the owner's lifestyle, or because owners regard repetitive behavior as an amusing eccentricity. Some evidence for the latter is the study of YouTube clips of repetitive behavior by Burn and colleagues,[12] in which owners and commenters regarded the behavior as funny and even inclined to encourage it. However, it has also been found that 89% of owners with dogs showing tail-chasing had tried to stop the behavior.[13] Although the differences in the findings between these studies could be due to recruitment biases in the study populations, there is also the implication that owners fail to recognize the influence of repetitive disorders until the problem is at a chronic and severe stage of development. Whatever the cause, we can still conclude that veterinarians should make efforts to actively detect cases at an early stage and educate people on the potential causes and implications of repetitive behaviors.

CLINICAL ASSESSMENT

The following assessment procedure presents a standardized way to describe the problem and to collect and organize the relevant information according to the different contributing factors.[14] It does not depend on a preestablished set of diagnostic categories, and it can be particularly useful to address problems such as repetitive disorders, where there is a lack of consensus regarding their cause, classification, and clinical interpretation. Information is organized in 5 categories or axes.

1. Functioning: This axis records information about the dog's ability to function in terms of his own welfare, his role as a pet, and his interactions with the environment, people, and other animals.
2. Behavior: This axis includes detailed descriptive information about the problem behavior, which could be used to create a descriptive diagnosis.
3. Health: To assess the influence on the animal's behavior, a review of the animal's past and present health would be included on this axis.
4. Environment: This axis would include the animal's environment and how it influences behavior.
5. Traits: This axis would include data on behavioral, temperamental, and personality traits that have been detected during the behavioral examination.

Functioning

This axis collects information about the quality of life of the dog and the family, and the dog's ability to function as a companion animal (in the family and in wider society).

Dysfunctional repetitive behaviors may indicate either a suboptimal environment, which results in poor welfare, or an underlying health problem. Some authors even consider dysfunctional repetitive behavior to be such a strong indicator of poor quality of life that they have argued for a "zero tolerance" policy when these behaviors are seen in zoo animals.[15] This suggests that we should not only prioritize repetitive behaviors in multiproblem cases but also that even the relatively low prevalence of repetitive behavior problems in the companion dog population is unacceptable and is an indication of widespread quality-of-life issues that should be addressed.

Mellor's model is a useful framework for assessing quality of life.[16] We should aim to provide the dog with a good life, in which the balance between positive and negative experiences and affective states is clearly positive. Repetitive behaviors directly interfere with the dog's ability to exhibit normal decision-making, to perform other normal behaviors, and to engage with the environment. They are therefore not only an indication of underlying environmental inadequacies that compromise well-being but also have an impact on the animal's behavior budget and represent an opportunity cost that directly affects quality of life.

In companion animals, one of the barriers to improving welfare is that the owner-perception of quality of life may be inaccurate. In a representative sample of 501 Spanish dog-owners, we found that owners who left their dogs alone for 10 or more hours per day and walked them just once per day gave their dogs a mean score of 9 out of 10, where 10 represented the best possible life for the dog.[17]

Behavior

Repetition forms an important part of normal functioning in animal behavior, from invertebrates to mammals.[18] For example, repeatedly practicing action-patterns enables the individual to acquire motor skills.[18] We see this in puppies that occasionally chase their tails within a display of playful behaviors.

To distinguish between normal and dysfunctional repetition, the first step is to obtain a detailed description of the repetitive behavior, together with a behavioral profile of the dog that includes information about the dog's general behavior, social relationships, and behavior problems.[14]

We need to fully characterize the repetitive behavior, including the following:

- A detailed description of the behavior, including its form, frequency, and duration of repetition, and the degree of variation/flexibility.

- The contexts, triggering stimuli, and targets for the behavior.
- Behavioral or emotional changes that precede or follow an episode of repetitive behavior.
- A timeline of the onset of the behavior, and how it has developed and changed over time.
- Information about the dog's level of arousal and awareness before, during, and after the episodes of repetitive behavior (including the dog's ability to respond to its environment and stimuli when it is performing the repetitive behavior).

According to Mason, the 3 main causes of repetition are disinhibition (which could broadly be thought of as difficulties resisting the initiation of the behavior or stopping it), reinforcement, and sustained elicitation by internal or external stimuli.[4] A detailed behavioral history should provide us with the information we need to evaluate these aspects of the problem.

We can then start to form a hypothesis about the nature of the problem: Is the behavior functional or not and what is the balance among medical, environmental, and temperamental factors?

Physical Health

After collecting a detailed description of the behavior, the next logical step is to identify medical conditions that could be involved in the development of the repetitive behavior.

There are 3 ways in which physical health interacts with repetitive behavior.

1. Primary physical health problems that directly cause the repetitive behavior (eg, sarcoptic mange).
2. Health problems that result from the repetitive behavior (eg, lick granuloma).
3. Physical health problems that contribute to the problem and help to maintain it but are not causal (eg, atopic disease). This could include secondary health problems from group 2.

Most of the repetitive behaviors described in **Table 1** could result from primary and secondary physical health problems. A preexisting primary illness can directly trigger the repetitive behavior either by directly affecting the central nervous system (eg, brain tumors and epilepsy) or by inducing peripheral changes in perception and/or sensation (eg, pain/numbness). Pain can also impair frontal cortical inhibitory control, which is essential for preventing repetitive behavior, through activation of the amygdala.[19]

ALD and tail-chasing are 2 very good examples of repetitive behaviors that can be related to a physical health problem. ALD, and other self-mutilation problems, can be related to dermatologic and neurologic problems, including neuropathies, allergies, infections, trauma, arthritis, neoplasia, and foreign bodies.[20,21] Similarly, tail-chasing can be related to intervertebral disk disease, gastrointestinal parasitism, focal seizures, and dermatologic conditions.[22] Health problems that are secondary to environmentally induced repetitive behavior are common and can aggravate and sustain the behavior, creating a vicious circle. For a more detailed discussion, with examples of the relationship between medical conditions and behavior problems, see Fatjó and Bowen[23] and Camps and colleagues.[24]

One of the most difficult challenges is determining the level of clinical investigation required to rule-out medical conditions while minimizing unnecessary, costly, or invasive tests. We should start with a review of the dog's clinical history, a thorough physical and neurologic examination and a standard hematology and biochemistry panel. Before proceeding to looking for new health problems, we should review the likely contribution of the dog's known problems, including chronic conditions such as epilepsy and painful orthopedic disease.

The following 5 questions can help to decide whether additional medical examinations are needed.

- Is the repetitive behavior associated with certain contexts and triggering stimuli?
- How easy is it to interrupt the behavior?
- How rigid, inflexible, and consistent is the behavior when it is repeated?
- Is the dog showing different patterns of repetitive behavior?
- Does the patient show other clinical signs that could indicate a physical disease?

In most cases, repetitive behaviors can be linked to a well-defined set of environmental situations and triggers. For example, in the article by Tiira and colleagues,[13] only 7% of owners of dogs with tail-chasing problems failed to connect the repetitive behavior with any immediate environmental factor. That minority of cases without environmental factors would be the ones with a greater likelihood of a primary physical health problem.

In general, most primary repetitive behaviors can be interrupted, although in certain cases, the dogs show a lower level of responsiveness. Dysfunctional repetitive behaviors can become emancipated from the environment but that is generally seen in chronic cases after a long period of development of the problem. The anamnesis of emancipated repetitive behavior usually reveals a past connection between the repetitive behavior and some environmental cues.

Although problematic repetitive behaviors are often described as invariable movement patterns, they do often show a degree of variation. For example, some patients show more than one pattern of repetitive behavior, such as tail-chasing combined with pacing[13] and tail-chasing can alternate between clockwise and counterclockwise motion. The less variation and flexibility in the behavior and the more the dog is insensible to its environment, the more we should suspect a primary physical health problem.

Age of onset and the development of the problem are also useful indicators. If the problem starts suddenly and fully formed in an adult animal that has no other history of behavior problems, this raises suspicions of a primary health problem.

Environment

Dysfunctional repetitive behavior disorders are frequently defined as maladaptive responses to an environment that the animal is unable to cope with. Unfortunately, this tends to focus on the animal's inability to cope rather than the environment's inadequacies.

Although dysfunctional repetitive behaviors have been observed in many different species, one common feature is that they are specifically associated with a captive environment, which is often compromised and deficient.

A good environment allows the activation of coping strategies to perceived threats, as well as the expression of behavioral needs linked to positive affective states. Good adaptation to the environment results in a system of behavior regulation that ensures a behavior repertoire that is both flexible and robust: always accommodating new strategies but reinforcing and fixing those behaviors that prove to be more beneficial.

Many of an animal's actions are clearly goal-oriented or triggered by environmental cues.[25] However, many behaviors performed by an animal are self-motivated activities that are spontaneously expressed, even in the absence of sensory triggers or external reward. Examples of self-motivated behaviors include grooming, prey seeking (and foraging), and locomotor exploration.[26]

Through the repetition of goal-directed behaviors that are orientated to the environment and achieving important outcomes, such as obtaining food through foraging and hunting, individuals acquire and perfect habitual responses that help them to reduce the cognitive load associated with the performance of everyday tasks. Essentially, habits enable the individual to perform those tasks without thinking too hard about them. Humans experience this in everyday life, such as when driving: Driving is initially cognitively challenging but becomes easier as components of the task, such as changing gear, become habitual responses. Complex behaviors are therefore a mosaic of functional habitual responses that can be recruited flexibly to achieve a successful outcome.

A bad environment lacks resources, is unpredictable and uncontrollable. An animal that lives in a bad environment is unable to predict, control, or avoid negative experiences, and it is unable to achieve its motivated expectations. The former primarily leads to anxiety and the latter to frustration, which contribute to an overall negative affective state and a reduced quality of life.

The set of habitual responses an animal acquires reflects the environment. In a good environment, the highly functional habitual responses the individual develops are so seamlessly integrated into everyday behavior that they are invisible. In a bad environment, habitual responses can form around meaningless contexts and triggers, becoming dysfunctional, repetitive, and increasingly prominent because they displace other behaviors.

Interestingly, self-motivated behaviors such as grooming or locomotion are often the source behavior for repetition. They are more likely to be performed in a barren or chaotic environment that lacks meaningful stimulation because they do not require an external trigger. The lack of opportunities to express other behaviors leaves the individual vulnerable to repeating self-motivated behaviors until they become increasingly irresistible habits. Hence, the repetitive pacing behaviors of captive species that would usually inhabit much larger home ranges. Historically, it was theorized that performing the repetitive behavior could help the animal to alleviate the stress derived from conflict and frustration.[27] This was supported by findings such as hens that paced due to frustration stopped their alarm calls once the pacing reached a high level.[28] More recent study in macaques has found that repetitive hairpulling but not repetitive locomotion (eg, pacing) was negatively associated with cortisol in situations of stress.[29] However, an alternative explanation was that blunting of hypothalamic–pituitary–adrenal (HPA)-axis sensitivity due to chronic stress led to a reduced basal cortisol and a reduced cortisol response to stress.[30] Ultimately, evidence for this stress-coping effects has been inconclusive and no mechanism for the proposed improvement in stress has been found. A more parsimonious explanation might be that repetitive behaviors are simply a desperate attempt to adjust to a dysfunctional environment, by regulating motivational and attentional mechanisms.

In carnivores, one of the main predictors of whether a species will exhibit stereotypical locomotion in captivity is wild home range size; species with larger home ranges, longer daily travel distances, and longer chase distances show more stereotypy in captivity.[31] In a study of dogs in Chile,[32] free-ranging owned dogs were found to have a mean home range size of 0.65 km^2 and a maximum travel from home of 1 km. Not only the home range size matters in terms of locomotion but also the size and complexity of the home range reflects the likelihood of accessing the physical and social resources that will allow the expression of behavioral needs. For dogs that live in homes without attached outdoor access, this suggests that walks and access to open spaces, and an enriched indoor environment, are particularly important. This is confirmed by evidence that repetitive behavior is more common in dogs that have less exercise and in homes without conspecifics.[33]

Free-ranging animals also have agency over the location of their home range and how they spend their time. We have to provide an environment that simulates this agency and goal-direction as much as is practical.

The early environment is particularly important for dogs. A poor rearing-environment can have consequences for the dog's adult temperament and resilience. Early separation from the mother has been linked to a less stress-resilient adult temperament and a greater likelihood of tail-chasing.[13] Better maternal-care during puppyhood is associated with less dependence on the mother and greater engagement with a novel environment,[34] and a reduced likelihood of tail-chasing.[13]

Repetitive behavior is just one way that an animal can react to an environment that does not allow good adaptation, and behavior is more likely to become dysfunctionally repetitive in dogs with certain temperamental predispositions.

To quickly summarize environmental deficiencies, we can ask 3 main questions.

- Does the environment provide the dog with enough space?
- Does the environment provide access to the social and physical resources that the dog requires to express a normal repertoire of goal-directed behavior?
- Is the environment predictable and does it enable the dog to experience agency and control?

The Vienna Framework gives us an insight into the quality of the environment, enabling us to compare the duration of benefits and degree of agency that experiences such as social play and getting treats provide.[35] For instance, just giving a dog food treat produces only a short-lasting positive affective state, whereas foraging for food in a garden or using a challenging puzzle/activity feeder not only produces a longer-lasting positive affect but also helps to satisfy the dog's need for goals and agency.[35] We can assess the overall quality of life of the dog by applying the Vienna Framework to what we know about its daily life and environment.

Traits

Not all dogs that are exposed to a poor-quality environment will go on to develop a repetitive behavior disorder. Some develop a repetitive disorder in an "average" environment that most dogs live in, as do some dogs that apparently experience highly enriched lifestyle.

Therefore, although the environment is crucial, individual differences also matter; individual dogs have combinations of traits that make them more, or less, vulnerable to developing dysfunctional repetitive behavior. The influence of traits in the development of behavior problems also helps us to understand patterns of comorbidity.

Anxiety, frustration, and arousal are states that are associated with the situational expression of repetitive behavior. The states of both anxiety and frustration are known factors in the development of repetitive behaviors, as well as triggers for episodes of repetitive behavior.[36] Excessive arousal impairs top–down behavioral inhibition, which reduces self-control and favors the expression of repetitive behaviors.[37]

These states have corresponding traits of anxiousness, frustration tolerance, and excitability. Although states are transient and situational, traits are stable across time and between different contexts, so they have more general and pervasive effects. They can be considered transdiagnostic when they are associated with multiple behavioral or psychiatric problems.

Dogs with increased traits of anxiousness or frustration will experience those emotions more often and across a wider range of environments. Anxiety and frustration set the scene for the problem to appear, and this is why compulsive disorders have been traditionally considered anxiety-related disorder.

Excitability relates to how easily the dog enters a state of high arousal and may be the equivalent of poor emotion regulation in people (the process by which individuals influence which emotions they have, when they have them, and how they experience and express these emotions).[38] However, something else is needed for an animal to develop a dysfunctional repetitive disorder.

Since the early 2010s, studies on human and animal models have identified the tendency toward habitual responding as an important trait in repetitive behaviors. This has become the focus of OCD research. For example, in a series of studies Gillan and colleagues found an inverse relationship between OCD severity and goal-directed control.[39] They also found an association between deficiency in goal-directed control and symptoms of other mental health problems that have been hypothesized to have impulsive and compulsive characteristics (addiction, eating disorders). The current evidence is, therefore, that in affected individuals, there is a defect within goal-directed behavior, which forces the individual to rely more heavily on the habitual responding that is at the root of compulsivity.[40]

In a key study neatly summarizes the concept, human respondents, with and without OCD, were given a button and shock-strap for each hand and instructed to press the corresponding button when a light appeared on the left or right of a screen.[41] An error would result in a shock. In the test phase of the experiment, one of the shock-straps was removed, devaluing that response so that pressing of the button for that side should extinguish. After overtraining, people with OCD continued to press the functionless button, indicating that they had developed enhanced avoidance habits that were difficult to throw off. They also reported having a strong urge to respond to the devalued on-screen stimuli (compulsion).

Although this defect in the balance between habitual and goal-directed responding has been extensively investigated and well established in humans and in animal models, specific evidence in companion dogs is lacking. However, reevaluation of existing work does provide some support. For example, evidence that repetitive behavior in dogs is associated with persistence and failure to respond to devaluation, which are characteristics of habitual responding.[42]

TREATMENTS AND PREVENTION
Owner Education

First, we need to make sure that the nature and influence of the problem on the dog's welfare is fully recognized by the owner. Being able to understand the affective state of the dog is a key factor influencing problem understanding and treatment adherence. We should adopt an emotion-based approach when communicating with the client, as opposed to one focused on biological explanations, for example, that the dog feels out of control or uncomfortable with its situation.

Environmental Modification

Environmental modification is the primary strategy in the prevention and treatment of repetitive disorders in captive animals in zoos, sanctuaries, laboratories, and agricultural production.

Environmental enrichment is important not only for providing opportunities for dogs to express behavioral needs but also for helping them in coping with potential stressors. The degree to which an animal is affected by a potential stressor and able to recover is referred to as resilience or psychological resilience. Studies conducted in different species indicate that general environmental enrichment enhances the individual resilience to stress.[43] There are many resources on environmental enrichment that readers will be familiar with. This section will only mention an approach to environmental modification that is specific to problem behavior, in this case dysfunctional repetitive behavior.

In this context, environmental modification can be thought of as having 3 levels.

1. *Meeting basic needs*: The starting point is to meet the basic requirements the dog has for space, resources, and activity but this is not enrichment.
2. *General enrichment*: Improvements that would improve the quality of life of any dog. This should consider the Vienna Framework, to ensure that enrichment produces long-term effects and agency for the dog.
3. *Therapeutic enrichment*: Using changes to the environment to modify behavior. The enrichment is tailored to the specific characteristics of the dog and planned to reduce problem behavior alongside behavior modification. In the case of dysfunctional repetitive behavior, this might include introducing many opportunities for goal-directed activity throughout the day (eg, training, puzzle-feeding, social interaction, exploration, and play), changing the environment to shield the dog from stressful triggers, and providing the dog with better avoidance opportunities.

In the following example, we apply this approach to feeding.

1. *Meeting basic needs*: Ensuring that the dog has appropriately sized regular meals of good quality food.
2. *General enrichment*: Upgrading the process of feeding from a bowl to giving some or all meals through activity feeders.
3. *Therapeutic enrichment*: Further upgrading the process of feeding to a range of carefully chosen, increasingly complex puzzles and feeders, as well as foraging activities and basic training at home and during walks, to maximize goal-directed behavior.

We can apply this approach to each aspect of the dog's activities and environment, including play, walks, social interaction with other dogs, interactions with the owner, resting places and toys. This must consider issues such as possessiveness and negative interactions with dogs.

Therapeutic enrichment helps to reduce the probability of expression of problem behavior but it is not actually focused on the specific problem behavior itself.

Different environmental enrichment interventions have different effects. For example, Hunt and colleagues measured signs of relaxation, alertness, and stress before and after 15-minute interventions that included spending time with a handler, an interactive toy, a food-stuffed toy, tug play with a handler, a bubble machine, conspecific play and time in a playhouse full of tunnels, slides and platforms with a handler providing encouragement.[44] They also found that conspecific play produced the largest and most reliable positive increases in relaxation signs and decreases in alert and stress behaviors. Time with a food-stuffed toy had the least beneficial effects. Being a pilot study in assistance dogs, we should not assume that the results can be generalized, and it is perhaps best to be guided by our patient's response to forms of enrichment.

In addition, repetitive behaviors may interfere with engagement with enrichments because the animal becomes locked into repetition in certain contexts. This is a potential barrier to the benefits of environmental enrichment, particularly when it is used without medication. Moreover, certain interventions that would enrich the environment of most individuals could be perceived as a source of frustration or stress by affected individuals.

Drug Treatment

As is the case in human compulsive disorders,[45,46] there are not that many highly effective treatments for repetitive behavior in dogs. The first-line pharmacologic treatment of repetitive disorders in dogs is the selective serotonin reuptake inhibitors (SSRIs), and fluoxetine (1–2 mg/kg q24) in particular. Serotonin is involved in the regulation of the function of many of the structures that have been involved in the neurophysiology of repetitive disorders, including the striatum and the frontal cortex.

SSRI drugs are not able to stop the behavior per se but seem to help in reversing the abnormal neurocircuitry behind compulsive behavior, including deficient information processing, lack of behavior flexibility, pathologic anxiety, and lack of impulse control.

In terms of learning processes, there is some evidence that fluoxetine can improve extinction learning, which could be very beneficial to support behavior modification techniques aimed to substitute the repetitive behavior by an alternative acceptable response.[47]

Clomipramine (1–2 mg/kg q12) has been also recommended to treat compulsive disorders in dogs.[48] Clomipramine shares with fluoxetine the ability to modulate the serotonin turnover but it is a less-specific drug that has also significant effects on other neurotransmitters.

Memantine (0.3–1 mg/kg q24), an N-methyl-D-aspartate (NMDA) receptor blocker, reduces glutamate neurotransmission, the main excitatory neurotransmitter in the brain, which has been implicated in the pathophysiology of many human mental-health problems, including OCD. In veterinary medicine, memantine has been proposed as either a single drug or an augmenting agent for refractory repetitive disorders that have shown little or no improvement after SSRI treatment.[49]

Although repetitive behavior problems could be considered to develop mostly from dysfunctions of behavioral regulation, they are frequently comorbid with emotional disorders such as separation-related anxiety or noise phobia. The addition of drugs that help SSRIs to regulate emotions and arousal could be beneficial in these cases. For example, clonidine (0.01–0.05 mg/kg q12) could be combined with an SSRI to reduce excitability and excessive arousal.

It is important to state that cause cannot be determined by drug response, and the use of medication does not indicate that the main source of the problem is within the animal. The fact that SSRI drugs have been successfully used to reduce repetitive behavior in zoo animals is an indication of the potential power of these drugs even in animals whose primary problem is an extremely compromised environment.

Behavior Modification

Although it is common to be prescriptive about behavior modification, the reality is that it is a complex process that must be adapted to the individual. It is not something that can be covered in a few paragraphs. Hewison and Mills provide a review of the current approach to behavior modification.[50] However, we can identify 4 main aspects of the treatment of repetitive behavior problems:

Treatment underlying emotional problems (eg, separation anxiety, noise phobia, or social conflict).

- Training to manage and control aspects of temperament, such as excitability or frustration (eg, training "wait" and "settle" commands).
- Training the dog alternative habits that replace the repetitive behavior (habitual responses to stimuli and contexts associated with the repetitive behavior).
- Correcting common mistakes: For example, not reinforcing problem behavior and stopping using punishment.

The veterinarian may not be in the position to deal with all these aspects of behavior modification but it is important to be aware of them and to be able to direct other professionals, such as nonveterinary behaviorists and trainers, who may be involved in treatment.

CLINICS CARE POINTS

- Repetitive behavior is, perhaps, the ultimate indicator that the dog's ability to function is severely impaired.
- We should actively detect cases at an early stage.
- It is important to educate people about the potential causes and implications of repetitive behaviors.
- Functional behaviors adapt to environmental changes and shifts in motivation but dysfunctional repetitive behaviors tend to become progressively more inflexible to change and indifferent to the environment over time.
- It is common for owners to ask whether certain kinds of repetitive behavior, such as tail-chasing, is normal in puppies. It is normal to see apparently nonfunctional behaviors such as this expressed in young animals that are experimenting with and rehearsing locomotor patterns as part of their development.
- If the behavior is not linked to contexts and triggering stimuli, a primary health cause is more likely.
- If the repetitive behavior is extremely difficult or almost impossible to interrupt, this strongly suggests a primary health cause.
- Further tests are justified if no preexisting health problem is considered causal in a case where a primary health problem is strongly suspected.
- Meaningful environments are required for meaningful behaviors to develop. Stimulation without structure and meaning is just noise.
- The quality of environmental enrichment can be assessed according to the Vienna Framework.
- Enrichment should provide dogs with goal-directed opportunities and agency as well as space and exercise.

REFERENCES

1. Luescher UA, McKeown DB, Halip J. Stereotypic or Obsessive-Compulsive Disorders in Dogs and Cats. Vet Clin North Am Small Animal Pract 1991;21:401–13.
2. Rapoport JL, Ryland DH, Kriete M. Drug Treatment of Canine Acral Lick: An Animal Model of Obsessive-compulsive Disorder. Arch Gen Psychiat 1992;49:517–21.
3. Goldberger E, Rapoport J. Canine acral lick dermatitis: response to the antiobsessional drug clomipramine. J Am Anim Hosp Assoc 1990;179–82.
4. Mason & G. Stereotypic behaviour in captive animals: fundamentals and implications for welfare and beyond. In Stereotypic animal behaviour: fundamentals and applications to welfare (2006).
5. Gough A, Thomas A, O'Neill D. Breed Predispositions to Disease in Dogs and Cats. 1–16 (2018) doi:10.1002/9781119225584.ch0.
6. Cuthbert BN, Insel TR. Toward the future of psychiatric diagnosis: the seven pillars of RDoC. BMC Med 2013;11:126.

7. Salonen M, Sulkama S, Mikkola S, et al. Prevalence, comorbidity, and breed differences in canine anxiety in 13,700 Finnish pet dogs. Sci Rep-uk 2020;10:2962.

8. Fatjó J, Ruiz-de-la-Torre J, Manteca X. The epidemiology of behavioural problems in dogs and cats: a survey of veterinary practitioners. Anim Welfare 2006;15:179–85.

9. Yamada R, KUZE-ARATA S, KIYOKAWA Y, et al. Prevalence of 25 canine behavioral problems and relevant factors of each behavior in Japan. J Vet Med Sci 2019;81:1090–6.

10. Powell L, Duffy DL, Kruger KA, et al. Relinquishing Owners Underestimate Their Dog's Behavioral Problems: Deception or Lack of Knowledge? Frontiers Vet Sci 2021;8:734973.

11. Dinwoodie IR, Dwyer B, Zottola V, et al. Demographics and comorbidity of behavior problems in dogs. J Vet Behav 2019;32:62–71.

12. Burn CCA. Vicious Cycle: A Cross-Sectional Study of Canine Tail-Chasing and Human Responses to It, Using a Free Video-Sharing Website. PLoS One 2011;6:e26553.

13. Tiira K, Hakosalo O, Kareinen L, et al. Environmental effects on compulsive tail chasing in dogs. PLoS One 2012;7(7):e41684.

14. Fatjó J, Bowen J. Making the Case for Multi-Axis Assessment of Behavioural Problems. Animals 2020;10:383.

15. Mason G, Clubb R, Latham N, et al. Why and how should we use environmental enrichment to tackle stereotypic behaviour? Appl Anim Behav Sci 2007;102:163–88.

16. Mellor DJ. Updating Animal Welfare Thinking: Moving beyond the "Five Freedoms" towards "A Life Worth Living.". Animals 2016;6:21.

17. Fatjó J, Bowen J. A clinical perspective of the human-animal bond. In: Proceedings of The Canine Science Forum Virtual Meeting, July 6-9 (Lisbon) (2021). 2021.

18. Langen M, Kas MJH, Staal WG, et al. The neurobiology of repetitive behavior: Of mice.... Neurosci Biobehav Rev 2011;35:345–55.

19. Ji G, et al. Cognitive impairment in pain through amygdala-driven prefrontal cortical deactivation. J Neurosci 2010;30:5451–64.

20. Denerolle P, White SD, Taylor TS, et al. Organic Diseases Mimicking Acral Lick Dermatitis in Six Dogs. J Am Anim Hosp Assoc 2014;43:215–20.

21. Bardagí M, Montoliu P, Ferrer L, et al. Acral Mutilation Syndrome in a Miniature Pinscher. J Comp Pathol 2011;144:235–8.

22. Low M. Stereotypies and behavioural medicine: confusions in current thinking. Aust Vet J 2003;81:192–8.

23. Fatjó J, Bowen J. Behavior and Medical Problems in Pet Animals. Adv Small Animal Care 2020;1:25–33.

24. Camps T, Amat M, Manteca X. A Review of Medical Conditions and Behavioral Problems in Dogs and Cats. Animals Open Access J Mdpi 2019;9:1133.

25. Khatib D, Morris G. Spontaneous behaviour is shaped by dopamine in two ways. Nature 2023;614:36–7.

26. Markowitz JE, Gillis WF, Jay M, et al. Spontaneous behaviour is structured by reinforcement without explicit reward. Nature 2023;614(7946):108–17.

27. Mason GJ. Stereotypies and suffering. Behav Process 1991;25:103–15.

28. Duncan IJH, Wood-Gush DGM. Thwarting of feeding behaviour in the domestic fowl. Anim Behav 1972;20:444–51.

29. Pomerantz O, Paukner A, Terkel J. Some stereotypic behaviors in rhesus macaques (Macaca mulatta) are correlated with both perseveration and the ability to cope with acute stressors. Behav Brain Res 2012;230:274–80.

30. Poirier C, Bateson M. Pacing stereotypies in laboratory rhesus macaques: Implications for animal welfare and the validity of neuroscientific findings. Neurosci Biobehav Rev 2017;83:508–15.

31. Kroshko J, Clubb R, Harper L, et al. Stereotypic route tracing in captive Carnivora is predicted by species-typical home range sizes and hunting styles. Anim Behav 2016;117:197–209.

32. Pérez GE, Conte A, Garde EJ, et al. Movement and home range of owned free-roaming male dogs in Puerto Natales, Chile. Appl Anim Behav Sci 2018;205: 74–82.

33. Sulkama S, Salonen M, Mikkola S, et al. Aggressiveness, ADHD-like behaviour, and environment influence repetitive behaviour in dogs. Sci Rep-uk 2022;12: 3520.

34. Guardini G, Mariti C, Bowen J, et al. Influence of morning maternal care on the behavioural responses of 8-week-old Beagle puppies to new environmental and social stimuli. Appl Anim Behav Sci 2016;181:137–44.

35. Rault J-L, Hintze S, Camerlink I, et al. Positive Welfare and the Like: Distinct Views and a Proposed Framework. Frontiers Vet Sci 2020;7:370.

36. Luescher AU. Diagnosis and management of compulsive disorders in dogs and cats. Vet Clin North Am Small Animal Pract 2003;33:253–67.

37. Bray EE, MacLean EL, Hare BA. Increasing arousal enhances inhibitory control in calm but not excitable dogs. Anim Cogn 2015;18:1317–29.

38. Gross JJ. The Emerging Field of Emotion Regulation: An Integrative Review. Rev Gen Psychol 1998;2:271–99.

39. Gillan CM, Kosinski M, Whelan R, et al. Characterizing a psychiatric symptom dimension related to deficits in goal-directed control. Elife 2016;5:e11305.

40. Gillan CM. In: Habits and goals in OCD, In: Pittinger C., *Obsessive-compulsive disorder: phenomenology, pathophysiology, and treatment.* New York: Oxford University Press; 2017. p. 161–70.

41. Gillan CM, Morein-Zamir S, Urcelay GP, et al. Enhanced avoidance habits in obsessive-compulsive disorder. Biol Psychiatry 2014;75(8):631–8.

42. Protopopova A, Hall NJ, Wynne CDL. Association between increased behavioral persistence and stereotypy in the pet dog. Behav Process 2014;106:77–81.

43. Ross M, Rausch Q, Vandenberg B, et al. Hens with benefits: Can environmental enrichment make chickens more resilient to stress? Physiol Behav 2020;226: 113077.

44. Hunt RL, Whiteside H, Prankel S. Effects of Environmental Enrichment on Dog Behaviour: Pilot Study. Animals 2022;12:141.

45. Irimajiri M, Luescher AU, Douglass G, et al. Randomized, controlled clinical trial of the efficacy of fluoxetine for treatment of compulsive disorders in dogs. J Am Vet Med Assoc 2009;235:705–9.

46. Stahl SM. Stahl's essential psychopharmacology: neuroscientific basis and practical applications. Cambridge: Cambridge University Press; 2021.

47. Pedraza LK, Sierra RO, Giachero M, et al. Chronic fluoxetine prevents fear memory generalization and enhances subsequent extinction by remodeling hippocampal dendritic spines and slowing down systems consolidation. Transl Psychiat 2019;9:53.

48. Seksel K, Lindeman M. Use of clomipramine in treatment of obsessive-compulsive disorder, separation anxiety and noise phobia in dogs: a preliminary, clinical study. Aust Vet J 2001;79:252–6.
49. Schneider BM, Dodman NH, Maranda L. Use of memantine in treatment of canine compulsive disorders. J Vet Behav Clin Appl Res 2009;4:118–26.
50. Hewison L, Mills DS. Small animal veterinary psychiatry. 123–141 (2021) doi:10.1079/9781786394552.0008.

The Effects of Fitness Training on Working Dog Behavior: Two Case Studies

Clara Wilson, BSc, MSc, PhD*, Dana Ebbecke, BA, Danielle Berger, Cynthia Otto, DVM, PhD, DACVECC, DACVSMR

KEYWORDS

- Fitness • Behavior • Conditioning • Working dog • Arousal • Training
- Operant conditioning

KEY POINTS

- Working dogs carry out a variety of complex tasks that require both physical and behavioral soundness.
- Training for fitness may improve both physical and behavioral outcomes.
- Integrating positive reinforcement fitness training can moderate arousal levels and improve performance outcomes in working dogs.

INTRODUCTION

Working, assistance, and therapy dogs have high inherent value because of their practical, operational, or commercial functions. As a result, these animals are generally expensive to purchase and to train. In addition, working dogs require a high level of care and close monitoring by their veterinarians because of their physical and behavioral demands. In line with the 2021 American Animal Hospital Association Guidelines,[1] the term working dog refers to either detection or protection dogs, trained for a specific purpose (eg, narcotics detection, search and rescue, and law enforcement). Assistance dog can refer to either a service dog (trained to accomplish specific tasks) or an emotional support dog (that provides support by their presence alone) to help persons with a diagnosed psychological or physical limitation that benefit from interaction with the dog.[1] A third category, therapy dogs, performs either animal-assisted activities or animal-assisted therapy, including duties such as goal-directed therapy, often directed by a health-care professional.[1] Although all of these roles for dogs can be considered "working," the focus of this article is on working dogs in the fields of detection, with principles applied to dogs working in protection disciplines as well as any canine athlete.

The Penn Vet Working Dog Center, 3401 Grays Ferry Avenue, Philadelphia, PA 19146, USA
* Corresponding author.
E-mail address: clarawil@vet.upenn.edu

Vet Clin Small Anim 54 (2024) 87–99
https://doi.org/10.1016/j.cvsm.2023.08.005
vetsmall.theclinics.com

Working dogs must achieve and maintain physical and behavioral fitness standards to meet the needs of their role. Detection dogs traverse a variety of surfaces and environments, whereas protection and apprehension dogs require high levels of strength and conditioning to work effectively (**Fig. 1**). A fitness and conditioning program to enhance core strength and flexibility may help prevent injury and increase working life span.[2,3] In addition, using operant conditioning to train physical fitness may have positive influences on the handler–dog bond and the dog's behavior. This article introduces the concept of fitness training influencing working dog behavior and describes 2 case studies of working dogs (with the roles of narcotics detection and medical detection/wilderness search and rescue) whose behavior were positively influenced by their fitness program training.

Both case studies describe dogs trained at The Penn Vet Working Dog Center (PVWDC).[4] This facility uses positive reinforcement training to encourage canines to participate in obedience, agility, husbandry, fitness, engagement, human scent detection, and odor detection (both in the field and in a laboratory setting on a "scent wheel"). The canines are trained Monday through Friday and are housed with foster families on evenings, weekends, and holidays. The canine fitness training program carried out at PVWDC was developed to help handlers, trainers, and organizations to build and assess working dog physical fitness in a simple, effective, and efficient manner.[2] The fundamental modalities of the fitness program are strength, stability, mobility, and proprioception (**Fig. 2**). Behaviors are taught using positive reinforcement (most commonly, the reward is represented by food) and range from simple stretches (eg, the dog turning to touch their nose to their flank) to intensive strength repetitions requiring core strength and stability (eg, performing squats on an elevated surface) (see Farr and colleagues[2]). This program has been shown to improve fitness assessment measures,[2] and increased physical fitness may decrease the risk of work-related injury and allow the dog to access an increased tissue range of motion.[5–8]

Less explored are the impacts of fitness training on behavioral outcomes in working dogs. Working dog training ranges from conditioning simple behaviors to highly

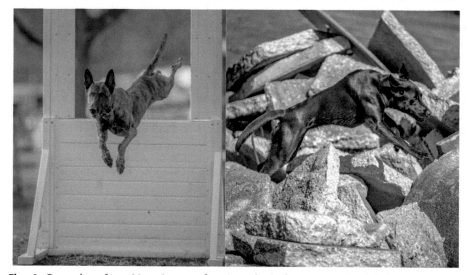

Fig. 1. Examples of working dogs performing physical activities. The left image shows a Dutch Shepherd jumping across a barrier, and the right image shows a Labrador Retriever traversing a rubble pile. (Image credit: (Left) Erik Larsson, (Right) Shelby Wise.)

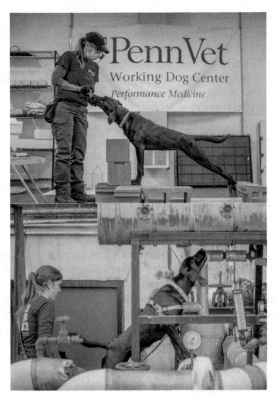

Fig. 2. A demonstration of how the plank exercise included in PVWDC Fitness program transfers to working environments, such as odor detection tasks. (Image credit: Shelby Wise.)

specific and complex behavioral sequences that capitalize on the abilities of dogs that humans lack, such as speed, agility, and an acute sense of smell. The effect of fitness on working dog behavior is likely multifaceted because increased fitness may improve the function and success of working dogs, which may in turn reduce frustration levels and/or improve confidence. Improving structural muscle mass and providing greater joint support may also reduce symptoms of pain, which is a well-documented significant influence on canine behavior.[9] Furthermore, additional operant training outside of the working environment may strengthen the handler/dog relationship. Finally, the skills learned during fitness training may be used in conjunction with working scenarios to facilitate improved concentration or task focus. These possibilities will be outlined in the case studies presented within this article.

Case Study One—Uzza: multipurpose narcotics, tracking, and evidence detection canine.

Signalment and History: Uzza is currently a 3-year-old Black Labrador Retriever (female, intact). Uzza arrived at PVWDC in 2019, at 8 weeks of age, where she began the foundation detection canine program.

Presentation Episodes: Several months into training, it was noted that Uzza was not progressing along a trajectory comparable to her siblings, and other dogs of a similar age and breed. On multiple occasions, she appeared to be unwilling to participate in scheduled training activities and was displaying behavioral challenges both at the training facility and at home with her foster family.

Behavioral and Training Observations

- Refusal to engage in tugging/toy play activities: would tug very briefly then let go and walk away and would not chase or retrieve toys.
- Displacement behaviors/stress signals during training: scratching, sniffing, biting and yawning, picking up inanimate objects, running away and destroying them.
- Slow to progress through agility foundation exercises.
- Laying down during training exercises.

Foster Family Observations

- Destructive.
- Restless.
- Difficult to walk on leash, pulling, biting leash, and picking up objects off ground and ingesting them.
- Poor bite inhibition; people, other pets, and objects.
- Tail suckling.

Original Examination Findings: At 4 months of age, Uzza was examined by PVWDC veterinary team to determine if there was a physical cause for her behaviors. During the examination, Uzza displayed a "bunny hop" gait as well as a "rounded spine." Her tail was wet and discolored due to suckling. She was unable to hold a sit or lie-down posture with the appropriate form[8] (eg, would shift her weight to either side) and was unable to climb across a low (1-foot) horizontal ladder. Uzza's body condition score (BCS) was a 5.5 out of 9, which is above the preferred score of 4 out of 9 for working dogs. No other remarkable findings were noted on Uzza's physical examination. Uzza was referred to the University of Pennsylvania, Matthew J. Ryan Veterinary Hospital for PennHIP radiographs at 5 months of age, rather than waiting until 12 months of age when the evaluation is typically performed. Diagnostic imaging revealed radiographically normal hips, with a distraction index (left hip 0.31 and right hip 0.30) associated with only a mild future osteoarthritis risk.

Initial Treatment Plan: Due to Uzza's age and the normal radiographs, it was decided to treat Uzza conservatively with gabapentin (12 mg/kg, q12 h) to address presumed neuropathic pain.[9–12] Additionally, a closely monitored modified training and fitness plan was introduced. The goal was to reduce the likelihood of injury, encourage a healthy BCS, increase flexibility and strength, strengthen muscles supporting the lower back, and decrease behavioral outbursts, while increasing levels of physical and mental performance.

Initial Treatment Details: Uzza's diet was temporarily changed from Purina Pro Plan Sport (Nestlé Purina Petcare Company, St. Louis, MO) to Purina Overweight Management (OM; Nestlé Purina Petcare Company, St. Louis, MO) to reduce caloric intake while promoting a healthy BCS. Correct posture, in the sit and down position, was encouraged at all times (**Fig. 3**).[8] This was done by reinforcing the sit and down position while using correct form, and withholding reinforcement and resetting her position if it was performed with an incorrect form. Uzza was restricted from jumping up on, or off, of any objects more than 1-foot high and was not permitted to climb unstable surfaces, slippery surfaces, or ladders. Uzza was still permitted to engage in obedience, agility, fitness, learn directional cues at a distance, odor work activities, and live human search while adhering to the restrictions in place.

Initial Treatment Response: During the initial phase of Uzza's treatment, the coronavirus disease 2019 pandemic occurred. As such, further diagnostics and treatment changes were temporarily delayed. Virtual (remote) care and support were provided to Uzza's foster family during this time. Uzza's weight, fitness, and training routine

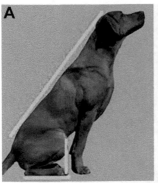
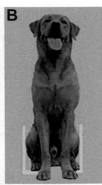
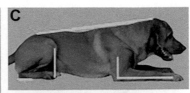
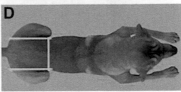

Fig. 3. The proper posture in the sit and down positions. (*A, B*) The proper sit position. Note the straight line from the head to the base of the tail. (*C, D*) The proper posture down position. Note the straight line from the head to the base of the tail. The forelimb is flexed at the elbow and shoulder. (All photos are original images taken by Kasey Seizova at the Penn Vet Working Dog Center.)

were closely monitored by her foster, with the support of PVWDC training and veterinary team. Uzza was making slight advancements; however, she was still not reaching the benchmarks required to continue on a working dog career trajectory. On return to "in-person" care, Uzza was reassessed by the veterinary and training team. Additional imaging was prescribed.

Diagnostic Workup and Findings: Radiographs and subsequent MRI of the lumbosacral area were obtained. Findings were consistent with lumbosacral instability and dynamic nerve compression.[13] Having obtained the final radiographs and MRI results, the veterinary and training teams were able to modify her training and treatment plan to accommodate her diagnosis.

Modified Treatment Plan: All previously mentioned training restrictions were continued, and special attention was provided to decrease the amount of pressure being directed toward the area of instability. Uzza's pain management and fitness plan was modified to address the lumbosacral instability and nerve compression. Gabapentin was increased to 15 mg/kg orally twice daily. Low-impact endurance exercises were introduced to enhance core muscular stability. Uzza's fitness program was tailored to meet her needs. For example, posture down to stand exercises were added to focus on building core stability and circuits of trotting over low obstacles (cavaletti poles) were incorporated to build strength in the muscles supporting the spine. Dietary restrictions with Purina OM (Nestlé Purina Petcare Company, St. Louis, MO) were continued to promote a heathy BCS. Additional manual passive range of motion daily stretches were prescribed, and a pain assessment was carried out each day.

Outcome: During the course of her treatment, Uzza's foster family reported that she became much more docile and less destructive in the home environment. Her BCS ranged between 3.5 and 4.5 and she was returned to her regular Purina Pro Plan Sport diet (Nestlé Purina Petcare Company, St. Louis, MO) (**Fig. 4**). It is important to note that we not only documented a lowered BCS but also documented, concurrently, an increased level of muscle mass. Increasing muscle mass in the back, abdomen, upper thighs, and gluteal areas offers greater spine stability and has been shown in several human studies to improve lower back pain,[14,15] with supportive preliminary findings but further research warranted in dogs.[16,17] Uzza's muscle mass increased in these areas because of the fitness program (**Fig. 5**). Her physical restrictions across all training platforms were progressively removed, with the exception of working in an

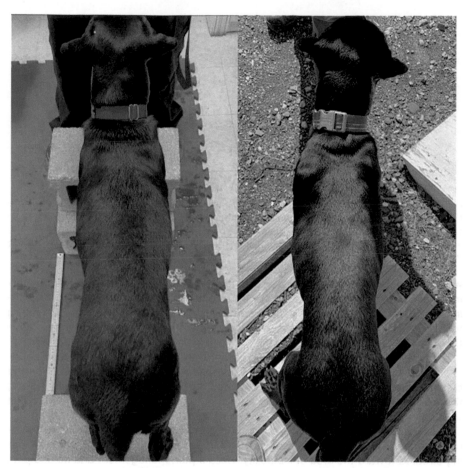

Fig. 4. A top–down view of Uzza standing. On the left, Uzza before engaging in her fitness modification program (BCS = 5.5/9). On the right, Uzza after engaging in her fitness program (BSC = 4/9). (Image credit: Lauren Filipe.)

urban rubble setting. The unstable surfaces and requirements for climbing, jumping, and crossing voids in a rubble pile could result in excessive strain to her lumbosacral spine; therefore, urban search and rescue was eliminated as a career option. Medications were discontinued and Uzza was permitted to continue engaging in odor detection training. Because of the modified fitness treatment plan, Uzza's overall performance improved dramatically, and her behavior outbursts became infrequent to the point of resolution. She became more willing to interact with handlers and trainers across all platforms of training. Uzza not only performed well but also exceeded the original expectations for strength, flexibility, endurance, and stamina. She graduated from PVWDC program as a multipurpose K9 (narcotics, tracking, and evidence search). During her transition to her working role, Uzza's handler was trained to implement the fitness regimen prescribed to support Uzza's current performance and comfort level. Since her graduation, Uzza's handler has reported multiple successes in both narcotics detection as well as locating missing persons. She is a revered part of the Clinton, Pennsylvania community and is frequently invited to participate in local outreach events where she performs demonstrations and socializes with the public.

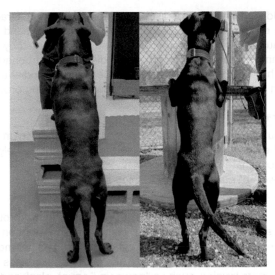

Fig. 5. Uzza performing a "paws up" exercise (one of the warm-up exercises within the fitness program). Left image shows Uzza at the beginning of her fitness training, Right image shows Uzza after completing her fitness training for several months. Image credit: Lauren Filipe.

Case Study Two—Vauk: wilderness search-and-rescue and biodetection dog.

Signalment and History: Vauk is currently a 2-year-old Labrador Retriever (female, spayed). She began her training in scent detection at 8 weeks of age and was trained in both live human scent detection and medical (bio) detection.

Examination: Vauk was initially trained on the mechanics of the scent wheel using Universal Detector Calibrant (UDC), a synthetic odor that allows dogs to learn the mechanics of an odor wheel before learning odors of academic interest.[18] This involves searching an 8-port wheel, where each port contains a discrete odor sample, including a target sample (the odor of interest), and distractor samples (eg, the type of gloves worn when handling samples, and so forth; **Fig. 6**). In March 2022, she began training on Chronic Wasting Disease (CWD), a prion disease that affects deer, elk, reindeer, moose, and sika deer.[19] Here, dogs were asked to detect low saliency odors from the feces of affected (target) and nonaffected (control) deer, and discriminate between

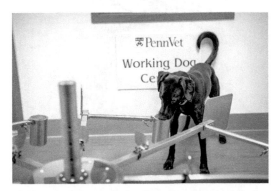

Fig. 6. Vauk performing a stand–freeze behavior over a target odor in a CWD biodetection research study. (Image credit: Shelby Wise.)

these odors, in addition to a variety of distractor odors.[20] During the transition to a lower saliency odor, in conjunction with an increased cognitive demand associated with discrimination, Vauk began to appear hyperaroused (as presented by increased vocalization, panting, and increased motor activity as displacement behavior—"fidgeting"). She appeared to have more difficulty following cues by her handler and needed more frequent breaks in between trials, thus slowing down the training process.

Behavioral and Training Observations

- Frequent bouts of frustration-related behaviors while training on the scent wheel.
- Searching the scent wheel at an accelerated pace, negatively influencing her ability to discriminate between odors.
- Increased levels of panting during training sessions.
- Barking throughout training sessions.

Treatment Plan: Vauk's handler observed the changes in her arousal and recommended that she engage in fitness activities before training (both on the scent wheel and in live-find scenarios), providing opportunities to stimulate her mentally and physically. The treatment plan included having her perform exercises from PVWDC's fitness program[2] before training, such as "paws up," squat, plank and pivot exercises, being cued and rewarded with food throughout the session (**Fig. 7**). Because of Vauk's high motivation for reward and tendency toward bouts of frustration barking, supporting behaviors were trained to aid in the performance of specific exercises. For example, the duration of a "nose target" behavior (rather than continuous food reinforcement) was trained, with increasing duration increments, during the plank exercise (**Fig. 8**). This behavior became integral in developing impulse control while simultaneously improving stamina in the physical position. Building impulse control via a

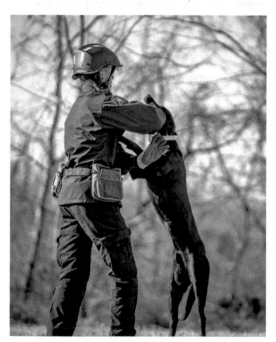

Fig. 7. Vauk performing a "paws up" exercise before a live human search. (Image credit: Shelby Wise.)

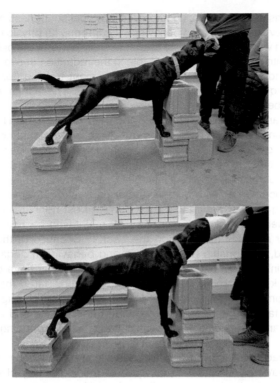

Fig. 8. Vauk holding a plank position using 2 examples of "nose target" behaviors. Top image shows a hand-touch behavior and bottom image shows a nose-in-bucket behavior (note there is no food or reward in the bucket, it is a nose touch that also reduces external visual stimuli). (Photo credit: Dana Ebbecke. Penn Vet Working Dog Center.)

reinforced nose hold behavior may have additionally aided in other aspects of Vauk's working career, such as freezing over the target odor in her biodetection training.

Outcome: Vauk's change in behavior during training and testing on the scent wheel was observed and her ability to focus on the scent wheel improved. In addition to lowering the frequency of less-desirable behaviors (such as vocalization during and in between trials, and undesired movement behaviors like fidgeting), a "pretraining" fitness session also improved the relationship between Vauk and her handler. Vauk's handler reports that she displayed fewer behaviors indicative of frustration during training sessions and felt as though Vauk's performance and overall well-being had improved since integrating fitness exercises before scent-training. In addition, the increased opportunities for improving fitness and reinforcement history of engaging in operant cues while being active also appeared to improve her performance in her secondary role as a wilderness search and rescue dog. Her search and rescue handler reported that since starting regular fitness training, she is better able to traverse the wilderness environment and has more confidence when navigating novel objects. Vauk now has a successful dual career in biodetection and wilderness search and rescue.

DISCUSSION

The 2 case studies presented describe scenarios in which fitness training was implemented and positively influenced working dog behavior. The main emerging themes from these studies are as follows: (1) improved physical soundness may address imbalances and alleviate pain-related behavioral symptoms, (2) physical fitness is a significant factor in a working dog's ability to successfully perform the behaviors required for their role, (3) fitness training can play a role in the reduction of overarousal in working scenarios, and (4) additional positive reinforcement training (for fitness training) may improve the quality of training in working scenarios. These themes are discussed in greater detail below.

Working dogs are expensive to purchase and train, require a high level of care, and require close monitoring by veterinarians due to their physical and behavioral demands. We have described the use of a fitness plan that improves physical fitness and decreases the risk of work-related injuries. Certain working dogs may develop medical issues, such as lumbosacral instability and/or dynamic nerve compression. Indeed, this is documented as one of the major causes of retirement in police[21] and military[22] working dogs. On diagnosis, the current best nonsurgical treatment options are management, including pain control, maintaining a healthy weight, and building stronger muscles that support the back.[16] Because of the complex, and well-documented, relationship between pain and behavior in dogs, it is important to consider the influences that even low levels of pain may have on working dog behavior and task engagement. In Uzza's case, it is considered that the alleviation of painful symptoms through appropriate fitness exercises and weight management is likely a major factor in her improved working performance and apparent enthusiasm in taking part in working activities without the need for ongoing pharmacologic intervention.

An important factor to consider when assessing the relationship between fitness training and behavioral outcomes is the type of training taking place. Current approaches for training animals are generally anchored in operant conditioning.[23] Operant conditioning can be classified into 4 categories: positive reinforcement, positive punishment, negative reinforcement, negative punishment. The categories of operant conditioning focused on in training likely influences behavioral outcomes. For example, Haverbeke, Laporte, Depiereux, Giffroy, and Diederich[24] found that military dogs had a lower performance score in an obedience trial test when exposed to a higher rate of positive punishment (the addition of aversive stimuli in efforts to reduce unwanted behavior). In addition to potentially reducing performance, the use of aversive stimuli has been linked to lower indices of welfare, and an increase in stress indicative behaviors and negative emotional states.[25–27]

Negative emotional states may further intersect with arousal levels and can greatly influence effectiveness of training and ability to recall operant tasks.[28–30] Arousal levels can be influenced by many factors, including the dog's environment, previous experiences, and the nature of the task or situation they are facing.[31,32] Fear, anxiety, and frustration can result in preparatory arousal, which may intersect with working performance and lower the thresholds required to display aggression.[33] As a result, dogs experiencing these states can become difficult, or dangerous, to handle in a working setting. Because problematic behaviors can be caused by, or result in, a manifestation of anxiety in dogs,[34] it is important to consider the use of operant conditioning in the training of working dogs, both directly related to their working role (eg, scent detection practice), and when using fitness training. Contrastingly, the application of positive reinforcement training can modify behavior in ways that benefit both the dog and handler.[35] Therefore, it is recommended that positive reinforcement is focused on in fitness training, both because of the reduced likelihood of welfare concerns, in addition to the basis of evidence linking reward-based training with improved working and affective outcomes.

The case studies presented highlight the less-explored influences of fitness training on behavioral outcomes in working dogs. Increased fitness may improve a working dog's function, working success, reduce frustration levels, and improve confidence. Additional operant training outside of the working environment may influence the handler–dog relationship positively. It should be emphasized that while PVWDC's fitness program[2] follows a progressive plan that includes the same exercises across dogs (eg, posture sit, posture down, "paws up," and so forth), each individual dog will experience tailored modification to each exercise depending on their physical fitness and previous training. What might be considered "moderate" for one dog may be extremely challenging for another dog; therefore, care needs to be taken when tailoring each exercise to ensure that the dog is able to be successful and progress in successive steps. Before engaging in a fitness regime, handlers should consult their veterinary professional and ensure that the exercises are both physically within their dog's capacity, and trained in such a way as to minimize a dog's frustration levels (eg, by rewarding frequently enough and building approximate steps toward complex behaviors) to create a positive and safe learning environment.

SUMMARY

This article presents 2 case studies of working dogs trained at PVWDC, whose behavior was positively impacted by their fitness program training. We conclude that fitness training can enhance the physical and behavioral fitness of working dogs, leading to positive effects on their behavior, reducing the risk of work-related injuries, and improving their work performance.

CLINICS CARE POINTS

- Including fitness and strengthening exercises into a working dog's training regimen may reduce the risk of injury and can be used to help rehabilitate from injuries and health conditions.
- Case studies suggest that the trained cues used in fitness exercises can additionally be used as an aid to modify and improve behavior in other areas of a working dog's role.
- Working dog handlers may find value in fitness training protocols to improve their dog's overall physical and behavioral state.
- Although the case studies presented focus on working dogs, the addition of fitness exercises should also be considered as a recommendation for nonworking patients to improve abnormal behaviors related to poor physical conditions.
- Physical exercises should be approved by a health professional and appropriate modifications should be made to ensure that the exercises are physically appropriate and taught in ways that facilitate improved behavior, rather than inducing frustration.

DISCLOSURE

The authors are employed at PVWDC where the described fitness program is used. The authors declare no conflict of interest.

REFERENCES

1. Otto CM, Darling T, Murphy L, et al. AAHA Working, Assistance, and Therapy Dog Guidelines. J Am Anim Hosp Assoc 2021;57(6):253–77.

2. Farr BD, Ramos MT, Otto CM. The penn vet working dog center fit to work program: a formalized method for assessing and developing foundational canine physical fitness. Front Vet Sci 2020;470.

3. Vitger AD, Stallknecht BM, Nielsen DH, et al. Integration of a physical training program in a weight loss plan for overweight pet dogs. J Am Vet Med Assoc 2016; 248(2):174–82.

4. The Penn Vet Working Dog Center. Penn Vet Working Dog Center Available at: https://www.vet.upenn.edu/research/centers-laboratories/center/penn-vet-working-dog-center. Accessed Feb 03, 2023.

5. Cline J, Reynolds A. Feeding the canine athlete. Nestle Purina Nutrition 2005; 9(1):1–7.

6. Safran MR, Seaber AV, Garrett WE. Warm-up and muscular injury prevention an update. Sports Med 1989;8(4):239–49.

7. Ramos MT, Otto CM. Canine Mobility Maintenance and Promotion of a Healthy Lifestyle. Vet Clin 2022;52(4):907–24.

8. Ramos MT, Farr BD, Otto CM. Sports medicine and rehabilitation in working dogs. Vet Clin Small Anim Pract 2021;51(4):859–76.

9. Mills DS, Demontigny-Bédard I, Gruen M, et al. Pain and problem behavior in cats and dogs. Animals 2020;10(2):318.

10. Moore SA. Managing neuropathic pain in dogs. Front Vet Sci 2016;3:12.

11. Mathews K. Physiologic and Pharmacologic Applications to Manage Neuropathic Pain. Analgesia and Anesthesia for the Ill or Injured Dog and Cat 2018;17. https://doi.org/10.1002/9781119036500.ch3.

12. Di Cesare F, Negro V, Ravasio G, et al. Gabapentin: Clinical Use and Pharmacokinetics in Dogs, Cats, and Horses. Animals 2023;13(12):2045.

13. Lampe R, Foss KD, Hague DW, et al. Dynamic MRI is reliable for evaluation of the lumbosacral spine in healthy dogs. Vet Radiol Ultrasound 2020;61(5):555–65.

14. Kim J, Gong W, Hwang B. The effects of resistivity and stability-combined exercise for lumbar muscles on strength, cross-sectional area and balance ability: exercises for prevention of lower back pain. J Phys Ther Sci 2011;23(2):247–50.

15. Marshall PW, Murphy BA. Evaluation of functional and neuromuscular changes after exercise rehabilitation for low back pain using a Swiss ball: a pilot study. J Manipulative Physiol Therapeut 2006;29(7):550–60.

16. Worth A, Meij B, Jeffery N. Canine degenerative lumbosacral stenosis: prevalence, impact and management strategies. Vet Med Res Rep 2019;169–83.

17. Henderson A, Hecht S, Millis D. Lumbar paraspinal muscle transverse area and symmetry in dogs with and without degenerative lumbosacral stenosis. J Small Anim Pract 2015;56(10):618–22.

18. Furton KG, Beltz K. Universal detector calibrant. Florida University, FIU: Google Patents; 2017.

19. Centers for Disease Control and Prevention. Chronic Wasting Disease (CWD) https://www.cdc.gov/prions/cwd/index.html. Accessed April 03, 2023.

20. Mallikarjun A, Swartz B, Kane SA, et al. Canine detection of chronic wasting disease (CWD) in laboratory and field settings. Prion 2023;17(1):16–28.

21. Worth A, Sandford M, Gibson B, et al. Causes of loss or retirement from active duty for New Zealand police German shepherd dogs. Anim Welf 2013;22(2): 167–74.

22. Evans RI, Herbold JR, Bradshaw BS, et al. Causes for discharge of military working dogs from service: 268 cases (2000–2004). J Am Vet Med Assoc 2007; 231(8):1215–20.

23. McGreevy P, Boakes R. Carrots and sticks: principles of animal training. NSW, Australia: Darlington Press; 2011.
24. Haverbeke A, Laporte B, Depiereux E, et al. Training methods of military dog handlers and their effects on the team's performances. Appl Anim Behav Sci 2008; 113(1–3):110–22.
25. Ziv G. The effects of using aversive training methods in dogs—A review. J Vet Behav 2017;19:50–60.
26. de Castro ACV, Fuchs D, Morello GM, et al. Does training method matter? Evidence for the negative impact of aversive-based methods on companion dog welfare. PLoS One 2020;15(12):e0225023.
27. Deldalle S, Gaunet F. Effects of 2 training methods on stress-related behaviors of the dog (Canis familiaris) and on the dog–owner relationship. Journal of Veterinary Behavior 2014;9(2):58–65.
28. Affenzeller N. Dog–human play, but not resting post-learning improve re-training performance up to one year after initial task acquisition in labrador retriever dogs: a follow-on study. Animals 2020;10(7):1235.
29. Affenzeller N, Palme R, Zulch H. Playful activity post-learning improves training performance in Labrador Retriever dogs (Canis lupus familiaris). Physiol Behav 2017;168:62–73.
30. Starling MJ, Branson N, Cody D, et al. Conceptualising the impact of arousal and affective state on training outcomes of operant conditioning. Animals 2013;3(2): 300–17.
31. Bray EE, MacLean EL, Hare BA. Increasing arousal enhances inhibitory control in calm but not excitable dogs. Anim Cognit 2015,18(6).1317–29.
32. Bray EE, MacLean EL, Hare BA. Context specificity of inhibitory control in dogs. Anim Cognit 2014;17:15–31.
33. Panksepp J. Affective neuroscience: the foundations of human and animal emotions. New York, NY: Oxford University Press; 2004.
34. Cobb M, Branson N, McGreevy P, et al. The advent of canine performance science: offering a sustainable future for working dogs. Behav Process 2015;110: 96–104.
35. Hiby E, Rooney N, Bradshaw J. Dog training methods: their use, effectiveness and interaction with behaviour and welfare. Anim Welf 2004;13(1):63–9.

Cognitive Changes Associated with Aging and Physical Disease in Dogs and Cats

Lena Provoost, DVM

KEYWORDS

- Cognition • Cognitive dysfunction • Aging • Senior pet

KEY POINTS

- Cognitive dysfunction can occur as a primary behavioral problem or sequela to primary medical problem.
- There is compelling evidence that cognitive dysfunction occurs secondary to chronic inflammatory states that should be differentiated from cognitive dysfunction syndrome to better identify preventions and treatments.
- Many factors can contribute to cognition and should be accounted for in future cognition studies.

INTRODUCTION

Cognition is a process of the mind acquiring knowledge and understanding through sense, experience, and thought. Cognition is classified as either social or nonsocial. Nonsocial cognition includes perceptual abilities, attention, learning, memory, and executive function (EF).[1] Social cognition explores the way in which individuals adapt and interact with conspecifics, as well as other species; some consider this emotional intelligence.[2] Unsurprising, current literature suggests there is overlap between social and nonsocial cognition due to shared neural circuits.[3] Cognition is also a vital aspect when studying normal aging and disease processes, often using dogs or cats as translational models. Because cognition plays such an integral role in everyday life, from decision-making to interactions, it follows that changes in any of these cognitive processes may manifest as a change in behavior.

Behavior changes are often the first clinical sign observed in companion animals to indicate physical disease. Such changes may be as subtle as no longer greeting the owner, stopping on walks or as marked as a loss of appetite and house soiling. In senior pets, each of these clinical signs can be a manifestation of cognitive dysfunction syndrome (CDS). However, it is necessary to rule out primary medical problems, such as renal disease. In similar manner, primary behavioral pathologic conditions, such as

Clinical Sciences & Advanced Medicine, University of Pennsylvania, 3900 Delancey Street, Philadelphia, PA 19104, USA
E-mail address: lenap@vet.upenn.edu

Vet Clin Small Anim 54 (2024) 101–119
https://doi.org/10.1016/j.cvsm.2023.08.002
0195-5616/24/© 2023 Elsevier Inc. All rights reserved.

thunderstorm phobia and separation anxiety, should be differentiated from secondary behavioral problems related to underlying medical causes, such as pain-related aggression.[4] It is our goal to review the evidence of how aging processes and disease states may alter cognition.

New approaches and methods to investigate cognition in companion pets have resulted in a marked increase of research and interest.[5] In pets, cognition is measured by owner response questionnaires. Two commonly used validated questionnaires are the canine dementia scale (CADES)[6] and canine cognitive dysfunction rating (CCDR).[7] Some postmortem studies have correlated the amount of beta amyloid deposition within the brain to severity of deficits noted by such screens.[8,9] In addition to the use of questionnaires, neurocognitive tasks are used in humans to identify ability and impairment, and modifications of such tasks have allowed us to evaluate animal cognition.

THE BRAIN AND COGNITIVE PROCESSES

The brain is responsible for sensory processing, movement, cognition, emotional processes, and regulating normal and social behaviors. Each part of the brain can be attributed with specific functions and most notable, for purposes of this article, is the forebrain. The forebrain contains centers for emotion and cognition, the prefrontal cortex (PFC) and amygdala.[10] For study purposes, cognition is divided into several domains including learning and memory, attention, and EF. Interestingly, EF seems to be the most sensitive to cognitive dysfunction because it is integral to synthesizing information to plan and make decisions.[11] Core EFs include inhibitory control, cognitive flexibility, working memory, and attention.[11]

As inhibition implies, it is the ability to control and selectively attend to relevant information in the environment, which can involve inhibiting impulses.[11,12] Cognitive flexibility allows an individual to adjust to changing demands and requires inhibition and working memory.[11] Working memory stores information for a short time and requires quick analysis and interpretation of information that is provided by EF.[13] Attention is the ability to attend to physical and/or social cues in an environment and considered central for goal-directed behaviors.[14] Sustained attention is the ability to maintain prolonged focus in order to complete a task, whereas selective attention is the ability to stay on task and ignore nonsalient information, which at times requires inhibition. In humans, declines in selective attention has been associated with mental health disease,[15] whereas declines in both sustained and selective attention occurs with age and associated with cognitive decline.[14]

The PFC, basal ganglia, and hippocampus work synergistically to control EF. The basal ganglia contain sites of dopamine production, which plays a major role in movement, memory, reward, and motivation.[16] Within the PFCs, both the medial PFC (mPFC) and the orbitofrontal PFC (OFC) participate in the regulation of EF, with the OFC responsible for inhibition and cognitive flexibility and the mPFC responsible for attention (**Table 1**). The PFC receives dopaminergic, noradrenergic, serotonergic, and cholinergic input. These neurotransmitters are key modulators of EF and declining levels are hallmarks of dysfunction.[17]

COGNITIVE DEVELOPMENT

Cognitive abilities of dogs change throughout life stages, increasing from juvenile to adult[21] and declining as seniors regardless of size or breed.[22] Studies using neurocognitive tests have reported younger dogs perform better on learning and executive function tasks when compared with older dogs. Furthermore, neurocognitive tests have been able to subclassify old dogs into cognitively versus noncognitively

Table 1
Effect of prefrontal cortex lesions on executive function

EF Domain	OFC Lesions	mPFC Lesions
Inhibitory control	Disrupted[16]	No effect[18]
Attention	No effect[17]	Disrupted[19]
Cognitive flexibility	Disrupted[18]	No effect[20]

impaired.[23] Aside from age being a determinant of cognitive faculty, some studies suggest differences in EF between small and large breed dogs based on brain volume, ~50g and ~120g respectively.[24] The cognitive development of cats has yet to be fully investigated.

Perinatal and early life experiences can also have a major influence on adult behavior and cognition.[25,26] For example, a study investigating the development of 8-week and 12+ week-old puppies ability to follow human pointing found that pups living in homes outperformed the shelter pups.[27] Puppies raised with early isolation show poor executive function on reversal learning tasks when compared with puppies with some human experience.[27,28] It has been suggested that emotional dysregulation or lack of self-control may be correlated with poor inhibitory control in humans.[29] However, in a group of candidate assistance puppies, it was found that puppies with more maternal care showed more perseveration and may perhaps lack inhibition.[30]

AGING

There are often marked physical changes when a pet enters its senior life stage including cognitive decline. Thus, the goal for senior pets should be successful aging that is defined as ensuring age-related changes are minimal, or at least, do not negatively influence quality of life.[31,32] When it comes to aging, body size and breed are particularly significant factors for predicted life span of dogs (**Table 2**).

Several studies have identified hematological and biochemical range variation among senior dogs and cats influenced by many factors, including the presence of systemic disease, diet, sex, and breed.[32] Those found to occur in both dogs and cats are decreased lymphocytes and increased alanine transaminase, *alkaline phosphatase*, and creatine kinase.[31–34]

A retrospective morbidity and mortality study in elderly dogs reported that degenerative lesions of the musculoskeletal system (ie, degenerative joint disease) and heart (ie, endocardial fibrosis and mineralization) were common morbidities, whereas neoplasia and cardiovascular and urinary pathologic conditions were frequent causes of death.[35] It is therefore imperative to be cognizant of not only age-related changes

Table 2
Designation of senior and geriatric stages in dogs and cats

		Senior	Geriatric
Dog			
Giant and large breed (≥22.7 –kg)		6–8 y[31]	≥ 9 y[31]
Medium and small breed (<22.7 kg)		7–10 y[31]	≥ 11 y[31]
	Mature	Senior	Geriatric
Cat	7–10 y[32]	11–14 y[32]	15+ y[32]

but also diseases that have a higher incidence in senior pets. Aging pets are likely to suffer from degenerative joint disease such as osteoarthritis that may manifest in a spectrum of behavior changes related to their discomfort.[4,32] The severity of periodontal disease increases with each passing year[36] and careful consideration should be given to oral health as periodontal disease has associations with systemic disease and chronic inflammation.[37] Senior pets are more likely to be affected by certain endocrinopathies; renal, cardiovascular, and pulmonary diseases; as well as sensory decline.[38] Along with these physical diseases, a myriad of nonspecific behavioral changes[39] can be observed (**Table 3**). Senior pets are also more likely to have skin lesions such as lipomas, cysts, and cancers.[31,32] Additionally, the nutritional needs of aging pets change due to reduced activity and reduced absorption abilities, requiring lower calorically dense foods that are highly digestible. Overfeeding can lead to obesity, poorly digestible protein can enhance sarcopenia, and chronic inflammation leads to cachexia. These changes drive the recommendation for senior pets to have biannual physical examinations, complete blood counts, biochemistries, fecal analysis, urinalysis, blood pressure readings (for cats), along with any other indicated diagnostics.[40,41]

Inflammation

There is an increasing body of evidence that has found an association between chronic inflammation and cognitive dysfunction.[49–51] As mentioned, senior pets are at risk for age-associated diseases associated with inflammation. Age-related decline of immune function is reported in both humans, cats, and dogs, this is termed immunosenescence[33,42] and can contribute to chronic inflammatory states, weakened immunity, and cancers. Immunosenescence is characterized by changes in B-cells; T-cells; immunoglobulin A, G, and M levels; and an upregulation of inflammatory cytokine production.[42] The changes in B-cell population and increased circulating levels of IgM, enhance inflammatory cytokine production, such as interleukin (IL)-6, IL-1, and tumor necrosis factor (TNF)-alpha.[42] These cytokines can lead to the release of acute phase proteins such as C-reactive protein. This cascade can slow resolution of inflammation and increase tissue damage and reactive oxygen species (ROS) leading to further oxidative damage of cells.[42] There are protective mechanisms in place to prevent protein damage, such as ROS scavenging enzymes, chaperone proteins, heat shock proteins, and antioxidants but, as animals age, the efficiency of these mechanisms declines.[52] Fundamentally, damage caused by ROS leads to age-related loss of physiologic function and perpetuates chronic inflammatory states.

Additionally, higher levels of serum cortisol levels[53] and reduced numbers of mineralocorticoid receptors (MRs) but not glucocorticoid receptors of the hippocampus have been found in aging versus young dogs.[54] Studies have reported that MRs of the hippocampus have neuroprotective effects that prevent glucocorticoid-mediated apoptosis of neurons[55] and preserve nonspatial memory in rats.[56] However, further studies are necessary to determine the effect of excess cortisol in regions with reduced MRs and its effect on cognition. Conversely, aldosterone bound to MRs expressed by immune cells have been associated with proinflammatory immune effects.[57] In humans, glucocorticoid excess, such as cortisol, is associated with loss of muscle, hypertension, osteopenia, visceral obesity, diabetes, and impaired recovery from stress.[58]

Obesity is common among pets, so it is worth noting that adipose tissue composition and function change with age. In humans and rodents, adipose tissue is redistributed to visceral compartments, brown adipose tissue activity is reduced, sex hormone levels are low, and abdominal adipose tissue expansion occurs. These changes

Table 3
Systemic changes in senior dogs and cats by body system and possible behavior changes

System	Dog	Cat	Possible Behavior Changes
Immune	Increased inflammaroty biomarkers such as: c-reactive protein, Immunoglobulin M, 8-hydroxy-2'deoxyguanosine, and glycoprotein, GlycA[42] Decreased Heat Shock Protein70[42] and lymphocytes[41,43]	Increased proinflammatory cytokines and IgA[41] Decreased lymphocytes[41]	Not reported but consider states of chronic inflammation may lead to activity, appetite, and social interaction changes; repetitive behaviors may be associated with localizable inflammation
Integument	Increased incidence of adenomas, cysts, papillomas, lipomas, and neoplasia[31,43]	Increased incidence of neoplasia[32]	Increased/decreased grooming, repetitive behavior (ie, self-licking), irritability. Consider gastrointestinal (GI) discomfort if licking is exclusive to abdomen
Oral/GI	Increased severity of periodontal disease (gingivitis, calculus deposition, bone resorption, tooth mobility, and loss) and oral tumors[43] Reduced liver function[43]	Increased severity of periodontal disease, stomatitis, and neoplasia[32,44] Slower GI transit[45]	Decreased: food ingestion and social interaction Increased: licking, chewing, vocalization, repetitive behavior (ie, lip licking, pawing, teeth chattering, jaw quiver, and pica), sleeping,[44] and aggression if face or abdomen touched
Musculoskeletal	Increased incidence of degenerative joint disease (DJD), osteopenia, obesity, sarcopenia[43]	Increased incidence of DJD, excessive sensitivity to touch may indicate central sensitization and hypersensitivity due to pain, obesity, sarcopenia,[32,44] and back pain (declawed cats)[46]	Decreased: activity and social interaction Increased: lethargy, night waking, vocalization, self-licking/grooming,[44] aggression, and house soiling[46]
Neurologic	Increased incidence: intervertebral disc disease and neoplasia[32,43] Decreased neurons and neurotransmitters[43]	Increased incidence: neoplasia[32]	Increased: vocalization, night waking, repetitive behaviors (ie, self-licking, self-scratching), aggression, irritability, house soiling, anxiety, and disorientation Decreased: activity, social interaction, and appetite

(continued on next page)

Table 3
(continued)

System	Dog	Cat	Possible Behavior Changes
Cardiac	Increased incidence of chronic valvular disease, and dilated cardiomyopathy[32,43]	Increased incidence of heart murmurs[44]	Decreased: activity, response to stimuli, and social interactions Increased: lethargy and changes in sleep–wake cycles, and confusion
Renal	Increased risk of chronic renal disease and urinary incontinence[43]	Increased risk of chronic renal disease[44]	Increased: house soiling, lethargy, irritability, anxiety, disorientation, aggression, and changes sleep–wake cycles Decreased: appetite
Respiratory	Increased risk of chronic bronchitis, pulmonary thromboembolism, tracheal collapse, laryngeal paralysis, and chronic rhinitis[43]	Feline calicivirus may be linked to gingivostomatitis in older cats[47]	Increased: anxiety, changes in sleep–wake cycles, and intraspecies aggression[48] Decreased: activity, social interactions, and appetite
Endocrine	Increased incidence of hypothyroidism and hyperadrenocorticism[43]	Increased incidence of hyperthyroidism[44] and hyperadrenocorticism[32]	Increased/decreased: activity and appetite Increased: house soiling, drinking,[44] vocalization, irritability, and lethargy
Sensory changes	Vision: Nuclear sclerosis (dense), cataracts, corneal degeneration and ulcers, and retinal degeneration[43] Hearing loss: due to chronic otitis, head trauma, and ototoxic drugs[43]	Vision: Nuclear sclerosis and blindness secondary to primary medical[44] (ie, hypertension) Hearing loss: due to head trauma, ototoxic drugs, and loud noise[44]	Increased: anxiety, aggression, and irritability Reduced: activity Changes in social interactions

influence secretion of adipokines that promote chronic low-grade systemic states of inflammation.[59,60] Ultimately, obesity can accelerate aging by increasing the risk of age-associated diseases and inflammation though this is yet to be identified in dogs or cats.[59]

PRIMARY PHYSICAL DISEASE ASSOCIATED WITH COGNITIVE DYSFUNCTION

As mentioned, many age-associated diseases can manifest with behavioral changes similar to CDS. Moreover, primary physical pathologic conditions have been associated with cognitive dysfunction or share similar features of CDS.

Neurologic

To optimally function, the brain requires adequate circulation to deliver oxygen and nutrients. Therefore, any disruption of circulation caused by brain tumors, vascular insufficiency, microhemorrhages, infarcts, or inflammation and edema secondary to head trauma can result in behavioral and cognitive changes. In cats, common sign of meningiomas is lethargy and behavioral changes[61] that may manifest as reduced activity and increased anxiety. Many dogs with primary tumors of the rostral cerebrum present for acute onset of seizures or behavioral changes described as dementia, aggression, and alterations to existing behavioral patterns or routines.[62]

In humans, vascular cognitive impairment (VCID) is the second leading cause of dementia and describes cognitive dysfunction caused by infarcts and microbleeds of various natures.[63] The severity of VCID cognitive impairment is not well understood and seems to be correlated with affected brain regions.[63] In dogs that have a history of stroke, MRI findings have confirmed the presence of infarcts,[64] whereas brain microhemorrhages were confirmed in dogs with hypertension.[65] Additional studies of these populations are needed to determine if they are at risk for or affected by CDS. One study has measured the interthalamic adhesion size and number of microhemorrhages between control dogs, noncognitively impaired geriatric dogs with brain microhemorrhages, and geriatric dogs with CDS. This study found that the noncognitively impaired dogs with brain microhemorrhages and dogs with CDS to be significantly different from clinically normal dogs.[66] A previous study confirmed that interthalamic adhesion size can quantify brain atrophy in dogs affected with CDS[67] and so the researchers postulated that these findings represent a distinct disease category.[66]

Early CDS[68,69] and increased anxiety[70] has been described in dogs with idiopathic epilepsy (IE). An analysis of owner reported behaviors in dogs with and without IE found memory impairment to be common in dogs with IE.[69] Furthermore when owners of IE affected dogs were asked to compare their dogs present behavior to 6 months ago, it was stable (ie, no signs of CDS progression) versus controls that had significant progression (ie, increased staring at walls, house soiling, difficulty finding dropped food, and problems recognizing familiar people).[69] The study also reported that dogs with IE had a higher risk of CDS at a young age (4–6 years) and those with a history of cluster seizures and high seizure frequency had more severe cognitive dysfunction.[69] For patients with epilepsy, dietary supplementation with medium chain triglycerides (MCTs) has shown positive effects on cognition.[68]

Gastrointestinal

Ingestive changes have been reported in dogs and cats with CDS, even though oral and metabolic disease should always be ruled out on a case-by-case basis before diagnosing this comorbidity. In a study of senior dogs with periodontal disease, dogs with higher CDS scores were more likely to have severe periodontal disease independent of age.[50] This may reflect cognitive dysfunction associated with chronic inflammation versus true CDS. Owners of senior cats describe behavioral changes during mealtime such as sniffing food and walking way without consuming their meal which may indicate gastrointestinal disease or oral pain as an association between dental disease and a higher liklihood of a matted coat and increased sleeping was observed in senior cats.[43]

BEHAVIORAL CHANGES ASSOCIATED WITH MEDICAL SYSTEMIC DISEASE

Although specific cognition studies have not been performed in companion pets affected with many common systemic diseases, behavior changes are frequently observed. **Table 3** reviewed systemic disease typical of senior pets and the associated behavior changes. However, similar changes can also be observed in younger dogs affected with systemic disease. Pets with metabolic diseases (renal insufficiency, hepatic insufficiency, and diabetes) and endocrinopathies (hypoadrenocorticism and hyperadrenocorticism; hyperthyroid and hypothyroid) may show irritability, lethargy, appetite changes, activity changes, increased anxiety, and house soiling.[39,71]

Pets with cardiovascular disease may be lethargic and withdrawn. These patients might be at higher risk of CDS due to poor blood flow and represent a distinctly different type of cognitive dysfunction; however, studies are needed to confirm this hypothesis.

Polyneuropathies, inherited or acquired, can result in repetitive behaviors, self-mutilation, and irritability. Polyneuropathies can be due to endocrinopathies that should be ruled out.[72]

Excessive licking can be diagnosed as a primary behavioral problem (ie, compulsive behavior and psychogenic alopecia) but it is important to rule out primary GI disease,[73] dermatologic problems, and pain.[39]

Finally, the painful pet may exhibit signs such as increased aggression when touched, excessive self-licking, increased vocalization, repetitive behaviors, changes in sleep–wake cycles, or reduced activity.[74] It is also important to also remember that sensory decline and drugs can cause a pet to seem confused, ataxic, lethargic, irritable, house soil, changes in sleep cycles, and altered response to stimuli.[71]

A BRIEF OVERVIEW OF COGNITIVE DYSFUNCTION SYNDROME

Because of its relevance in formulating a differential diagnostics for behavioral and cognitive changes observed in senior dogs, we will provide here a brief overview of CDS. For a comprehensive review, please see chapter 4.

Expected behavior changes in aging pets include reduced activity levels, less active interaction with but closer proximity to their owner.[75] These changes should undoubtedly raise concern for CDS. CDS is a primary neurobehavioral syndrome considered an analog of human Alzheimer disease (AD). It is characterized by the pathologic accumulation of beta amyloid plaques in brain tissue resulting in behavioral and progressive cognitive changes.[76] The severity of impairment ranges from mild to severe and is correlated with the degree of beta amyloid plaque formation in the hippocampus and cortex. It is a diagnosis of exclusion since confirmation can only be performed postmortem. However, new technologies are investigating alternative modalities to identify and confirm CDS, as reviewed below. Clinical signs include learning and memory deficits, habit changes (sleep, activity, and interactions), motivational changes, and increased fears and anxiety.[77,78] A simple way to screen for CDS is using the acronym DISHAAL: disorientation, interaction changes with owners or pets, sleep–wake cycle changes, house soiling, alterations in activity and anxiety, and learning and memory changes; as well as increased vocalization for cats.[79]

There is a linear relationship between age and increasing risk of CDS.[80,81] Clinical signs in dogs are noticed between 8 and 11 years of age.[80,82] As expected in aging pets, sensory decline is a common comorbidity.[80] Clinical signs of CDS in cats may be noticed between 7 and 11 years of age.[80,83] In cats common signs of CDS at 11 to 14 years are changes in interaction, whereas cats aged older than 15 years exhibit excessive vocalization and aimless wandering.[84]

Pathology

CDS is characterized by beta amyloid deposition in brain tissue, declining neurotransmitters, mitochondrial dysfunction, ventricular dilation, hippocampal and cortex atrophy, and compromised cerebrovascular flow due to microhemorrhages, infarcts, or arteriosclerosis.[78,85] Vascular insufficiency leads to inadequate levels of nutrition and exchange of wastes within the brain, creating a toxic environment with high levels of ROS, oxidative damage, and inflammation. As a result, neuronal degeneration and mitochondrial dysfunction occurs leading to impaired energy production and increased inflammation.[78]

Diagnostics

Because CDS is a diagnosis of exclusion, a thorough history, physical examination, CDS questionnaire, complete blood counts, biochemistry panel, urinalysis, fecal, blood pressure (for cats), and any additional testing based on history and examination findings are warranted. This may include endocrine testing, evaluating Feline Leukemia Virus (FeLV) and Feline Immunodeficiency Viurs (FIV) status, heartworm and tick panels, imaging (abdominal ultrasound, radiographs, and MRI/computed tomography), and microscopic evaluation of skin samples.

New Diagnostics on the Horizon

There has been a boon of promising research that may be helpful in confirming a CDS diagnosis using biomarkers. Neurofilament light chain (NfL) can be measured in cerebral spinal fluid and serum. It is a neuronal cytoplasmic protein found only in large caliber myelinated axons and increased levels found in cerebrospinal fluid (CSF) or blood serum are proportional to the degree of axonal damage. In humans, NfL is used as a diagnostic and prognostic indicator of neurologic disorders, including inflammatory, neurodegenerative, traumatic, and cerebrovascular diseases.[85] A recent study reported a significant increase of serum NfL of mildly cognitively impaired dogs as indicated by CADES screening; as well as elevated AST and ALT.[8] A second study using both CADES and CCDR screens, neurocognitive tasks, and NfL levels to quantify CDS in dogs aged 9 to 13 years reported NfL levels and CDS severity were correlated with performance on inhibitory control.[86] They also reported that severely affected dogs were not able to perform the neurocognitive tasks,[86] which has been reported elsewhere.[23] A different group of investigators looked into the use of electroencephalogram (EEG) to identify differences in dogs categorized as normal, at risk of CDS, and CDS impaired have reported EEG differences in both dogs at risk and impaired CDS dogs.[87]

Risk/Protective Factors

Several studies using CADES or CCDR screens have reported that diet, activity, and sensory loss may affect cognition. A 3-year longitudinal study of laboratory dogs reported protective cognitive effects of a diet high in antioxidants and enrichment on age-matched controls.[88] For dogs, high activity seems to be a protective factor because dogs classified as not active had a 6.47 times greater odds of having CDS versus dogs classified as very active.[81] Similarly, another study reported a significant association between high levels of activity and less cognitive impairment in dogs.[89] Age is the most consistent risk factor with the odds of CDS increasing by 52% with each passing year.[81] Additionally, dogs with neurologic, eye, and ear disorders have a higher odds of having CDS.[81] A recent study using neurocognitive tasks confirmed that executive function is significantly decreased in elderly dogs with hearing loss with severe CDS being associated with worse hearing.[90]

TREATMENT OF COGNITIVE AND BEHAVIOR CHANGES

In comparison to human medicine, there is a lack of comprehensive literature on the maintenance or enhancement of cognitive health in companion animals. Based on the available knowledge, a primary goal should be to ensure companion animals receive adequate medical care throughout their life. This includes preventative care as well as disease screening to allow for early identification and treatment of medical conditions to minimize disease progression, whether physical or cognitive. Along with addressing medical care, obtaining information regarding the patients' environment and their response to stressors is important to understand because anxieties and fears can negatively affect health and life span.[91]

Interventions for cognitive impairment can be classified into pharmaceuticals, nutrition, and enrichment. Two classes of pharmaceuticals have shown clinical efficacy in reducing signs of CDS in dogs, monoamine oxidase inhibitors, and cholinergic drugs. Selegiline (also known as L-deprenyl or Anipryl), a monoamine oxidase inhibitor, is an FDA-approved treatment of CDS in dogs that has been shown to slow progression and increase life span by 6 months.[76] Selegiline prevents the catabolism of dopamine, serotonin, epinephrine, and norepinephrine and is thought to have neuroprotective, antioxidant, and anti-inflammatory effects.[92] However, response to selegiline varies, and in an early study, it proved effective in improving visuospatial working memory in aged dogs but failed to improve performance in young dogs.[93] Interestingly, selegiline has been found to improve operant conditioning, as well as attention, in young dogs.[94] These differing results may indicate an age effect on different cognitive domains, as well as a population effect. Serotonergic medications, such as selective serotonin reuptake inhibitors (SSRIs) and tricyclic antidepressants (TCAs), should not be used in combination with selegiline due to the risk of serotonin toxicity. Drugs that target the cholinergic system, such as acetylcholinesterase inhibitors and butyrylcholinesterase inhibitors, function by reducing the catabolism of choline-based esters. A preliminary study investigating the efficacy of a butyrylcholinesterase inhibitor for the treatment of CDS in dogs found a marked improvement for CADES score and performance on neurocognitive tasks.[95] However, improvement and slowed progression was only observed for moderately impaired dogs.[95] Finally, treatment of pain and systemic disease to increase quality of life is warranted. Medications that may be useful for treating pain and sleep disruptions include gabapentin, amantadine, nonsteroidal anti-inflammatories, and benzodiazepines.[96] Although both classes of medications may be helpful to ensure a restful night, paradoxic effects can be observed with either so trial before use is recommended. If selegiline is not used for cognitive health, due to contraindication, cost, poor response, or adverse reactions, SSRIs can be considered to treat fears and anxieties in senior cats and dogs.[4] Care should be taken when using medications with anticholinergic side effects, such as TCAs.

Nutritional interventions have been shown to be beneficial in improving and delaying cognitive impairment in aged dogs.[97-100] There are 2 types of diets marketed to improve brain function and cognitive health, and both have anti-inflammatory effects but essentially there are those high in antioxidants and those that are ketogenic, which supply mitochondria with a glucose alternative.[97,100] The major antioxidants used in such diets are often: vitamin C, vitamin E, L-carnitine, omega-3, and alpha-lipoic acid.[97] There is evidence to show that senior laboratory dogs fed a diet with high levels of antioxidants perform better on neuropsychological tasks than aged-matched controls.[98-100] The same study also found a lower amount of beta-amyloid accumulation in the parietal cortex[101] and an additive effect when senior dogs also received enrichment.[98,100] However, a more recent study failed to find a similar effect; however, there were difference in the antioxidant ingredients used, population, and duration of the study.[102] Interestingly a few studies report that L-carnitine and alpha-lipoic acid need to be supplemented together to have any positive effect on cognition.[103] However, care should be taken when recommending antioxidant supplementation use in dogs and cats because they are not always indicated for both species. For instance, low doses of alpha-lipoic acid can be toxic to cats and should generally be avoided.[104] The goal of antioxidants is to minimize oxidative damage, reduce ROS, and decrease inflammation. The second type of diet, ketogenic, contains MCTs, which are converted by the liver to form ketones. There is a concern that the brain may have trouble acquiring adequate nutrition due to reduced cerebral blood flow that occurs naturally with age. Thus, the goal of ketogenic diets is to ensure that the brain is provided with an alternative fuel source that does not interfere with existing glucose use. Diets fortified with MCTs and antioxidants (that include vitamin B complex) have been shown to improve cognitive performance on neuropsychological tasks in senior laboratory dogs[100] and dogs affected with CDS.[105]

A nutritional supplement containing phosphatidylserine, ginkgo biloba, vitamin B6, vitamin E, and resveratrol (Senilife) was reported to be effective in reducing signs of cognitive dysfunction as described by owners during a period of 84 days; however, only 8 dogs were included in the study.[82] In humans, gingko biloba has been found to be effective only if the patient has circulatory problems[13] but no formal studies have been done in dogs or cats. Another supplement with some evidence of efficacy in humans with VCID and AD is Huperzine A, a compound found in Chinese club moss that inhibits acetylcholinesterase.[106,107] To date no studies have been published on efficacy for CDS in dogs or cats. Supplements may also have a positive influence on patients experiencing changes associated with aging or cognitive impairment, such as joint, liver, bladder, and renal supplements, provided there are no interactions with existing medications.

S-adenosylmethionine (SAMe) is a molecule synthesized within the body and involved in many anabolic reactions such as methyl group transfer. In veterinary medicine, it is used for liver support and in human medicine, treats depression (increasing dopamine and serotonin levels), liver disease, and osteoarthritis.[108,109] SAMe tosylate can be supplemented to companion animals, and one study reports executive function improvement in nonseverely impaired senior dogs (100 mg/day for dogs <10 kg; 200 mg/day for dogs 10–20 kg) and cats (100 mg/cat/day).[110]

Finally, enrichment with exercise and mental stimulation has been shown to have some neuroprotective effects in dogs. The aging process causes a variety of changes including cortical atrophy, ventricular dilation, and thus a reduction in the number of neurons. In a study noted above, the effect of enrichment (2 additional 15-minute exercise sessions per week, sets of toys alternated weekly, and regular cognitive evaluation/testing) modified neuronal loss within the hilus of the brain and improved cognitive performance on neuropsychological tasks.[98] A pilot study found that a 4-week positive reinforcement training class may have slowed CDS progression for dogs that participated in the course versus dogs that did not.[111]

Owner education regarding the care and expectations of senior companion animals can be helpful to ensure that clinical signs are reported. Reduced mobility, sensory decline, and a higher incidence of systemic disease are anticipated changes in senior pets and a driving factor to promote frequent wellness visits and to consider physical therapy when appropriate. Environmental changes at home may be helpful for any senior companion animal and should focus around meeting their functional needs. Companion animals should have a comfortable space dedicated to them to sleep and relax. As companion animals age, they lose their ability to thermoregulate efficiently, so it is important they can stay warm during cold times and keep cool when hot. They should be able to navigate their home with ease that will allow them to easily access resources such as food and places to eliminate. For instance, traction on slippery flooring (ie, carpets, runners) can reduce fear associated with slipping in companion animals affected with neurologic or musculoskeletal disease. Consider providing steps or low shelving to get to elevated surfaces more easily. There are commercial products but at home, items may be just as useful, such as linen-filled suitcases or old sofa cushions strategically placed.[112] Moreover, consider low-lipped and easy entry litterboxes for cats.

Physical and social needs should be met, which include high-quality diets fortified with antioxidants, regular short bouts of exercise, social interaction with owners and conspecifics provided they are positive, and a variety of mental stimulation. Ensure that types of mental stimulation provided are appropriate for the patient and that a variety of food options are provided to owners, particularly if there are dietary restrictions. Owners should be encouraged to continue or initiate positive reinforcement training with verbal, light, or vibration cues in anticipation of sensory decline.

SUMMARY

The role and interaction between life factors, aging, disease, and inflammation should be considered when treating senior patients. There is a need for more evidence-based studies to differentiate cognitive dysfunction in veterinary patients that may stem from different causes when compared with CDS because prevention, treatment, and progression may differ. The implications of biological mechanisms and their driving factors on cognition can contribute to improved welfare in various aspects including prevention and treatments.

CLINICS CARE POINTS

- As evidenced in human medicine, cognitive dysfunction in pets is likely to have more than a single etiology which may present an opportunity for enhanced treatment options. However, further research is needed regarding the prevalence and pathogenesis of cognitive dysfunction associated with chronic disease states.

- Aging pets are at a higher risk for cognitive dysfunction and medical disease necessitating routine behavioral and physical screens and record keeping for early identification and treatment.

- Behavioral changes in senior pets should not be readily discounted as cognitive decline as they can often be a clinical sign of other medical conditions. Equally important is determining the cognitive and behavioral health of patients suffering from chronic medical conditions (ie IE, cardiovascular disease, and inflammation) to provide behavioral treatment.

- Optimization of cognitive health should include a quality diet that provides adequate nutrition and antioxidants to the brain, mental enrichment, physical exercise (depending on tolerance), and special considerations given to reduce inflammation, stress, and anxiety.
- Treatment of cognitive dysfunction syndrome should be aimed at improving the patient's quality of life with a focus on the limitations that aging may have, slowing progression, alleviating emotional and physical discomfort of the patient, while maintaining the human-animal bond.

DISCLOSURE

There are no commercial or financialconflicts.

REFERENCES

1. Tulsky DS, Price LR. The joint WAIS-III and WMS-III factor structure: development and cross-validation of a six-factor model of cognitive functioning. Psychol Assess 2003;15(2):149.
2. Brabec CM, Gfeller JD, Ross MJ. An exploration of relationships among measures of social cognition, decision making, and emotional intelligence. J Clin Exp Neuropsychol 2012;34(8):887–94.
3. Rodríguez-Rajo R, García-Rudolph A, Sánchez-Carrión R, et al. Social and nonsocial cognition: Are they linked? A study on patients with moderate-to-severe traumatic brain injury. Appl Neuropsychol: Adultspan 2020;1–10. https://doi.org/10.1080/23279095.2020.1845171.
4. Landsberg G, Araujo JA. Behavior problems in geriatric pets. Veterinary Clinics: Small Animal Practice 2005;35(3):675–98.
5. Aria M, Alterisio A, Scandurra A, et al. The scholar's best friend: Research trends in dog cognitive and behavioral studies. Anim Cognit 2021;24:541–53.
6. Madari A, Farbakova J, Katina S, et al. Assessment of severity and progression of canine cognitive dysfunction syndrome using the CAnine DEmentia Scale (CADES). Appl Anim Behav Sci 2015;171:138–45.
7. Salvin HE, McGreevy PD, Sachdev PS, et al. The canine cognitive dysfunction rating scale (CCDR): a data-driven and ecologically relevant assessment tool. Vet J 2011;188(3):331–6.
8. Vikartovska Z, Farbakova J, Smolek T, et al. Novel diagnostic tools for identifying cognitive impairment in dogs: behavior, biomarkers, and pathology. Front Vet Sci 2021;7:551895.
9. Colle MA, Hauw JJ, Crespeau F, et al. Vascular and parenchymal Aβ deposition in the aging dog: correlation with behavior. Neurobiol Aging 2000;21(5):695–704.
10. Bower JM, Parsons LM. Rethinking the "lesser brain". Sci Am 2003;289(2):50–7.
11. Diamond A. Executive functions. Annu Rev Psychol 2013;64:135–68.
12. Filley CM. The neuroanatomy ofa ttention. Semin Speech Lang 2002;23(2):89–98.
13. Reisberg D. Cognition: exploring the science of the mind. New York: W.W. Norton & Company; 2019.
14. Staub B, Doignon-Camus N, Després O, et al. Sustained attention in the elderly: What do we know and what does it tell us about cognitive aging? Ageing Res Rev 2013;12(2):459–68.

15. Green MF, Horan WP, Lee J. Social cognition in schizophrenia. Nat Rev Neurosci 2015;16(10):620–31.
16. Kitamura T, Ogawa SK, Roy DS, et al. Engrams and circuits crucial for systems consolidation of a memory. Science 2017;356(6333):73–8.
17. Logue SF, Gould TJ. The neural and genetic basis of executive function: attention, cognitive flexibility, and response inhibition. Pharmacol Biochem Behav 2014;123:45–54.
18. Eagle DM, Baunez C, Hutcheson DM, et al. Stop-signal reaction-time task performance: role of prefrontal cortex and subthalamic nucleus. Cerebr Cortex 2008;18(1):178–88.
19. Maddux JM, Holland PC. Effects of dorsal or ventral medial prefrontal cortical lesions on five-choice serial reaction time performance in rats. Behav Brain Res 2011;221(1):63–74.
20. McAlonan K, Brown VJ. Orbital prefrontal cortex mediates reversal learning and not attentional set shifting in the rat. Behav Brain Res 2003;146(1–2):97–103.
21. Bray EE, Gruen ME, Gnanadesikan GE, et al. Dog cognitive development: a longitudinal study across the first 2 years of life. Anim Cognit 2021;24:311–28.
22. Watowich MM, MacLean EL, Hare B, et al. Age influences domestic dog cognitive performance independent of average breed lifespan. Anim Cognit 2020;23: 795–805.
23. Adams B, Chan A, Callahan H, et al. Use of a delayed non-matching to position task to model age-dependent cognitive decline in the dog. Behav Brain Res 2000;108(1):47–56.
24. Horschler DJ, Hare B, Call J, et al. Absolute brain size predicts dog breed differences in executive function. Anim Cognit 2019;22:187–98.
25. McMillan FD. Behavioral and psychological outcomes for dogs sold as puppies through pet stores and/or born in commercial breeding establishments: Current knowledge and putative causes. Journal of veterinary behavior 2017;19:14–26.
26. Zaine I, Domeniconi C, Wynne CD. The ontogeny of human point following in dogs: When younger dogs outperform older. Behav Process 2015;119:76–85.
27. Fuller JL. Transitory effects of experiential deprivation upon reversal learning in dogs. Psychonomic Sci 1966;4:273–4.
28. Thompson WR, Heron W. The effects of restricting early experience on the problem-solving capacity of dogs. Canadian Journal of Psychology/Revue canadienne de psychologie 1954;8(1):17.
29. Carlson SM, Wang TS. Inhibitory control and emotion regulation in preschool children. Cognit Dev 2007;22(4):489–510.
30. Bray EE, Sammel MD, Cheney DL, et al. Effects of maternal investment, temperament, and cognition on guide dog success. Proc Natl Acad Sci USA 2017; 114(34):9128–33.
31. Bellows J, Colitz CM, Daristotle L, et al. Defining healthy aging in older dogs and differentiating healthy aging from disease. J Am Vet Med Assoc 2015;246(1): 77–89.
32. Bellows J, Center S, Daristotle L, et al. Evaluating aging in cats: How to determine what is healthy and what is disease. J Feline Med Surg 2016;18(7):551–70.
33. Puurunen J, Ottka C, Salonen M, et al. Age, breed, sex and diet influence serum metabolite profiles of 2000 pet dogs. R Soc Open Sci 2022;9(2):211642.
34. Radakovich LB, Pannone SC, Truelove MP, et al. Hematology and biochemistry of aging—evidence of "anemia of the elderly" in old dogs. Vet Clin Pathol 2017; 46(1):34–45.

35. Dias-Pereira P. Morbidity and mortality in elderly dogs–a model for human aging. BMC Vet Res 2022;18(1):1–8.
36. Harvey CE, Shofer FS, Laster L. Association of age and body weight with periodontal disease in North American dogs. J Vet Dent 1994;11(3):94–105.
37. Dos Santos JDP, Cunha E, Nunes T, et al. Relation between periodontal disease and systemic diseases in dogs. Res Vet Sci 2019;125:136–40.
38. Keijser SFA, Meijndert LE, Fieten H, et al. Disease burden in four populations of dog and cat breeds compared to mixed-breed dogs and European shorthair cats. Prev Vet Med 2017;140:38–44.
39. Frank D. Recognizing behavioral signs of pain and disease: a guide for practitioners. Veterinary Clinics: Small Animal Practice 2014;44(3):507–24.
40. Dhaliwal R, Boynton E, Carrera-Justiz S, et al. 2023 AAHA Senior Care Guidelines for Dogs and Cats. J Am Anim Hosp Assoc 2023;59(1):1–21.
41. Day MJ. Ageing, immunosenescence and inflammageing in the dog and cat. J Comp Pathol 2010;142:S60–9.
42. Alexander JE, Colyer A, Haydock RM, et al. Understanding how dogs age: longitudinal analysis of markers of inflammation, immune function, and oxidative stress. J Gerontol: Series A 2018;73(6):720–8.
43. Mosier JE. Effect of aging on body systems of the dog. Vet Clin Small Anim Pract 1989;19(1):1–12.
44. Dowgray N, Pinchbeck G, Eyre K, et al. Aging in cats: Owner observations and clinical finding in 206 mature cats at enrolment to the cat prospective aging and welfare study. Front Vet Sci 2022;9:351.
45. Peachey SE, Dawson JM, Harper EJ. Gastrointestinal transit times in young and old cats. Comp Biochem Physiol Mol Integr Physiol 2000;126(1):85–90.
46. Martell-Moran NK, Solano M, Townsend HG. Pain and adverse behavior in declawed cats. J Feline Med Surg 2018;20(4):280–8.
47. Fernandez M, Manzanilla EG, Lloret A, et al. Prevalence of feline herpesvirus-1, feline calicivirus, Chlamydophila felis and Mycoplasma felis DNA and associated risk factors in cats in Spain with upper respiratory tract disease, conjunctivitis and/or gingivostomatitis. J Feline Med Surg 2017;19(4):461–9.
48. Asproni P, Cozzi A, Verin R, et al. Pathology and behaviour in feline medicine: Investigating the link between vomeronasalitis and aggression. J Feline Med Surg 2016;18(12):997–1002.
49. Schütt T, Toft N, Berendt M. Cognitive function, progression of age-related behavioral changes, biomarkers, and survival in dogs more than 8 years old. J Vet Intern Med 2015;29(6):1569–77.
50. Mastinu A, Bonini SA, Rungratanawanich W, et al. Gamma-oryzanol prevents LPS-induced brain inflammation and cognitive impairment in adult mice. Nutrients 2019;11(4):728.
51. Dewey CW, Rishniw M. Periodontal disease is associated with cognitive dysfunction in aging dogs: A blinded prospective comparison of visual periodontal and cognitive questionnaire scores. Open Vet J 2021;11(2):210–6.
52. Holbrook NJ, Ikeyama S. Age-related decline in cellular response to oxidative stress: links to growth factor signaling pathways with common defects. Biochem Pharmacol 2002;64(5–6):999–1005.
53. Choi JH, Hwang IK, Lee CH, et al. Immunoreactivities and levels of mineralocorticoid and glucocorticoid receptors in the hippocampal CA1 region and dentate gyrus of adult and aged dogs. Neurochem Res 2008;33:562–8.

54. Jaqueline Szriber S, Santana Novaes L, Barreto Dos Santos N, et al. Imbalance in the ratio between mineralocorticoid and glucocorticoid receptors and neurodegeneration in the dentate gyrus of aged dogs. Vet World 2022;15(11).

55. Almeida OFX, Conde GL, Crochemore C, et al. Subtle shifts in the ratio between pro-and antiapoptotic molecules after activation of corticosteroid receptors decide neuronal fate. Faseb J 2000;14(5):779–90.

56. Ferguson D, Sapolsky R. Mineralocorticoid receptor overexpression differentially modulates specific phases of spatial and nonspatial memory. J Neurosci 2007;27(30):8046–52.

57. Muñoz-Durango N, Vecchiola A, Gonzalez-Gomez LM, et al. Modulation of Immunity and Inflammation by the Mineralocorticoid Receptor and Aldosterone. Biomed Res Int 2015;2015:652738. https://doi.org/10.1155/2015/652738.

58. Yiallouris A, Tsioutis C, Agapidaki E, et al. Adrenal aging and its implications on stress responsiveness in humans. Front Endocrinol 2019;10:54.

59. Mancuso P, Bouchard B. The impact of aging on adipose function and adipokine synthesis. Front Endocrinol 2019;10:137.

60. Swanson KS, Belsito KR, Vester BM, et al. Adipose tissue gene expression profiles of healthy young adult and geriatric dogs. Arch Anim Nutr 2009;63(2): 160–71.

61. Adamo PF, Forrest L, Dubielzig R. Canine and feline meningiomas: diagnosis, treatment, and prognosis. Compendium 2004;26:951–66.

62. Foster ES, Carrillo JM, Patnaik AK. Clinical signs of tumors affecting the rostral cerebrum in 43 dogs. J Vet Intern Med 1988;2(2):71–4.

63. Helman AM, Murphy MP. Vascular cognitive impairment: Modeling a critical neurologic disease in vitro and in vivo. Biochim Biophys Acta (BBA) - Mol Basis Dis 2016;1862(5):975–82.

64. Arnold SA, Platt SR, Gendron KP, et al. Imaging ischemic and hemorrhagic disease of the brain in dogs. Front Vet Sci 2020;279.

65. Kerwin SC, Levine JM, Budke CM, et al. Putative cerebral microbleeds in dogs undergoing magnetic resonance imaging of the head: a retrospective study of demographics, clinical associations, and relationship to case outcome. J Vet Intern Med 2017;31(4):1140–8.

66. Dewey CW, Rishniw M, Johnson PJ, et al. Interthalamic adhesion size in aging dogs with presumptive spontaneous brain microhemorrhages: a comparative retrospective MRI study of dogs with and without evidence of canine cognitive dysfunction. PeerJ 2020;8:e9012.

67. Noh D, Choi S, Choi H, et al. Evaluation of interthalamic adhesion size as an indicator of brain atrophy in dogs with and without cognitive dysfunction. Vet Radiol Ultrasound 2017;58(5):581–7.

68. Berk BA, Packer RMA, Law TH, et al. Medium-chain triglycerides dietary supplement improves cognitive abilities in canine epilepsy. Epilepsy Behav 2021; 114:107608.

69. Packer RM, McGreevy PD, Salvin HE, et al. Cognitive dysfunction in naturally occurring canine idiopathic epilepsy. PLoS One 2018;13(2):e0192182.

70. Watson F, Packer RMA, Rusbridge C, et al. Behavioural changes in dogs with idiopathic epilepsy. Vet Rec 2020;186(3):93.

71. Denenberg S, Liebel FX, Rose J. Behavioural and medical differentials of cognitive decline and dementia in dogs and cats. Canine and Feline Dementia 2017;13–58.

72. Mathews KA. Neuropathic pain in dogs and cats: if only they could tell us if they hurt. Vet Clin Small Anim Pract 2008;38(6):1365–414.

73. Bécuwe-Bonnet V, Bélanger MC, Frank D, et al. Gastrointestinal disorders in dogs with excessive licking of surfaces. Journal of Veterinary Behavior 2012; 7(4):194–204.
74. Camps T, Amat M, Manteca X. A review of medical conditions and behavioral problems in dogs and cats. Animals 2019;9(12):1133.
75. Landsberg GM, Nichol J, Araujo JA. Cognitive dysfunction syndrome: a disease of canine and feline brain aging. Veterinary Clinics: Small Animal Practice 2012; 42(4):749–68.
76. Ruehl WW, Entriken TL, Muggenburg BA, et al. Treatment with L-deprenyl prolongs life in elderly dogs. Life Sci 1997;61(11):1037–44.
77. Chapman BL, Voith VL. Behavioral problems in old dogs: 26 cases (1984-1987). J Am Vet Med Assoc 1990;196(6):944–6.
78. Dewey CW, Davies ES, Xie H, et al. Canine cognitive dysfunction: pathophysiology, diagnosis, and treatment. Veterinary Clinics: Small Animal Practice 2019;49(3):477–99.
79. Černá P, Gardiner H, Sordo L, et al. Potential causes of increased vocalisation in elderly cats with cognitive dysfunction syndrome as assessed by their owners. Animals 2020;10(6):1092.
80. Neilson JC, Hart BL, Cliff KD, et al. Prevalence of behavioral changes associated with age-related cognitive impairment in dogs. J Am Vet Med Assoc 2001;218(11):1787–91.
81. Yarborough S, Fitzpatrick A, Schwartz SM, et al. Evaluation of cognitive function in the Dog Aging Project: associations with baseline canine characteristics. Sci Rep 2022;12(1):13316.
82. Osella MC, Re G, Odore R, et al. Canine cognitive dysfunction syndrome: prevalence, clinical signs and treatment with a neuroprotective nutraceutical. Appl Anim Behav Sci 2007;105(4):297–310.
83. Sordo L, Gunn-Moore DA. Cognitive dysfunction in cats: Update on neuropathological and behavioural changes plus clinical management. Vet Rec 2021; 188(1):e3.
84. Moffat KS, Landsberg GM. An investigation of the prevalence of clinical signs of cognitive dysfunction syndrome (CDS) in cats. J Am Anim Hosp Assoc 2003; 39(512):10–5326.
85. Gaetani L, Blennow K, Calabresi P, et al. Neurofilament light chain as a biomarker in neurological disorders. J Neurol Neurosurg Psychiatr 2019;90(8): 870–81.
86. Fefer G, Panek WK, Khan MZ, et al. Use of cognitive testing, questionnaires, and plasma biomarkers to quantify cognitive impairment in an aging pet dog population. J Alzheim Dis 2022;1–12.
87. Mondino A, Gutiérrez M, González C, et al. Electroencephalographic signatures of dogs with presumptive diagnosis of canine cognitive dysfunction. Res Vet Sci 2022;150:36–43.
88. Milgram NW, Head E, Zicker SC, et al. Long-term treatment with antioxidants and a program of behavioral enrichment reduces age-dependent impairment in discrimination and reversal learning in beagle dogs. Exp Gerontol 2004; 39(5):753–65.
89. Bray EE, Raichlen DA, Forsyth KK, et al. Associations between physical activity and cognitive dysfunction in older companion dogs: Results from the Dog Aging Project. GeroScience 2023;45(2):645–61.

90. Fefer G, Khan MZ, Panek WK, et al. Relationship between hearing, cognitive function, and quality of life in aging companion dogs. J Vet Intern Med 2022; 36(5):1708–18.

91. Dreschel NA. The effects of fear and anxiety on health and lifespan in pet dogs. Appl Anim Behav Sci 2010;125(3–4):157–62.

92. Ostadkarampour M, Putnins EE. Monoamine oxidase inhibitors: a review of their anti-inflammatory therapeutic potential and mechanisms of action. Front Pharmacol 2021;12:676239.

93. Head E, Hartley J, Kameka AM, et al. The effects of L-deprenyl on spatial short term memory in young and aged dogs. Prog Neuro Psychopharmacol Biol Psychiatr 1996;20(3):515–30.

94. Mills D, Ledger R. The effects of oral selegiline hydrochloride on learning and training in the dog: a psychobiological interpretation. Prog Neuro Psychopharmacol Biol Psychiatr 2001;25(8):1597–613.

95. Zakošek Pipan M, Prpar Mihevc S, Štrbenc M, et al. Treatment of canine cognitive dysfunction with novel butyrylcholinesterase inhibitor. Sci Rep 2021;11(1): 18098.

96. Horwitz DF, editor. Blackwell's five-minute veterinary consult clinical companion: canine and feline behavior. New Jersey: John Wiley & Sons; 2018.

97. Milgram NW, Zicker SC, Head E, et al. Dietary enrichment counteracts age-associated cognitive dysfunction in canines. Neurobiol Aging 2002;23(5): 737–45.

98. Milgram NW, Head E, Zicker SC, et al. Learning ability in aged beagle dogs is preserved by behavioral enrichment and dietary fortification: a two-year longitudinal study. Neurobiol Aging 2005;26(1):77–90.

99. Nippak PMD, Mendelson J, Muggenburg B, et al. Enhanced spatial ability in aged dogs following dietary and behavioural enrichment. Neurobiol Learn Mem 2007;87(4):610–23.

100. Pan Y, Larson B, Araujo JA, et al. Dietary supplementation with medium-chain TAG has long-lasting cognition-enhancing effects in aged dogs. Br J Nutr 2010;103(12):1746–54.

101. Pop V, Head E, Hill MA, et al. Synergistic effects of long-term antioxidant diet and behavioral enrichment on β-amyloid load and non-amyloidogenic processing in aged canines. J Neurosci 2010;30(29):9831–9.

102. Chapagain D, Wallis LJ, Range F, et al. Behavioural and cognitive changes in aged pet dogs: No effects of an enriched diet and lifelong training. PLoS One 2020;15(9):e0238517.

103. Snigdha S, de Rivera C, Milgram NW, et al. Effect of mitochondrial cofactors and antioxidants supplementation on cognition in the aged canine. Neurobiol Aging 2016;37:171–8.

104. Hovda LR, Brutlag A, Poppenga RH, et al, editors. Blackwell's five-minute veterinary consult clinical companion: small animal toxicology. New Jersey: John Wiley & Sons; 2016.

105. Pan Y, Landsberg G, Mougeot I, et al. Efficacy of a therapeutic diet on dogs with signs of cognitive dysfunction syndrome (CDS): a prospective double blinded placebo controlled clinical study. Front Nutr 2018;5:127.

106. Xu ZQ, Liang XM, Zhang, et al. Treatment with Huperzine A improves cognition in vascular dementia patients. Cell Biochem Biophys 2012;62:55–8.

107. Zhang Z, Wang X, Chen Q, et al. Clinical efficacy and safety of huperzine Alpha in treatment of mild to moderate Alzheimer disease, a placebo-controlled, double-blind, randomized trial. Zhonghua Yixue Zazhi 2002;82(14):941–4.

108. Carpenter DJ. St. John's Wort and S-Adenosyl Methionine as" Natural" Alternative to Conventional Antidepressants in the Era of the Suicidality Boxed Warning: What is the Evidence for Clinically Relevant Benefit? Alternative Med Rev 2011;16(1).
109. De Silva V, El-Metwally A, Ernst E, et al. Evidence for the efficacy of complementary and alternative medicines in the management of osteoarthritis: a systematic review. Rheumatology 2011;50(5):911–20.
110. Araujo JA, Faubert ML, Brooks ML, et al. NOVIFIT®(NoviSAMe®) Tablets Improve Executive Function in Aged Dogs and Cats: Implications for Treatment of Cognitive Dysfunction Syndrome. International Journal of Applied Research inVeterinary Medicine 2012;10(1):90.
111. O'Brian ML, Herron ME, Smith AM, et al. Effects of a four-week group class created for dogs at least eight years of age on the development and progression of signs of cognitive dysfunction syndrome. J Am Vet Med Assoc 2021; 259(6):637–43.
112. Siracusa C. Understanding the Behavior of Geriatric Patients to Enhance their Welfare. In: Gardner M, McVety D, editors. Treatment and care of the geriatric veterinary patient. New Jersey: John Wiley & Sons; 2017. p. 257–68.

Cat Inappropriate Elimination and its Interaction with Physical Disease

Amy Learn, VMD[a],*, Debra Horwitz, DVM[b]

KEYWORDS

- Behavior • Cat • Defecation • Health • Inappropriate elimination • Marking • Stress
- Urination

KEY POINTS

- Stress may affect physical and behavioral health.
- Inappropriate elimination is normal elimination behavior in an unacceptable location.
- Marking is a behavior related to territorial delineation and social stress.
- All potential health issues must be identified, treated, or ruled out in order to change unwanted elimination behavior.
- Treatments include identifying sources of social stress, increasing enrichment, appropriate cleaning of soiled areas, providing the patient with litter boxes to meet their needs, and possible psychotropic medications.

INTRODUCTION

In the United States as well as in other countries, inappropriate elimination disorders (also known as periuria/perichezia) are the most frequently treated behavioral disorders in cats. According to the National Council of Pet Population Study and Policy 72% of cats that are surrendered to shelters each year are euthanized due to house soiling problems. Estimates such as this one would result in euthanasia of approximately 10,000 cats per day.[1] House soiling, inappropriate elimination, and behavioral periuria are vague terms that often require clarification to be fully understood and used. Some authors have suggested a more precise label of "unacceptable elimination" as a catch all term for the entire category.[2] Elimination is a normal, natural, and necessary function that is intrinsically reinforcing; therefore, it is not necessarily inappropriate but often the location may be unacceptable to human household members when it occurs outside of the litter box.

[a] Animal Behavior Wellness Center, 1130 Wilkinson Road, Richmond VA 23227, USA;
[b] Veterinary Behavior Consultations, 321 Carlyle Lake Drive, St Louis, MO 63141, USA
* Corresponding author. Animal Behavior Wellness Center, 1130 Wilkinson Road, Richmond VA 23227.
E-mail address: alearn2@hotmail.com

Vet Clin Small Anim 54 (2024) 121–134
https://doi.org/10.1016/j.cvsm.2023.07.002
0195-5616/24/© 2023 Elsevier Inc. All rights reserved.
vetsmall.theclinics.com

Because feline elimination problems are pervasive and often have medical components involved, practitioners must first rule out the possible contribution of a current or historical medical component (**Table 1**). Different body systems contribute to thirst and appetite, and disorders in these systems may lead to changes in elimination patterns of urine and feces. Because physical disease cannot truly be separated from changes in behavioral patterns, this article will outline how to evaluate symptoms of behavioral and physical disease in order to make the correct diagnosis and formulate treatment plans. Behavior change may be one of the first or only signs of a health issue for clients and, therefore, may act as a sentinel for illnesses.

DISCUSSION

There is a well-established link between illness or disease and stress, and the effects of stress on the body and behavior has been documented. Stress is the body's physiologic and behavioral response to an aversive or challenging stimulus to attempt restoring the homeostasis (neutral). Stressors can be classified as physical in nature or social, and the latter may be either intraspecific or interspecific.[3] The aversive object, condition, or event itself is not inherently the problem but rather it is the individual's perception of that event, which determines how it affects the individual patient.[3] A normal individual can usually handle low levels of stress and easily return to a baseline normal state. Stress can even be beneficial in small amounts (called eustress) and helps the brain to focus or the body fine tune its response to similar events. This might be more obvious when observing the high arousal associated with the reunion of a pet with his owner. In comparison, abnormal or chronic stress is labeled distress and can have more detrimental effects on the body and an individual's welfare. The way any individual perceives or manages stress can be variable and based on several factors: genetics, perinatal stress, neonatal illness, inadequate socialization, and traumatic experiences. Each of these can impair the individual's resiliency or ability to cope.[4] Houpt noted that poor maternal nutrition and inadequate socialization may have a dynamic effect on problem behavior in cats.[5]

SYSTEMIC EFFECT OF STRESS

Stress activates both the sympathetic adrenomedullary system (SAM) and the hypothalamic pituitary adrenal axis (HPA). The SAM facilitates the fight, flight, or fidget

Table 1
Medical rule outs for unacceptable elimination

Behavior	System	Condition
Urination	Degenerative	Arthritis, cognitive dysfunction
	Metabolic	Diabetes mellitus, renal disease, hepatopathy, hyperthyroidism, diabetes insipidus
	Neurologic	Loss of control
	Inflammatory	LUTD and pandora
Defecation	Degenerative	Arthritis and pelvic pain
	Metabolic	Hyperthyroidism
	Infectious/inflammatory	Colitis and parasitism
	Other	Diarrhea, constipation, and rectal stricture
Marking	Acquired	Anal gland impaction and urolithiasis
	Metabolic	Chronic kidney disease (CKD), hyperadrenocorticism, LUTD, and hormonal
	Neurologic	Fecal incontinence

Data from Stelow E. Behavior as an Illness Indicator. Veterinary Clinics: Small Animal Practice. 2020: 50(4):695-706.

responses by quickly releasing epinephrine and norepinephrine. These cathecol-amines prepares the body to physiologically respond to danger by causing increased cardiac output and respiratory rate, peripheral vasoconstriction to nonessential systems, and release of energy stores.[6] The HPA axis triggers the release of glucocorticoids such as cortisol in order to help the body protect itself on a longer-term basis. Glucocorticoids can cause both anti-inflammatory and proinflammatory effects at different time of the acute stress response, and catabolic changes, all of which ultimately assist in survival during a temporary stressful episode.[6,7]

Any changes in the household routine, feeding, or health of the cat may cause stress and secondarily result in behavioral changes, for example, hiding and loss of appetite (**Table 2** Differential diagnoses for behavior change). These protective responses to threats may also have negative effects on many body systems especially with extreme or chronic stress. These effects may result in immune suppression, decreased healing, infertility, gastrointestinal (GI) disruption, enhanced pain or itch sensitivity, increased blood pressure and risk of stroke, dry skin, poor coat, decreased concentration/

Table 2
Differential diagnoses for common behavior changes

Behavior Change	Differential Diagnoses
Decreased activity	Lack of enrichment, conflict, fear, weakness, musculoskeletal or neurologic disease, cardiovascular or respiratory disease, pain, obesity, hypothyroidism, and hyperadrenocorticism
Increased activity	Hyperthyroidism and metabolic disease
Inappetence	Conflict, inaccessibility, kidney disease, enteropathy, dental/oral disease, Central nervous system (CNS) disease, and systemic illness
Polyphagia	Endocrine disease (diabetes mellitus, hyperadrenocorticism, hyperthyroidism), exocrine pancreatic insufficiency, enteropathy, endoparasites, and negative energy balance
Decreased water intake	Conflict, inaccessibility, oral disease, fear, whisker fatigue, CNS disease, and nausea
Polydipsia	Diabetes mellitus, diabetes insipidus, hyperthyroidism, hyperadrenocorticism, kidney disease, hepatic disease, and hypercalcemia
Restlessness	Illness, pain, and distress
Sleeping more	Illness, pain, distress, and hypothyroidism
Undergrooming	Obesity, musculoskeletal or neurologic disease, and systemic disease
Overgrooming	Dermatologic, pain, distress, and ectoparasites
Decreased mobility	Musculoskeletal or neurologic disease, cardiovascular or respiratory disease, social conflict, and obesity
Increased vocalization	Hyperthyroidism, cognitive dysfunction, hypertension, distress, sensory decline, fear, or anxiety
Decreased vocalization	Distress and lethargy
Altered elimination	FLUTD, inaccessibility, musculoskeletal or neurologic disease, conflict, distress, poor hygiene, aversion, and enteropathy
Avoidance of people	Pain, illness, fear, and changes in routine or environment
Increased clinginess	Pain, illness, fear, and changes in routine or environment
Aggression	Pain, illness, fear, social conflict, and CNS disease

Data from Horwitz DF. Common feline problem behaviors: Urine spraying. Journal of feline medicine and surgery. 2019;21(3):209-19.

memory, and irritability. Additionally, stress specifically adversely affects the bladder by increasing bladder lining permeability, which impairs bladder integrity through activation of inflammatory processes.[7] Cats with lower urinary disease may have an increased activation of their stress response and decreased adrenocortical activity.[8]

NATURAL FELINE BEHAVIORS AND THEIR RELATIONSHIP TO STRESS

Cats are solitary hunters but due to their small stature may also be considered potential prey. Survival of any prey species relies on preserving health and the appearance of fitness at all costs. Cats will use scent and other territorial marking strategies to avoid conflict with other individuals, thereby reducing injury and hiding signs of illness until they are unable to compensate.[9]

In a multicat or multipet environment, one animal will inevitably affect others through the course of their regular routines and interactions. Some of these effects may be negative or stress inducing. The household may be divided into specific groups of cats, each with their respective territories or core areas within the same territory. Individual groups can be identified based on affiliative behaviors: which cats rub on each other, groom each other, rest near each other, and share resources.[10] Some of these group boundary lines are created with scent from facial rubbing, interdigital scent glands, or marking with urine or feces. However, when there is confusion about the boundary, or resources are not well distributed, or when individuals are added or subtracted, then discord and stress may occur.

DIAGNOSTIC CATEGORIES
Periuria

Behavioral periuria denotes a cat(s) who is depositing urine outside of the box or the ideal location for urine to be deposited.[11] There are 2 main categories of periuria: inappropriate latrining or toileting (emptying the bladder and bowel) versus marking or spraying. Each category has its own motivation that precipitates the behavior. Therefore, it is essential to determine the motivation for the periuria before creating a treatment plan. Several differentiating factors must be investigated to determine whether a cat is marking or toileting. These include whether the surface where urine is found is horizontal or vertical (not definitively diagnostic on its own); the amount of urine; the location of urination; whether the litter box is ever used; and what actions precede, follow, or correlate with the urination activity[12] (**Table 3** Taking a behavioral history).

Marking

Urine marking, a normal scent marking behavior of cats, is generally unacceptable to the human caretakers and thus may strain the human–animal bond. Cats use various methods of scent deposits as a primary source of communication. These scents may include secretions from facial, interdigital, and perianal glands as well as from urine and feces.[12] In a multiple cat household, members may define access to resources and safe spaces using facial expressions and body language to communicate, allorubbing (when a cat rubs against another to create or strengthen a social bond), and allogrooming. However, it is speculated that cats may not use submissive or reconciliation signals to foster harmony the way dogs do.[10] Social groups are variable but can include 2 or more cats that comfortably share territory and resources, groom each other, and rest near each other. More than one group can exist within the environment, although these groups may or may not coexist harmoniously.[13] Scent marking may be valuable in this type of environment. Scents can be recognized at a temporal and geographic distance, effectively acting as messages that are traded without face-

Table 3
Taking a behavior history: Important information to gather

Question	Relevance
Urination or defecation or both outside of the litter box	Suggests continence or neurologic issue vs metabolic vs a choice that is made about where to eliminate
Horizontal or vertical surface	Marking vs toileting
When did it start: Was there a trigger: move to new home, addition of new pet, and change in diet	Causes of stress, anxiety, or conflict, change in box hygiene, and inability to access box
Where does it occur	Always in the same location, always on the same surface type, never in the litter box may indicate a preference or aversion
Stance and behavior during elimination	Posture: digging in the box or nearby surface, squatting in the box or on the edge, covering, balancing on the sides, vocalization
Which cat	In multicat households, 1 or more cats may be involved and identifying which may the treatment more effective
Number of boxes and locations	Are they accessible, are there enough, are they spaced apart, are they too far away
Previous interventions	Punishment may cause more anxiety and exacerbate a problem

to-face interaction. This allows for delineation of territorial boundaries and individual presence in a conflict-free manner. Urine marks can convey several bits of information including sex, reproductive status, and degree of familiarity of the marker as well as how recently the area was marked.[14]

Studies suggest that approximately one-third of cats that are eliminating in an unacceptable location are urine marking.[15] One study found that 10% of males and 5% of females frequently urine-marked regardless of the age at which they were gonadectomized.[16] The frequency of marking can be dramatically different between sexes as well. Some reports state that the frequency of marking increases as the number of cats in a household increase.[17]

The body posture typically associated with urine marking is very distinctive and when present, differentiates it from other types of periuria. The marking cat stands with the tail extended vertically above the body, backs up to a vertical surface (usually while twitching the tail) treads the rear paws, and ejects a variable amount of urine that may hit the vertical surface and drip downward onto the horizontal surface. Alternatively, some cats may squat-mark on a horizontal surface. The targets of marking may be socially significant locations, around entryways such as windows or doors, or objects such as shoes or visitor's possessions, which may carry new, unfamiliar scents.[9]

Toileting

In a domestic situation where cats are primarily indoors, humans provide the location and substrate where urine should be deposited. This contrasts with cats in the wild, who choose their own toileting location based on ease of access, substrate quality, and safety. Toileting usually occurs away from food and resting areas and the behavior may have a series of choreographed steps including sniffing, digging, posturing, and covering.[18] Although the purpose of these actions is unclear, they may serve to uncover other previous scents, add new personal scents, identify the preferred location for eliminating, or to hide the excrement to prevent parasite infection. However, neither do all cats have a set elimination pattern before horizontal elimination nor do they follow all or some of these steps. Some authors have found that cats who eliminate in unacceptable locations are also less likely to dig or cover in their litter boxes.[19,20] However, cats who are reluctant to dig or cover may not like the substrate offered or may have some type of pain associated with the activity, such as with declawed or arthritic cats.[21,22]

Perichezia

Defecation outside of the litter box (perichezia) is a less common behavioral problem but is more likely to be seen in cats that also urinate outside the box. Causes of perichezia can be related to litter box aversions or preferences, marking (middening), or medical illness.[23]

Perichezia can result from any condition that causes cats to have malabsorption or maldigestion, GI pain, constipation, or loose stools. Additionally, non-GI causes can include hyperthyroidism, cognitive dysfunction, sensory decline, musculoskeletal pain, or neurologic dysfunction. Cats with disorders resulting in diarrhea or constipation may learn either to avoid the box due to chronic discomfort or to misplace the excrement because they do not have full control of when it occurs.[24]

The health of the microbiome affects the function of the GI system as well as many body systems and consequently disruptions in the population of the microbiome may result in conditions such as inflammatory bowel disease, allergy, and obesity.[25] A gut–brain axis has been recognized in several species signifying communication between the brain and intestinal tract via biochemical mediators (cytokines, bacterial metabolites, and precursors of neurohormones...) and direct vagal connection.[26] Studies have shown differences in populations of gut bacteria between dogs classified as normal, aggressive, or anxious. As such, restoring a healthy multispecies microbiome may improve GI, systemic, and mental health also in cats.

Litter Boxes Litter Box Location, Type, and Distribution

In some feline households, choosing a location for litter boxes is not an easy decision. Location may be a factor within a multiple cat household perhaps creating stressful situations about when the litter box can be accessed or who may be in the way when the cat tries to approach. Additional decisions such as size or type of box, or the substrate provided inside must also be made. Each of these decisions can affect the cat and create stress. Different studies have explored litter box details and the generally accepted (but perhaps arbitrary) criteria for litter boxes is that they should be big enough for a cat to explore (1.5 times the length of the cat); have a fine particulate, clumping, nonscented litter; contain approximately 4 inches deep litter bed; lack a cover; and be easily accessible.[19,27,28] Accessibility reflects the number of boxes within a household and where they are placed. The unproven standard is to provide one more litter box than the number of cats in the home to allow easier access or so that a cleaner litter box might be available if one has already been used.[28] However, when all litter boxes are within one location, this is just one toileting site and still may trigger litter box avoidance due to social conflict or poor hygiene. Ideally, there should be multiple locations for litter boxes especially in larger homes. Litter box hygiene is also a matter of great importance. Cats may choose a cleaner area if the box itself either has an unpleasant odor or appearance or is filled with elimination deposits.[29]

Cats may develop an aversion to a litter box, the location of it, or the type of litter if perceived as unpleasant for some reason. Causes of an aversion may include a box that is too small, litter texture or odor that is unacceptable, and scary noises (even if perceived as benign to the owner); social stresses such as fear of or bullying by another pet; or difficulty physically accessing the box, perhaps due to an aggressive housemate blocking it, or an arthritic cat having difficulty getting to or into the box. Similarly, some cats have particular preferences for their litter box expectations and if the box does not meet their standards, they choose a different location that does. They may have a substrate preference for a different-feeling particle, or soft or smooth surfaces. Location preferences may involve the attraction of a retained previous odor, a safer location where they are not attacked or can visualize other cats approaching, or an area appealing to the cat for some other reason.[21,24,28,30]

CONTRIBUTION OF PHYSICAL DISEASE

Alternatively, any number of physical diseases can contribute to depositing urine outside the litter box. Various authors have found laboratory or historical illness or abnormalities in cats that are marking with urine and those that have unacceptable toileting issues suggesting that physical illness may be present in periuria even when the cats seem healthy[16,30,31] (**Fig. 1** Feline Unacceptable Elimination).

Any illness that causes increased thirst will likely cause increased urination either in frequency or in volume. This may result in a cat that may not be able to get to the box frequently enough or be unable to find a clean place in the box to comfortably urinate if cleaned infrequently. Increased frequency may affect not only the ill cat but create a dirty box that results in other cats avoiding the box. Discomfort of the urinary tract may also result in either an urgent need to urinate or a negative association with the box because it was uncomfortable to "go" there previously, causing the cat to avoid returning.[32] Accessing the box may also be problematic if there is any reason for

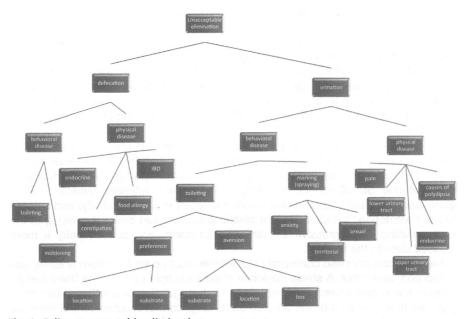

Fig. 1. Feline unacceptable elimination.

cognitive decline, altered perception, or difficulty getting to the box due to neurologic or musculoskeletal impairment.

PAIN

Any type of pain may contribute to changes in behavior including unacceptable elimination, changes in activity or mobility, or self-grooming.[33] In recent years, degenerative joint disease (DJD) or inflammation of any joint has been more commonly recognized in cats.[34] Since 2010, multiple studies report a majority of cats (74%–91%), especially those aged older than 5 years have radiographic evidence of DJD, even if lameness is not observed.[35,36] This suggests orthopedic pain is difficult to diagnose in cats based on traditional observations or physical examination metrics. Consequently, practitioners should be vigilant to identify seemingly unrelated behavioral changes such as litter box avoidance, which may be a sign of DJD.

Given that pain is difficult to assess in cats, Gruen and colleagues used a clinical pain medication trial and subsequent discontinuation of pain medication to assess whether owner observations of their cats' activity level, ambulation, and mood might help facilitate diagnoses.[37,38] Results indicated that when compared with placebo some owners were able to detect an acute response to the analgesic, whereas others were better able to discern a regression once the medication was discontinued.[39] Because our feline patients may provide challenges to diagnosing pain, this study suggests that we may be better able to diagnose painful conditions in cats through the use of appropriate client education and using client observations of pain medication trials and their results.

FELINE LOWER URINARY TRACT DISEASE

Feline lower urinary tract disease (FLUTD) is a broad category of urinary conditions including idiopathic cystitis (FIC), a common condition in cats. Clinical signs of FLUTD are not pathognomonic for any disease but can include stranguria, hematuria, dysuria, polyuria, and pollakiuria and may contribute to a negative association or disuse of the litter box.

As many as 30% of cats may experience an episode of FIC in their lifetime.[40] Separate articles suggest that stress or upregulation of the HPA axis may have a detrimental effect on bladder health and contribute to FIC.[41,42] Furthermore, sickness behavior, inflammation, changes in mood and sensitivity to pain can all vary based on specific qualities of a stressor, the animal's general health condition, and its individual resilience to stressors.[43] Additionally, cats with lower urinary tract signs often have other comorbid disorders.[44]

Cats with FIC generate a more intense stress response than healthy cats, possibly due to increased arousal and release of norepinephrine after environmental experiences.[43] The bladder is controlled by sympathetic, parasympathetic, and somatic nervous systems. Stimulation of the sympathetic system releases substance P (a neuropeptide), causing pain, inflammation, increased wall permeability, and smooth muscle contraction.[45] Repeated sympathetic activation can cause a rewiring of the brain, resulting in progressive sensitivity to stressors and subsequently a more diseased state in the bladder.

Over time, the scientific community has learned that no body system is totally detached from any other. A stress response affects multiple parts of the body and an illness in one organ system may contribute to dysregulation of another. It has been proposed that disorders of the skin, GI tract, lung, cardiovascular, central nervous, endocrine, or immune systems contribute to chronic lower urinary signs in some cats.[42] The integration of these systems and their response to stress underscore the importance of using a wholistic approach to stress and illness. There have been improvements in severity or frequency of clinical signs of FIC, for example, with implementation of anxiety management techniques and/or environmental enrichment.

CLINICAL RELEVANCE

Diagnosing and treating elimination disorders are often not clear or straightforward. The causes of elimination disorders are varied and complicated. Research indicates that only two-thirds of general practice veterinarians correctly diagnose elimination problems yet more than half of all cat owners seek advice for house soiling.[1] It is important for clinicians to understand what medical issues to pursue as differential diagnoses. Then they should be able to differentiate between the types and causes of unacceptable elimination to facilitate a diagnosis and formulate the appropriate treatment plan.

THERAPEUTIC OPTIONS

A thorough workup should be pursued for every elimination problem. This includes gathering a complete history, performing a comprehensive examination, and evaluating laboratory diagnostics including complete blood count, serum biochemistry, thyroid panel, urinalysis (with culture when specified), and blood pressure measurement. Other diagnostics such as ultrasound may be indicated in some situations. Once the diagnosis or diagnoses are made, the next focus is creating a therapeutic plan to improve or resolve the problem.

Addressing and Treating Stress

Multimodal environmental modification (MEMO) is a method of providing enrichment for cats (or any species) to decrease stress. MEMO focuses on adjusting the environment to allow the expression of more natural behaviors. Clients must be educated about the most ideal ways to decrease stress and improve welfare for their cats.[8] The Buffington MEMO plan[8] includes avoid any form of punishment; institute or ensure appropriate litter box factors and hygiene; provide climbing structures and perches, scratching posts, and sensory stimulation; increase individual interaction, and work to resolve any intercat conflict.

Probiotics

As previously discussed, the microbiome is important not only in GI health but also in overall health. Supplementation of probiotics is one way to balance the gut flora that ultimately may improve systemic health as well as resolve some causes of diarrhea or constipation.

Nutritional Interventions

The dietary recommendations in the MEMO study included increasing water intake and transitioning from dry to a canned food diet for cats that are willing to change. The patient's diagnosis may lead to considerations of various diets designed to change urine acidity, adjust mineral composition, and/or increase water intake thereby reducing the risk of urolithiasis.[46] Some of these diets have also been shown to decrease stress and may include ingredients that help calm the patient. Other diets such as those designed for sensitive systems or food allergies can decrease inflammation in the GI tract and enhance proper digestion, which often increases patient comfort.[47]

Environmental Considerations

Cats have different preferences for types of boxes or litter so it may be useful to offer a variety boxes and litter types and allow the cat to choose. Caregivers can note which box is used most and copy that style in multiple locations. Next, consider the size of the box. Most standard boxes available in the store are much too small for modern cats. One study shows that a box of 86 cm in length (approximately 3 feet) is preferred to smaller boxes.[48] This allows enough space for cats to sniff, dig, eliminate, and cover.

However, if a cat prefers a specific location to eliminate, then a box may be placed in that area—once it is used reliably there, it can be moved in short increments (on a scale of inches) per day to a more ideal location. Alternatively, that area can be repurposed. Placing a feeding or resting station there may discourage the cat from eliminating in the same location but works best when associated with enhanced litter box hygiene and addressing other issues.

Poor litter box hygiene has been associated with litter box avoidance. Daily removal of waste materials is essential to encourage regular box use.[49] Although cats generally prefer uncovered litter boxes, one study showed a tolerance toward a covered box if it was larger and kept clean.[11]

Medications

Some cats that suffer from comorbid behavior issues including generalized anxiety, or a social conflict (stress related to agonistic encounters between cats) may benefit from psychopharmacological intervention. Medication options range from antidepressants to supplemental products. All medical conditions, including possible pain, should be appropriately treated with their respective medications (**Table 4** Psychopharmacologic choices).

Several studies have investigated how to treat unacceptable elimination and marking behavior. Multiple medications have been shown to help in this area but only one is labeled for use in cats for elimination problems. This medication, Clomicalm (clomipramine), is labeled in Australia for feline inappropriate elimination (the same drug is labeled in the United States for dogs with separation anxiety). Studies show that Clomicalm reduces urine spraying in most cats by 16 weeks of use.[50] In another study, 80% of cats on Clomicalm improved by 75% with treatment.[51]

Fluoxetine (an off-label usage) has also been shown to decrease spraying in cats when compared with placebo.[50,52] Improved litter box hygiene was also shown to decrease urine marking.[53] Many cats responded within 8 weeks and continued to improve through 16 weeks but regressed when treatment was discontinued.

Table 4 Common psychopharmacologic choices, dose, and use		
Product	**Dose**	**Use**
Fluoxetine	0.5–1.5 mg/kg q 24h	Spraying
Clomipramine (Clomicalm)	0.25–0.5 mg/kg q 24h	Spraying and elimination
Buspirone	0.5–1 mg/kg q 12–24h	Spraying
F3 feline facial pheromones	Diffuser or spray	Spraying
Alpha-casozepine	15–30 mg/kg q 24h	Anxiety
L-theanine	5–10 mg/kg q 12h	Anxiety

Data from Refs.[28,50,52,54–56]

An early study of buspirone reported an improvement in both spraying and toileting behavior in cats.[54] Buspirone is not as effective in single cat households and only shows improvement in approximately 50% of cats treated.

The 2 most common nutritional supplements used for behavior problems in cats are alpha-casozepine and L-theanine.[55,56] These supplements help to decrease anxiety, which may contribute to unacceptable elimination in the home.

SUMMARY

Many elimination behavior problems have an underlying medical problem or may be due to the influence of stress. For the best outcomes, a practitioner should strive to identify and treat any medical problems in addition to focusing on the behavioral problems. Treatment should include enrichment, management of the environment, diminishment of stressors, provision of appropriate resources, dietary considerations, as well as any medication or supplements needed to reduce anxiety.

CLINICS CARE POINTS (BULLETED PEARLS AND PITFALLS)

- Performing a comprehensive physical examination and appropriate laboratory testing is the cornerstone of correctly diagnosing a behavioral problem.
- Stress may play a significant role in physical and mental health.
- Any illness that causes an increase in thirst or urination or GI upset may contribute to elimination problems.

CONFLICT OF INTEREST

Nil.

REFERENCES

1. Carney H, Sadek T, Curtis T, et al. AAFPand ISFM Guidelines for diagnosing and solving house-soiling behavior in cats. J Feline Med Surg 2014;16(7):579-98.
2. Seksel K. Preventive behavioural medicine for cats. In: BSAVA manual of canine and feline behavioural medicine. 2nd edition. BSAVA Library; 2009. p. 75–82. Horwitz and Mills.
3. Amat M, Camps T, Manteca X. Stress in owned cats: behavioural changes and welfare implications. J Feline Med Surg 2016;18(8):577–86.
4. Koolhaas JM, Korte SM, De Boer SF, et al. Coping styles in animals: current status in behavior and stress-physiology. Neurosci Biobehav Rev 1999;23:925e935.
5. Houpt KA, Zicker S. Dietary effects on canine and feline behavior. Veterinary Clinics: Small Animal Practice 2003;33(2):405–16.
6. Levine ED. Feline fear and anxiety. Vet Clin Small Anim Pract 2008 Sep;38(5): 1065–79.
7. Kunz-Ebrecht SR, Mohamed-Ali V, Feldman PJ, et al. Cortisol responses to mild psychological stress are inversely associated with proinflammatory cytokines. Brain Behav Immun 2003;17(5):373–83.
8. Buffington CT, Westropp JL, Chew DJ, et al. Clinical evaluation of multimodal environmental modification (MEMO) in the management of cats with idiopathic cystitis. J Feline Med Surg 2006;8(4):261–8.

9. Shreve KR, Udell MA. Stress, security, and scent: The influence of chemical signals on the social lives of domestic cats and implications for applied settings. Appl Anim Behav Sci 2017;187:69–76.
10. Bradshaw JW. Sociality in cats: A comparative review. Journal of veterinary behavior 2016;11:113–24.
11. Grigg E, Pick L, Nibblett B. Litter box preference in domestic cats: covered versus uncovered. J Feline Med Surg 2012;15(4):280–4.
12. Borchelt PL, Voith VL. Elimination behavior problems in cats. Compend Continuing Educ Pract Vet 1986;8:197–207.
13. Heath S. Common feline problem behaviours: unacceptable indoor elimination. J Feline Med Surg 2019;21(3):199–208.
14. Hart B, Hart L. Feline behavioral problems and solutions. In: Turner DC, Bateson P, Bateson PP, editors. The domestic cat: the biology of its behaviour. 3rd edition. Cambridge University Press; 2000. p. 201–12.
15. Frank D, Erb H, Houpt K. Urine spraying in cats: presence of concurrent disease and effects of a pheromone treatment. Appl Anim Behav Sci 1999;61(3):263–72.
16. Hart BL, Cooper L. Factors relating to urine spraying and fighting in prepubertally gonadectomized cats. J Am Vet Med Assoc 1984;184:1255–8.
17. Barcelos A, McPeake K, Affenzeller N, et al. Common risk factors for urinary house soiling (periuria) in cats and its differentiation: The sensitivity and specificity of common diagnostic signs. Front Vet Sci 2018;5:108.
18. McGowan RT, Ellis JJ, Bensky MK, et al. The ins and outs of the litter box: A detailed ethogram of cat elimination behavior in two contrasting environments. Appl Anim Behav Sci 2017;194:67–78.
19. Horwitz DF. Behavioral and environmental factors associated with elimination behavior problems in cats: a retrospective study. Appl Anim Behav Sci 1997; 52(1–2):129–37.
20. Sung W, Crowell-Davis S. Elimination behavior patterns of domestic cats (Felis catus) with and without elimination behavior problems. Am J Vet Res 2006;67: 1500–4.
21. Martell-Moran NK, Solano M, Townsend HG. Pain and adverse behavior in declawed cats. J Feline Med Surg 2018;20(4):280–8.
22. Monteiro BP, Steagall PV. Chronic pain in cats: recent advances in clinical assessment. J Feline Med Surg 2019;21(7):601–14.
23. Wright JC, Amoss RT. Prevalence of house soiling and aggression in kittens during the first year after adoption from a humane society. J Am Vet Med Assoc 2004;224(11):1790–5.
24. Stelow E. Behavior as an Illness Indicator. Veterinary Clinics: Small Animal Practice 2020;50(4):695–706.
25. Wernimont SM, Radosevich J, Jackson MI, et al. The effects of nutrition on the gastrointestinal microbiome of cats and dogs: impact on health and disease. Front Microbiol 2020;11:1266.
26. Sampson TR, Mazmanian SK. Control of brain development, function, and behavior by the microbiome. Cell Host Microbe 2015;17(5):565–76.
27. Borchelt PL. Cat elimination behavior problems. Vet Clin Small Anim Pract 1991; 21(2):257–64.
28. Neilson J. Thinking outside the box: feline elimination. J Feline Med Surg 2004; 6(1):5–11.
29. Ellis JJ, McGowan RT, Martin F. Does previous use affect litter box appeal in multi-cat households? Behav Process 2017;141:284–90.

30. Horwitz DF. Common feline problem behaviors: Urine spraying. J Feline Med Surg 2019;21(3):209–19.
31. Ramos D, Reche-Junior A, Mills DS, et al. A closer look at the health of cats showing urinary house-soiling (periuria): A case-control study. J Feline Med Surg 2019;21(8):772–9.
32. Frank D. Recognizing behavioral signs of pain and disease: a guide for practitioners. Veterinary Clinics 2014;44(3):507–24.
33. Klinck MP, Frank D, Guillot M, et al. Owner-perceived signs and veterinary diagnosis in 50 cases of feline osteoarthritis. Can Vet J 2012;53(11):1181.
34. Benito J, Gruen ME, Thomson A, et al. Owner-assessed indices of quality of life in cats and the relationship to the presence of degenerative joint disease. J Feline Med Surg 2012;14(12):863–70.
35. Lascelles BD, Henry JB III, Brown J, et al. Cross-sectional study of the prevalence of radiographic degenerative joint disease in domesticated cats. Vet Surg 2010; 39(5):535–44.
36. Kimura T, Kimura S, Okada J, et al. Retrospective radiographic study of degenerative joint disease in cats: Prevalence based on orthogonal radiographs. Front Vet Sci 2020;7:138.
37. Evangelista MC, Watanabe R, Leung VS, et al. Facial expressions of pain in cats: the development and validation of a Feline Grimace Scale. Sci Rep 2019;9(1): 19128.
38. Enomoto M, Lascelles BD, Robertson JB, et al. Refinement of the Feline Musculoskeletal Pain Index (FMPI) and development of the short-form FMPI. J Feline Med Surg 2022;24(2):142–51.
39. Gruen ME, Griffith E, Thomson A, et al. Detection of clinically relevant pain relief in cats with degenerative joint disease associated pain. J Vet Intern Med 2014; 28(2):346–50.
40. Olm DD, Houpt KA. Feline house-soiling problems. Appl Anim Behav Sci 1988; 20(3–4):335–45.
41. Westropp JL, Buffington CT. Feline idiopathic cystitis: current understanding of pathophysiology and management. Veterinary Clinics: Small Animal Practice 2004;34(4):1043–55.
42. Buffington C. Idiopathic cystitis in domestic cats: beyond the lower urinary tract. J Vet Intern Med 2011;25:784–96.
43. Strouse TB. The relationship between cytokines and pain/depression: a review and current status. Curr Pain Headache Rep 2007;11:98–103.
44. Stella JL, Lord LK, Buffington CT. Sickness behaviors in response to unusual external events in healthy cats and cats with feline interstitial cystitis. J Am Vet Med Assoc 2011;238(1):67–73.
45. Seawright A, Casey R, Kiddie J, et al. A case of recurrent feline idiopathic cystitis: the control of clinical signs with behavior therapy. J Vet Behav 2008;3(1):32–8.
46. Kerr KR. Companion Animals Symposium: dietary management of feline lower urinary tract symptoms. J Anim Sci 2013;91(6):2965–75.
47. Landsberg G, Milgram B, Mougeot I, et al. Therapeutic effects of an alpha-casozepine and L-tryptophan supplemented diet on fear and anxiety in the cat. J Feline Med Surg 2017;19(6):594–602.
48. Guy NC, Hopson M, Vanderstichel R. Litterbox size preference in domestic cats (Felis catus). Journal of Veterinary Behavior 2014;9(2):78–82.
49. Ellis JJ, McGowan RT, Martin F. Does previous use affect litter box appeal in multi-cat households? Behav Process 2017;141:284–90.

50. Hart BL, Cliff KD, Tynes VV, et al. Control of urine marking by use of long-term treatment with fluoxetine or clomipramine in cats. J Am Vet Med Assoc 2005; 226(3):378–82.
51. Landsberg GM, Wilson AL. Effects of clomipramine on cats presented for urine marking. J Am Anim Hosp Assoc 2005;41(1):3–11.
52. Pryor PA, Hart BL, Cliff KD, et al. Effects of a selective serotonin reuptake inhibitor on urine spraying behavior in cats. J Am Vet Med Assoc 2001;219(11):1557–61.
53. Pryor PA, Hart BL, Bain MJ, et al. Causes of urine marking in cats and effects of environmental management on frequency of marking. J Am Vet Med Assoc 2001; 219(12):1709–13.
54. Hart BL, Eckstein RA, Powell KL, et al. Effectiveness of buspirone on urine spraying and inappropriate urination in cats. J Am Vet Med Assoc 1993;203(2):254–8.
55. Beata C, Beaumont-Graff E, Coll V, et al. Effect of alpha-casozepine (Zylkene) on anxiety in cats. Journal of Veterinary Behavior 2007;2(2):40–6.
56. Dramard V, Kern L, Hofmans J, et al. Clinical efficacy of L-theanine tablets to reduce anxiety-related emotional disorders in cats: a pilot open-label clinical trial. J Vet Behav 2007;2:85–6.

Skin Disease and Behavior Changes in the Cat

M. Leanne Lilly, DVM, DACVB[a],*,
Carlo Siracusa, DVM, MS, PhD, DACVB, DECAWBM[b]

KEYWORDS

- Cat • Compulsive behavior • Hyperesthesia • Overgrooming • Skin • Stress
- Psychogenic alopecia • Tail chasing

KEY POINTS

- Skin and behavioral health in cats are connected.
- Overgrooming is one of the main behaviors through which cats manifest stress.
- Stress can be influenced by internal (temperament, physical health) and external (home environment) factors.
- Overgrooming can cause lesions of the skin and coat such as alopecia, scratches, ulcers, and self-mutilation.
- Treatment of problems related to overgrooming must be multimodal and address the underlying internal and external factors.

INTRODUCTION

Any illness that includes among its signs an observable action the animal repeats frequently is at risk of being declared a "behavioral problem" and approached solely as such, regardless of the underlying cause(s). In most cases, however, this is not the case. Repetitive grooming behaviors directed toward the coat and skin of cats such as self-directed licking, chewing, barbering, and scratching are no exception to this common misconception, as often they are signs of an underlying physical disease.

Here we examine the evidence-based approach to examination, diagnosis, and management of the most common categories of repetitive behaviors directed to the skin and coat in the cat.

- Excessive self-directed licking/grooming
- Excessive self-directed chewing or sucking
- Self-directed scratching
- Self-directed biting

[a] Department of Clinical Sciences, College of Veterinary Medicine, The Ohio State University, 601 Vernon L Tharp Street, Columbus, OH 43210, USA; [b] Department of Clinical Sciences and Advanced Medicine, School of Veterinary Medicine, University of Pennsylvania, 3800 Spruce Street, Philadelphia, PA 19104, USA
* Corresponding author. 601 Vernon L Tharp Street, Columbus, OH 43210.
E-mail address: lilly.136@osu.edu

Vet Clin Small Anim 54 (2024) 135–151
https://doi.org/10.1016/j.cvsm.2023.09.004
0195-5616/24/© 2023 Elsevier Inc. All rights reserved.
vetsmall.theclinics.com

SKIN PHYSIOLOGY AND BEHAVIOR

As the largest contiguous organ in the body, it is perhaps no great surprise that the skin and brain are interconnected. In fact the skin is a major target of the most commonly listed stress mediators: corticotropin releasing hormone, adrenocorticotropic hormone, cortisol, catecholamines, prolactin, and substance P. Moreover, keratinocytes can release substances classically associated with the nervous system like the neurotransmitters glutamate and dopamine.[1,2] Opioid peptides such as enkephalin, endorphin, and dynorphin have long been implicated in pruritus in humans[3], and morphine-induced itch has been documented in cats.[4] The skin-brain connection seems to be reciprocal both at the neurochemical level and at the full body level. Keratinocytes have the capacity to release both cortisol and oxytocin.[5,6] Depression and anxiety can be both sequalae of, or worsen pruritus.[7]

Pain and itch are nominally distinct and separate sensations, but they share a significant amount of overlap. Both sensations induce a specific, adaptive reflex: pain induces withdrawal, and itch induces scratching. Both sensations and their reflexes can be induced by a multitude of triggers, and many pruritogens such as histamine and capsaicin also produce pain.[8] Interestingly, both sensations seem prone to sensitization, and recognition that itch, like pain, can be or become neuropathic is on the rise.[9] Potentially contributing to this propensity in felines, is the relatively high concentration of Merkel's discs, Ruffinian corpuscles, and slow-adapting receptors in the skin of cats, making them particularly sensitive to touch.[10] Interestingly, Merkel's discs have serotonergic synapses with Aβ fibers, and both the electrophysiologic and behavioral responses to tactile stimuli are serotonin dependent.[11]

When all these elements are taken together, it becomes evident that the patient with a skin-directed repetitive behavior must be approached from a dermatologic, neurologic, endocrinologic, and behavioral standpoint.

TAKING A HISTORY

The evaluation of any behavior starts with the same approach as any other symptom set: taking a thorough, detailed history. The treating clinician needs to collect accurate and descriptive information of the behavior displayed. This information is sometimes challenging to obtain, as clients are prone to providing interpretations of behavior that may be inaccurate. There is also the risk of clients telling veterinary staff what they think we want to hear, especially if leading questions are used. Wading through client information can be aided through questionnaires; check boxes regarding observed behaviors can expedite some of this process and prime the client for types of things to watch for and report. Asking what the feline patient in question "looks like" or "does" may be more rewarding than "how" question such as "how is the licking going?" With the advent of smart phones, recording tablets, and laptops, requesting video is more readily accommodated than ever before.

The clinician needs a thorough understanding of the following:

The behavior(s) happening; any changes to those behaviors over time (and in response to prior treatment); where (specific anatomic area) the behavior is directed; when and how often the behavior occurs; the environment the cat resides in (household composition interms of animals and humans, home and surrounding area); and what triggers the behavior.

This last question is often challenging for clients to answer. Cat caregivers may report that a behavior is "unprovoked" or "out of the blue" because the stimuli that 'trigger' a stress and/or tactile response may not be immediately obvious to a client as such. This is when video recordings and written logs of the environment and behavior can be very useful. The client can be asked to record a daily log of information on the external and internal environment such as the weather outside, the presence of other pets in the area, frequency of self-scratching, etc (**Table 1**).

DIFFERENTIAL DIAGNOSES

The differential diagnosis for repetitive overgrooming behavior and possible related skin disease varies slightly by both behavioral symptomatology, location involved, and evaluation of the skin itself. For any patient where the skin or hair has been damaged, the following dermatologic diagnoses *must* be considered even if they do not turn out to be the sole causative factors:[12-15]

- Infections: bacterial, fungal, viral, or parasitic (this may be secondary contributing etiologies)
- Hypersensitivity allergic reactions: flea, contact, or food
- Neoplasia, particularly mast cell tumors or feline paraneoplastic alopecia and dermatitis
- Pain: local to the skin, the underlying area, or a nearby, but inaccessible body part (eg, anal glands in an obese cat or bladder pain below abdominal skin)
- Metabolic/endocrine causes such as cutaneous adverse drug reaction
- Idiopathic facial oral pain syndrome

To further complicate the evaluation, these diagnoses are not inherently mutually exclusive, and excessive grooming may come with other comorbidities such as pica.[16]

Behavioral dermatoses, that is, skin conditions that have a significant behavioral or emotional component, can be divided in to 3 types.

- Excessive self-directed licking/grooming (termed *psychogenic alopecia* when the primary cause is stress behavior)
- Chewing/suckling/biting, self-mutilation
- Excessive self-directed scratching

We will walk through the pathogenesis, differentials, and nuances of approach to each of these.

SELF-LICKING/GROOMING

Licking and grooming are adaptive and normal behaviors which serve to maintain cleanliness, remove parasites, and may also be cooling.[17] Housed cats may spend up to 30% of their day in comfort behaviors such as grooming and stretching.[18] Face and head grooming is normally a repetitive behavior sequence, stereotyped in its form but with an adaptive function. The cat sits, applies saliva to the medial aspect of the front limb while holding said limb horizontally, the limb is swept from caudal to rostral across the head/face with a circular and upward motion, with each pass stretching the forelimb further rostral.[17] The remainder of grooming is not stereotypic with various body parts licked in various orders. Grooming proceeds, typically in the direction of the fur, with various numbers of long licks. Cats who are prevented from grooming with an Elizabethan collar, will groom more when the collar is removed than they did prior to collar application, suggesting an inherent drive to perform this behavior regardless of other external factors (ie visible 'dirt').[18] Cats may also groom themselves as an acute response to stress, a displacement behavior.[19,20] Displacement behaviors (fidgeting) are one of the 4 primary coping strategies associated with stress response activation of the hypothalamic-pituitary-adrenal and sympathetic-adreno-medullary axes; fight, flight, and freeze being the other 3.[21] It is worth noting that anticipation of a

Table 1
Example of behavior log for caregivers of cats with overgroming behavior. Log must be adapted to the specific signs the patient is showing

Cat	Day	Time	Environment		Behavior in the Household		Overgrooming Behaviors						
			Indoor	Outdoor	With People	With Animals	Lick	Scratch	Suck	Self-Bite	Skin Twitch/Roll	Lesions	Vocalization
Ginger	9/14	8:00 PM	Quiet	Very noisy (roadwork)	Normal	Hissing at Roger (cat)	X	-	-	X (3)	-	Wet/broken hairs	-

stressor (anxiety) and fear of specific stimuli in the moment are both physiologic states that act as stressors.[22] Recognition that stress may trigger grooming as a displacement behavior, or be a component of compulsive disorder likened to trichotillomania in humans or compulsive washing, has elucidated our understanding of feline care.[13] However, focusing solely on this component may drive a clinician toward inappropriate behavioral diagnoses.

While the focus of this section is on excessive grooming, it is worth noting that decreased or lack of grooming is a recognized 'sickness behavior' and may be an early sign of any feline disease or external stressor.[23,24] Allogrooming contributes to the maintenance of group scent or colony odor, and cats who allogroom are more likely to sleep together and less likely to flee or hiss.[19,25] Consequently in multi-cat households the presence of allogrooming, changes in, or lack thereof are key parts of the history. Interestingly, excessive grooming of other cats as a sole complaint is rarely reported (personal observation).

Feline patients with excessive licking or grooming are likely to have areas of skin with any or all of the following.

- Alopecia (**Fig. 1**)
- Hypotrichosis with broken hairs of varying lengths, broken hairs in short tufts of uniform lengths, or hook-liked coiled hairs[26]
- Erythema, especially in the face of secondary infections

Cats of any age, sex, or breed can be affected with psychogenic alopecia. There may be genetic predispositions as the tightly related color-point breeds Siamese,

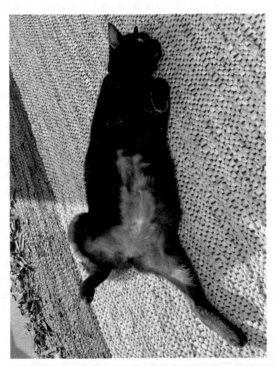

Fig. 1. Cleo, a female domestic shorthair, presents alopecia and hypotrichosis secondary to excessive licking in ventral areas of her body. (*Courtesy of* Dr. Anna Mukhina, DVM.)

Burmese, and Himalayans, and the Abyssinian (not a color-point breed) are overrepresented in cases.[27]

As a diagnosis of exclusion, it is most likely still overused. In 21 cases already 'diagnosed' with psychogenic alopecia, only 2 (9.5%) had no other underlying etiology, while 76.5% (16) had purely medical underlying etiologies.[28] Of the cats with medical causes, over half of those had multiple medical causes. One of the key diagnostic delineators was the presence of inflammation on biopsy—all cats with histologic evidence of inflammation had an underlying medical condition. However, the reverse failed to hold 4 of the cats without inflammation on histologic evaluation had environmental hypersensitivity, adverse food reaction, or both. At the very least, the bar to diagnose psychogenic alopecia requires the findings of a skin biopsy to rule out primary inflammatory disease and a complete chemistry with thyroid screen, as excessive grooming has been observed in association with hyperthyroidism.

In order to rule out the variety of medical underpinnings for excessive licking, the diagnostic plan will follow the history and symptomatology. However, a core evaluation requires the following:

- Physical examination, including evaluation of the structures below the affected area
- Dermatologic examination (skin impression, scraping, flea comb, trichogram, biopsy)
- Basic neurologic examination, especially if lesions/signs are not symmetric or the behavior is directed at the tail
- Complete blood cell count, chemistry panel, thyroid, and urinalysis
- Additional evaluation of underlying structures (location dependent)
  - Orthopedic and radiographic examination for lesions directed over a joint or joints
  - Urinalysis, fecal, abdominal ultrasound for licking directed at ventral abdomen
- Analgesic trial
- Consider gastrointestinal disease, especially if
  - Licking is also directed at surfaces or fabrics (wool sucking). While we lack the variety of research present in dogs, abnormal oral behaviors are increasingly associated with gastrointestinal abnormalities also in cats[16,29–31]
  - Concurrent vomiting or diarrhea, even at rates that do not concern the owner, as concurrent pruritus is common in feline food sensitivity[32]

The astute practitioner will remain aware that finding a physical cause may not mean finding the only cause. Follow up on progress and integration of the history are needed to identify and manage those cats with both physical and behavioral contributions to their disorder.

Treatment always requires addressing the underlying physical disease. If there is suspicion or confirmation of a behavioral component as well, concurrent or slightly staggered treatment is necessary. Short term, the use of an Elizabethan collar or clothing may prevent licking. However, it may also add to frustration by preventing all grooming and interfere with normal jumping. Rebound grooming is to be expected when the Elizabethan collar or the clothing is removed even without an underlying excessive licking component, and the client must be warned of this if utilizing one.[18]

All stressors for the specific patient should be mitigated. See the later section on environmental and behavioral modifications for recommendations that span the different presentations. If Elizabethan collars or clothing are utilized, adaptive changes in the environment should be implemented to account for the inability or unwillingness to jump, decreased echolocation, and visual impairment. This is especially important in households with multiple cats, since temporospatial separation is a primary peace-keeping behavior.[25,33,34] Cats wearing Elizabethan collars should not be outdoors for safety reasons.

SCRATCHING SELF-TRAUMA

Pruritus of any cause can trigger scratching and self-excoriations. A full dermatologic work up is always necessary with scratching-induced trauma. Culture and sensitivity is warranted as well, because not only standard skin bacteria may be found, but also environmental bacteria or fungi can be driven into deep wounds, especially *Sporo-thrix.*[15] In addition, a core evaluation requires the following.

- Physical examination, including evaluation of the structures below the affected area
- Dermatologic examination (skin impression, scraping, flea comb, trichogram, biopsy)
  - Due to the high distribution of mast cells in the ear, chin, and neck, scratching of these areas is a common sole sign of atopic dermatitis[35]
- Basic neurologic examination, especially if lesions are not symmetric or the behavior is directed at the tail. Consistent recruitment of a single limb with repetitive movement must be differentiated from a psychomotor seizure[36]
- Complete blood cell count, chemistry panel, thyroid, and urinalysis
- Additional evaluation of underlying structures (location-dependent)[12–15]
  - Head and neck-otoscopic, oropharyngeal, dental, cervical spine
  - Facial/muzzle-nasal passage, upper dental arcade, sinuses
  - Chin feline eosinophilic granulomatous complex is rarely itchy without secondary infections
  - Ear tips solar dermatitis in white cats may become pruritic and painful when chronic
  - Shoulders/axillae/elbows-spine, shoulder and elbow orthopedic evaluation, axillary lymph node evaluation. Cats can often reach the cranial aspects of these areas with their tongues so mixed licking and scratching may occur

Underlying causes for scratching trauma may also lie well below the skin—orthopedic pain or underlying organ discomfort. In the head and neck area, ear infections, polyps, dental disease, cervical pain can all result in scratching. Drug-induced pruritus caused by methimazole may affect any area, but most commonly results in head and neck scratching.[37,38]

Additionally, there is a rare syndrome in cats called feline behavioral ulcerative dermatitis (FBUD).[39] Previously described as idiopathic, this disorder is characterized by non-healing ulcerative lesions on the dorsal or lateral aspect of the neck, or on the interscapular area due to scratching, with an average age of onset of 19 months.[15,39] Presentation is not pathognomonic and overlaps with many other dermatologic condition (mycotic, bacterial, allergic hypersensitivity, or neoplasia).[14,15] Rarely lesions of the face, and of the rostral area in particular, are reported. If these are the only area of lesions, other syndromes or underlying disease processes such as dental pain may be at play.[40] Unlike the other differentials for ulcerative lesions in this area, FBUD is associated with other indicators of poor welfare beyond the wounds to the head and neck, such as frustration or stress associated with lack of control of the access to valuable resources, hiding spaces, perching/observation spaces, and human-cat or cat-cat social interactions.[39] As such, FBUD responds most commonly to environmental modification and modification of the human-cat interactions rather than medications, including steroids to which FBUD frequently becomes refractory.[39,40]

Another rare syndrome the clinician must keep in mind specifically for lesions on the rostral face and lips is feline orofacial pain syndrome (FOPS). Most commonly in Burmese, FOPS is characterized by episodic scratching of the head and lips, often with exaggerated licking or chewing movements, sometimes unilaterally.[41] Unilateral chewing behaviors must be differentiated from psychomotor seizures.[36] Severe cases may be accompanied by intra-oral mutilation to the togue, buccal mucosa, and lips.[41] 16% of cats show onset of signs starting with eruption of permanent teeth and 12% are euthanized as a consequence of this syndrome. It is a complex syndrome that can be devastating to feline and guardians alike. Sharing many of the symptomatology of trigeminal neuralgia in humans, including onset of attacks from benign stimuli such as eating or drinking, FOPS does not appear responsive to nonsteroidal anti-inflammatory drugs, steroids, or opioids.[41] This may also be a serotonergic mediated syndrome: a subgroup of serotonergic neurons in the dorsal raphe is highly activated with oral-buccal movements of chewing, licking, and grooming and by sensory stimuli in the head, neck, and face.[42]

BITING SELF-TRAUMA

Self-injurious biting may be directed at any part of the body that the cat can reach. Some areas of the body are associated with different underlying causes or processes. From the original localized processes, the behavior could then expand and become emancipated (ie, independent from the original causes), more diffused, and persistent and thus be classified as compulsive. The areas most commonly affected and the respective localized causes are as follows.

- Appendages: rule out musculoskeletal or neuropathic pain
- Hips, perineal area: musculoskeletal pain, neuropathic pain, anal gland problems, previous or current tail bite abscess
- Tail directed:
  o May start as play behavior, however the inflammation and associated pain can create a neuropathy increasing a persistent drive to try to relieve those sensations[13]
  o Can be secondary to underlying orthopedic disease or spinal pain

The other syndrome to recognize with self-directed biting is that of feline hyperesthesia. This syndrome goes by many names including "rolling skin syndrome", "twitching cat disease", or "atypical neurodermatitis". Hyperesthesia syndrome is associated with a variety of comorbidities: dermatologic pain, pruritus, localized or systemic infections, parasite infestations, partial seizures, spinal disease and other neuropathies, and musculoskeletal discomfort (from different causes including systemic infection and inclusion body myopathies).[43–45] Independent of underlying neurodermatologic abnormalities, episodes may appear as displacement behaviors triggered by any period of high arousal (play, fear, conflict, or anticipation).[44] Hallmark signs include rippling, twitching and spasm of the epaxial and trunk muscles, tail twitching, other signs of arousal such as mydriasis and vocalizing, estrus-like rolling, running, and redirected aggression.[10,13] Onset may be between 1 and 6 years of age, and may be more prevalent in males, based on a small retrospective study[45]. In this retrospective, the most successful treatment modalities included the administration of gabapentin alone or in combination with a variety of other drugs (anti-inflammatory or immunomodulatory medications, anti-seizure medications, and/or amitriptyline).

TREATMENT

Because of the intricate relationship between underlying physical conditions and behavior abnormalities, and the fact that self-injurious overgrooming behaviors are chronic problems with a cumulative stress effect, behavioral treatment must be incorporated even in the face of confirmed physical components.

Environmental Management

All stressors identified in the history should be mitigated to the best of the ability to create a predictable, safe, and enriched environment. This will in turn decrease frustration, sympathetic arousal, and stress. A cat-friendly house should include a plethora of safe spots for resting and perching that will vary by cats (hiding under furniture, perching or hiding on top of furniture). All natural behaviors should also have appropriate outlets: scratching, stretching, "hunting" simulated preys like toys of food-filled devices, and interactive playtime. Because play is an abbreviated and ritualized predatory cycle, even short sessions (5–10 minutes) should end with a consummatory phase (edible treats or kibble) to prevent frustration.[46–49] Caution should be used in considering laser pointers, and they may cause frustration and generate stress-related behavior problems.[50] Olfactory stimulation (catnip, silver vine, valerian) and modulation (pheromones) are readily available adjunct environmental management strategies for stress mitigation.[51–55]

Social conflict, between cats or with other animals or humans, is a common source of stress for cats. Avoidance such as hiding or time-sharing are common coping tactics among cats that are less readily recognized than overt aggression such as hissing, spitting, yowling, swatting or biting.[24,25,39] Each cat and individual animal should have their own safe core area with all essential resources (food, water, litter box, sleeping/scratching outlets) arranged. Cats that tend to spend prolonged time together and show affiliative behaviors like rubbing each other and sleeping in contact could have overlapping safe core areas. Otherwise, all cats must have separate and non-overlapping areas. In the event of overt aggression (hissing, swatting, stalking pouncing, biting), individuals must be separated by a barrier and behavioral modification specifically implemented to change that relationship.[56]

Behavioral Management

Inadvertent reinforcement of behavior must be evaluated by the clinician and stopped, keeping in mind that the learner (cat) determines if an intervention is reinforcing or not.[57] Punishment, "reprimands" or "discipline", even as benign as clapping or saying a stern "no'", must be avoided due to increasing stress without addressing the underlying issue. This is particularly important for behaviors such as self-injurious repetitive overgrooming for which increased stress is a relevant contributor. Instead, behavior modification should utilize desensitization and counter conditioning that use appropriate stimuli and cues combined with positive reinforcement for desirable behaviors.[58,59] Interactions that the cat may find unpleasant, even if desirable for the client (forced hugging, lifting, unsolicited petting), should be discontinued.[39,60] When cats are engaging in a self-injurious overgrooming behavior, current environmental contexts should be noted for monitoring and follow up, and the cat should be engaged in alternate rewarding activities. Cue words for alternate behaviors such as "go to your mat/tree" or "come/touch" can be used as the distraction cue. Walking away during the undesirable behavior may or may not facilitate a decreased occurrence of the undesired behavior, depending on its cause and the previous experience of the cat.[61]

Pharmacologic Management (Including Nutraceuticals)

The decision to reach for psychotropic medications should be based on history and clear identification of a behavioral component. Psychotropic medication must be considered for animals that have problems regulating their emotional response and are therefore in a chronic state of distress, fear, anxiety, or heightened reactivity. However, when the stress that a cat experiences is primarily caused by an inadequate environment, psychotropic medication may not be the first choice. For many of the diagnoses (FBUD, alopecia/excessive grooming with a psychogenic component) primary management of the environment including social interactions may be as, if not more, effective than psychotropics.[28,39] If the behavioral triggers cannot be sufficiently modulated or avoided, or are unpredictable (sounds from neighbors in an apartment building), then anxiety-relieving pharmacologic agents are warranted for appropriate welfare, to ease panic, fear, and allow for more effective behavior modification. Utilization early in treatment plan may be warranted when the risk of relinquishment or euthanasia is high even in the face of mild-to-moderate severity and their support tapered after the household is no longer in crisis mode.

It is important for the clinician to remember that, despite the increasingly common use of behavior modification medications, no behavior medications are licensed in the United States for such use in cats and disclosure of off-label usage is needed.

Rapid acting medications

These pharmacologic interventions take effect within 1 to 3 hours but also wear off within a few hours (typically, between 4 and 8 hours). They can be started as 'crisis busters' or prior to triggering events. Among the rapid acting medications, gabapentin can be used for its analgesic, anti-anxiety, and sedative effect[62–65] *Liquid gabapentin for humans commonly contains xylitol, caution must be considered in scripting liquid gabapentin out for feline households that contain dogs.*[66] Benzodiazepines are true anti-panic medications and can be considered when fear and anxiety are thought to have a major role in the development of the overgrooming behavior. They are selected based on duration needed and metabolism. Diazepam may case fulminant hepatic necrosis in cats when given per os and should be avoided[67,68]; both clorazepate and chlordiazepoxide share the entire metabolic pathway with diazepam so are best avoided in cats as well. *Due to the risk of disinhibition and agitation, benzodiazepines are less frequently used when there is also aggression.* Trazodone, a serotonin antagonist reuptake inhibitor (SARI), is used for its anti-anxiety and mild-to-moderate sedative effect. Onset time of action appears variable in cats, ranging from 60 minutes to 3 hours[69,70]. It is metabolized by the liver, cleared by the kidneys, and has been documented in healthy cats to decrease systolic blood pressure with no echocardiographic or heart rate changes.[71] Buprenorphine, a mixed opioid agonist, should be considered as needed when sedation and analgesia can be beneficial in managing the self-injurious behavior.[72]

Long lasting/daily options

Administered regularly regardless of behavior or events, these drugs may take days or weeks to reach therapeutic effects. The medications meeting this criteria fall into 3 categories in cats: SSRIs (fluoxetine, sertraline, and paroxetine), tricyclic-antidepressants (clomipramine, amitriptyline), and azapirone (buspirone). All of the diets for stress mitigation (Hills c/d series, Royal Canine Calm therapeutic diet), Purina Calming Care, and L-theanine have been studied in long-term contexts (days to weeks to effect), with Hills c/d multi care stress being the only 1 to specifically report on overgrooming decreases.[73–98]

For a short list of commonly used drugs, see **Table 2**.

Table 2
Commonly used drugs for overgrooming behavior

	Serotonergic Y/N	Dose Range	Frequency	Time to Effect
Fluoxetine	Y	0.5–1.5 mg/kg	Q24H	4–6 wk
Clomipramine	Y	0.25–1.3 mg/kg	Q24H	3–5 wk
Trazodone	Y	50–100 mg/cat	PRN	30 min-4H
Alprazolam	N (GABA)	0.0125–0.25 mg/kg	PRN or Q8H	30–60 min
Lorazepam	N (GABA)	0.03–0.08 mg/kg	PRN or Q12H	30–60 min
Gabapentin	N	3–20 mg/kg	PRN or Q8-24H	60–120 min

Combination of 2 serotonergic drugs is not recommended in cats. All drugs are administered PO. Time of effect: Fast 1-3 hours; Slow, between 1 and 4 wk. *There are no peer reviewed studies on repeated dosing in cats
GABA, gamma-aminobutyric acid; PRN, pro re nata.

PROGNOSIS

The prognosis is variable, dependent on the underlying causes, complicating factors, and the ability to manage stressors that may not be under client or clinician control. Interdisciplinary approaches are often needed, and patients may benefit from recruitment of multiple specialists, at least initially, to determine the causes. When underlying behavioral factors predominate and can be controlled or removed, signs may be fully resolved. This level of success may also be found when underlying medical factors respond well to medical management. However, most cases require long-term management to some degree, and relapses are to be expected occasionally. Appropriate education of the client and client-centered communication can help minimize the impact on the human-animal bond and facilitate success.[99]

CLINICS CARE POINTS

- Collect a thorough and descriptive behavior history of the environment where the cat lives
- Determine is the cat has an anxious, fearful, or reactive temperament that could be influencing his response to environmental stressors
- Ask the owner to video record the behavior of the cat in their presence and absence and use these videos to identify possible triggers
- Screen for systemic and localized disease that could affect the overgrooming behavior
- Cautiously explore (include palpation) all the areas of the body to identify all skin lesions possibly covered by the coat (eg, crusts on the tip of the tail)
- Identify and remove as many stressors as possible
- Address all the physical and behavioral causes of the overgrooming
- Do a thorough and consistent follow up to support the owner and monitor the progression of the behavior problem

DISCLOSURE

No conflict of interest to disclose.

REFERENCES

1. Arck PC, Slominski A, Theoharides TC, et al. Neuroimmunology of Stress: Skin Takes Center Stage. J Invest Dermatol 2006;126(8):1697–704.
2. Denda M. Epidermis as the "Third Brain". Dermatol Sin 2015;33(2):70–3.
3. Ko MC. Roles of Central Opioid Receptor Subtypes in Regulating Itch Sensation. In: Carstens E, Akiyama T, editors. *Itch: Mechanisms and treatment.* Frontiers in neuroscience. CRC Press/Taylor & Francis; 2014. Available at: http://www.ncbi.nlm.nih.gov/books/NBK200928/. Accessed March 11, 2023.
4. Evangelista MC, Steagall P, Garofalo NA, et al. Morphine-induced pruritus after epidural administration followed by treatment with naloxone in a cat. JFMS Open Rep 2016;2(1). https://doi.org/10.1177/2055116916634105. 2055116916634105.
5. Takei K, Denda S, Kumamoto J, et al. Low environmental humidity induces synthesis and release of cortisol in an epidermal organotypic culture system. Exp Dermatol 2013;22(10):662–4.
6. Denda S, Takei K, Kumamoto J, et al. Oxytocin is expressed in epidermal keratinocytes and released upon stimulation with adenosine 5'-[γ-thio]triphosphate in vitro. Exp Dermatol 2012;21(7):535–7.
7. Tey HL, Wallengren J, Yosipovitch G. Psychosomatic factors in pruritus. Clin Dermatol 2013;31(1):31–40.
8. Han L, Dong X. Itch Mechanisms and Circuits. Annu Rev Biophys 2014;43: 331–55.
9. Oaklander AL. Neuropathic Itch. In: Carstens E, Akiyama T, editors. *Itch: Mechanisms and treatment.* Frontiers in neuroscience. CRC Press/Taylor & Francis; 2014. Available at: http://www.ncbi.nlm.nih.gov/books/NBK200940/. Accessed March 11, 2023.
10. Overall KL. Manual of clincial behavioral medicine for dogs and cats. Elsevier; 2013.
11. Chang W, Kanda H, Ikeda R, et al. Merkel disc is a serotonergic synapse in the epidermis for transmitting tactile signals in mammals. Proc Natl Acad Sci USA 2016;113(37):E5491–500.
12. Tapp T, Virga V. Behavioural disorders. BSAVA Man Canine Feline Dermatol. Published online 2012. https://www.bsavalibrary.com/content/chapter/10.22233/9781905319886.chap31.
13. Landsberg G, Hunthausen W, Ackerman L. Stereotypic and compulsive disorders. In: Handbook of behavior problems of the dog and cat. Saunders Elsevier; 2013. p. 163–79.
14. Medleau L, Hnilica KA. Small animal dermatology: a color atlas and therapeutic guide. 2nd edition. Saunders Elsevier; 2006.
15. Muller WH, Griffin CE, Campbell KL. Muller and kirk's small animal dermatology. 7th edition. Elsevier Mosby; 2013. Available at: https://www.us.elsevierhealth.com/muller-and-kirks-small-animal-dermatology-9781416000280.html. Accessed May 4, 2023.
16. Demontigny-Bédard I, Beauchamp G, Bélanger MC, et al. Characterization of pica and chewing behaviors in privately owned cats: a case-control study. J Feline Med Surg 2016;18(8):652–7.
17. Houpt KA. Aggression and Social Structure. In: Domestic animal behavior for veterinarians and animal scientists. 5th ed. Wiley-Blackwell; 2012. p. 25–49.
18. Houpt KA. Biological Rhythms and Sleep and Stereotypic Behavior. In: Domestic animal behavior for veterinarians and animal scientists. 5th edition. Wiley-Blackwell; 2012. p. 51–81.

19. Crowell-Davis SL, Barry K, Wolfe R. Social behavior and aggressive problems of cats. Vet Clin North Am Small Anim Pract 1997;27(3):549–68.
20. van den Bos R. Post-conflict stress-response in confined group-living cats (Felis silvestris catus). Appl Anim Behav Sci 1998;59(4):323–30.
21. Stress, anxiety and neurodevelopmental disorders. In: Physiology of behavior. 11th edition. Pearson; 2012. p. 5XX–XXX.
22. Tynes VV. The physiologic effects of fear. Vet Med 2014;109(8):274–6, 279-280.
23. Beaver BV. Chapter 10 - feline grooming behavior. In: Feline behavior. 2nd Edition. W.B. Saunders; 2003. p. 311–21. https://doi.org/10.1016/B0-72-169498-5/50011-3.
24. Stella JL, Lord LK, Buffington CAT. Sickness behaviors in response to unusual external events in healthy cats and cats with feline interstitial cystitis. J Am Vet Med Assoc 2011;238(1):67–73.
25. Elzerman AL, DePorter TL, Beck A, et al. Conflict and affiliative behavior frequency between cats in multi-cat households: a survey-based study. J Feline Med Surg 2020;22(8):705–17.
26. Scarampella F, Zanna G, Peano A, et al. Dermoscopic features in 12 cats with dermatophytosis and in 12 cats with self-induced alopecia due to other causes: an observational descriptive study. Vet Dermatol 2015;26(4):282, e63.
27. Sawyer LS, Moon-Fanelli AA, Dodman NH. Psychogenic alopecia in cats: 11 cases (1993-1996). J Am Vet Med Assoc 1999;214(1):71–4.
28. Waisglass SE, Landsberg GM, Yager JA, et al. Underlying medical conditions in cats with presumptive psychogenic alopecia. J Am Vet Med Assoc 2006;228(11):1705–9.
29. Bradshaw JWS, Neville PF, Sawyer D. Factors affecting pica in the domestic cat. Appl Anim Behav Sci 1997;52(3):373–9.
30. Bécuwe-Bonnet V, Bélanger MC, Frank D, et al. Gastrointestinal disorders in dogs with excessive licking of surfaces. J Vet Behav Clin Appl Res 2012;7(4):194–204.
31. Frank D, Bélanger MC, Bécuwe-Bonnet V, et al. Prospective medical evaluation of 7 dogs presented with fly biting. Can Vet J 2012;53(12):1279–84.
32. Guilford WG, Markwell PJ, Jones BR, et al. Prevalence and causes of food sensitivity in cats with chronic pruritus, vomiting or diarrhea. J Nutr 1998;128(12):2790S–1S.
33. Horn JA, Mateus-Pinilla N, Warner RE, et al. Home range, habitat use, and activity patterns of free-roaming domestic cats. J Wildl Manag 2011;75(5):1177–85.
34. Secret life of the cat: What do our feline companions get up to? *BBC News.*//www.bbc.co.uk/news/science-environment-22567526. Published June 12, 2013. Accessed May 13, 2023.
35. Foster AP. A Study of the number and distribution of cutaneous mast cells in cats with disease not affecting the skin. Vet Dermatol 1994;5(1):17–20.
36. Kline KL. Seizure disorders and treatment options. Consult Feline Intern Med 2006;517–26. https://doi.org/10.1016/B0-72-160423-4/50058-5.
37. Felimazole (methimazole) Coated Tablets Package Insert. Published online 2015. Available at: https://www.dechra-us.com/Files/Files/ProductDownloads/US/felimazole-25mg-pack-insert.pdf. Accessed May 13, 2023.
38. Ioannou A, Mahony O. Clinician's brief: feline hyperthyroid treatment causing pruritus. Clinician's Brief 2022. Available at:.
39. Titeux E, Gilbert C, Briand A, et al. From feline idiopathic ulcerative dermatitis to feline behavioral ulcerative dermatitis: grooming repetitive behaviors indicators of poor welfare in cats. Front Vet Sci 2018;5:81.

40. Spaterna A, Mechelli L, Rueca F, et al. Feline Idiopathic Ulcerative Dermatosis: Three Cases. Vet Res Commun 2003;27(1):795–8.
41. Rusbridge C, Heath S, Gunn-Moore DA, et al. Feline orofacial pain syndrome (FOPS): A retrospective study of 113 cases. J Feline Med Surg 2010;12(6):498–508.
42. Fornal CA, Metzler CW, Marrosu F, et al. A subgroup of dorsal raphe serotonergic neurons in the cat is strongly activated during oral-buccal movements. Brain Res 1996;716(1):123–33.
43. Carmichael KP, Bienzle D, Mcdonnell JJ. Feline Leukemia Virus-associated Myelopathy in Cats. Vet Pathol 2002;39(5):536–45.
44. Ciribassi J. Understanding Behavior- Feline Hyperesthesia Syndrome. In: Compendium continuing education for veterinarians. VetFolio; 2009. Available at: https://www.vetfolio.com/learn/article/understanding-behavior-feline-hyperesthesia-syndrome. Accessed May 20, 2023.
45. Amengual Batle P, Rusbridge C, Nuttall T, et al. Feline hyperaesthesia syndrome with self-trauma to the tail: retrospective study of seven cases and proposal for an integrated multidisciplinary diagnostic approach. J Feline Med Surg 2019;21(2):178–85.
46. Strickler BL, Shull EA. An owner survey of toys, activities, and behavior problems in indoor cats. J Vet Behav 2014;9(5):207–14.
47. Herron ME, Buffington CAT. Environmental Enrichment for Indoor Cats: Implementing Enrichment. Compend Contin Educ Vet 2012;34(1):E3.
48. Delgado MM, Han BSG, Bain MJ. Domestic cats (Felis catus) prefer freely available food over food that requires effort. Anim Cognit 2022;25(1):95–102.
49. Dantas LM, Delgado MM, Johnson I, et al. Food puzzles for cats: Feeding for physical and emotional wellbeing. J Feline Med Surg 2016;18(9):723–32.
50. Kogan LR, Grigg EK. Laser Light Pointers for Use in Companion Cat Play: Association with Guardian-Reported Abnormal Repetitive Behaviors. Animals 2021;11(8):2178.
51. Bol S, Caspers J, Buckingham L, et al. Responsiveness of cats (Felidae) to silver vine (Actinidia polygama), Tatarian honeysuckle (Lonicera tatarica), valerian (Valeriana officinalis) and catnip (Nepeta cataria). BMC Vet Res 2017;13(1):70.
52. Ellis SLH, Wells DL. The influence of olfactory stimulation on the behaviour of cats housed in a rescue shelter. Appl Anim Behav Sci 2010;123(1):56–62.
53. De Jaeger X, Meppiel L, Endersby S, et al. An Initial Open-Label Study of a Novel Pheromone Complex for Use in Cats. Open J Vet Med 2021;11(03):105–16.
54. Gunn-Moore DA, Cameron ME. A pilot study using synthetic feline facial pheromone for the management of feline idiopathic cystitis. J Feline Med Surg 2004;6(3):133–8.
55. Griffith CA, Steigerwald ES, Buffington CAT. Effects of a synthetic facial pheromone on behavior of cats. J Am Vet Med Assoc 2000;217(8):1154–6.
56. Ramos D. Common feline problem behaviors: Aggression in multi-cat households. J Feline Med Surg 2019;21(3):221–33.
57. Mazur JE. Learning & behavior. 8th Edition. 7th edition. Routledge; 2013.
58. Hammerle M, Horst C, Levine E, et al. 2015 AAHA Canine and Feline Behavior Management Guidelines. J Am Anim Hosp Assoc 2015;51(4):205–21.
59. Overall KL, Rodan I V, Beaver BV, et al. Beaver B, et al. Feline behavior guidelines from the American Association of Feline Practitioners. J Am Vet Med Assoc 2005;227(1):70–84.
60. Amat M, Camps T, Manteca X. Stress in owned cats: behavioural changes and welfare implications. J Feline Med Surg 2016;18(8):577–86.

61. Landsberg GM, Hunthausen WL, Ackerman LJ. Behavior Modification Techniques. In: Behavior problems of the dog and cat. 3rd editin. Saunders Elsevier; 2013. p. 97–112.
62. Guedes AGP, Meadows JM, Pypendop BH, et al. Assessment of the effects of gabapentin on activity levels and owner-perceived mobility impairment and quality of life in osteoarthritic geriatric cats. J Am Vet Med Assoc 2018;253(5):579–85.
63. Pankratz KE, Ferris KK, Griffith EH, et al. Use of single-dose oral gabapentin to attenuate fear responses in cage-trap confined community cats: a double-blind, placebo-controlled field trial. J Feline Med Surg 2017. https://doi.org/10.1177/1098612X17719399. Published online July 1.
64. van Haaften KA, Forsythe LRE, Stelow EA, et al. Effects of a single preappointment dose of gabapentin on signs of stress in cats during transportation and veterinary examination. J Am Vet Med Assoc 2017;251(10):1175–81.
65. Kruszka M, Graff E, Medam T, et al. Clinical evaluation of the effects of a single oral dose of gabapentin on fear-based aggressive behaviors in cats during veterinary examinations. J Am Vet Med Assoc 2021;1:1–7.
66. American Veterinary Medical Association. Eliminate xylitol from canine prescriptions. American Veterinary Medical Association. Published May 30, 2017. https://www.avma.org/blog/eliminate-xylitol-canine-prescriptions. Accessed August 25, 2021.
67. Center SA, Elston TH, Rowland PH, et al. Fulminant hepatic failure associated with oral administration of diazepam in 11 cats. J Am Vet Med Assoc 1996; 209(3):618–25.
68. Hughs D, Moreau RE, Overall KL, et al. Acute Hepatic Necrosis And Liver Failure Associated With Benzodiazepine Therapy In Six Cats, 1986–1995. J Vet Emerg Crit Care 1996;6(1):13–20.
69. Orlando JM, Case BC, Thomson AE, et al. Use of oral trazodone for sedation in cats: a pilot study. J Feline Med Surg 2016;18(6):476–82.
70. Stevens BJ, Frantz EM, Orlando JM, et al. Efficacy of a single dose of trazodone hydrochloride given to cats prior to veterinary visits to reduce signs of transport- and examination-related anxiety. J Am Vet Med Assoc 2016;249(2):202–7.
71. Fries RC, Kadotani S, Vitt JP, et al. Effects of oral trazodone on echocardiographic and hemodynamic variables in healthy cats. J Feline Med Surg 2019;21(12): 1080–5.
72. KuKanich B, Papich MG. Opioid Analgesic Drugs. In: Veterinary pharmacology and therapeutics. Wiley-Blackwell; 2017. p. 165–449.
73. Beata C, Beaumont-Graff E, Diaz C, et al. Effects of alpha-casozepine (Zylkene) versus selegiline hydrochloride (Selgian, Anipryl) on anxiety disorders in dogs. J Vet Behav 2007;2(5):175–83.
74. Beata C, Beaumont-Graff E, Coll V, et al. Effect of alpha-casozepine (Zylkene) on anxiety in cats. J Vet Behav 2007;2(2):40–6.
75. Makawey A, Iben C, Palme R. Cats at the Vet: The Effect of Alpha-s1 Casozepin. Animals 2020;10(11):2047.
76. Pereira GDG, Fragoso, S., Pires, Eduarda. Effect of Dietary Intake of L-Tryptophan Supplementation on Multi-Housed Cats Presenting Stress Related Behaviours. In: Proceedings of the 53rd British Small Animal Veterinary Congress. ; 2010. https://www.vin.com/members/cms/project/defaultadv1.aspx?id=4419847&pid=11304&. Accessed March 12, 2022.
77. Landsberg G, Milgram B, Mougeot I, et al. Therapeutic effects of an alpha-casozepine and L-tryptophan supplemented diet on fear and anxiety in the cat. J Feline Med Surg 2017;19(6):594–602.

78. Miyaji K, Kato M, Ohtani N, et al. Experimental Verification of the Effects on Normal Domestic Cats by Feeding Prescription Diet for Decreasing Stress. J Appl Anim Welf Sci 2015;18(4):355–62.
79. Kruger JM, Lulich JP, MacLeay J, et al. Comparison of foods with differing nutritional profiles for long-term management of acute nonobstructive idiopathic cystitis in cats. J Am Vet Med Assoc 2015;247(5):508–17.
80. Meyer HP, Bečvářová I. Effects of a Urinary Food Supplemented with Milk Protein Hydrolysate and L-tryptophan on Feline Idiopathic Cystitis – Results of a Case Series in 10 Cats. Int J Appl Res Vet Med 2016;14(1):59–65.
81. Naarden B, Corbee RJ. The effect of a therapeutic urinary stress diet on the short-term recurrence of feline idiopathic cystitis. Vet Med Sci 2020;6(1). https://doi.org/10.1002/vms3.197.
82. DePorter T, Bledsoe D, Conley J, Warner CW, Linn E, Griffin D. Case report series of clinical effectiveness and safety of Solliquin® for behavioral support in dogs and cats. Presented at: August 5, 2016; San Antonio, TX. https://www.research-gate.net/profile/Theresa-Deporter/publication/306274188_Case_report_series_of_clinical_effectiveness_and_safety_of_SolliquinR_for_behavioral_support_in_-dogs_and_cats/links/57b5cbcf08aede8a665bb058/Case-report-series-of-clinical-effectiveness-and-safety-of-SolliquinR-for-behavioral-support-in-dogs-and-cats.pdf.
83. Lappin M. Colorado State University Study Evaluates Probiotic for Calming Effects in Cats. https://files.brief.vet/2021-06/Purina%20Nutrition%20Exchange,%20July_optimized.pdf.
84. DiCiccio VK, McClosky ME. Fluoxetine-induced urinary retention in a cat. JFMS Open Rep 2022;8(2). https://doi.org/10.1177/20551169221112065. 20551169221112064.
85. Ogata N, Dantas LM de S, Crowell-Davis SL. Selective Serotonin Reuptake Inhibitors. In: Veterinary psychopharmacology. Second edition. Wiley-Blackwell; 2019. p. 103–28.
86. Hart BL, Cliff KD, Tynes VV, et al. Control of urine marking by use of long-term treatment with fluoxetine or clomipramine in cats. J Am Vet Med Assoc 2005; 226(3):378–82.
87. Ciribassi J, Luescher A, Pasloske KS, et al. Comparative bioavailability of fluoxetine after transdermal and oral administration to healthy cats. Am J Vet Res 2003;64(8):994–8.
88. Lilly ML. Animal Behavior Case of the Month. J Am Vet Med Assoc 2020;257(5): 493–8.
89. Landsberg GM, Hunthausen WL, Ackerman LJ, et al. Pharmacologic intervention in behavior therapy. In: Behavior problems of the dog and cat. 3rd edition. Saunders Elsevier; 2013. p. 113–38.
90. Crowell-Davis SL. Tricyclic Antidepressants. In: Veterinary psychopharmacology. 2nd edition. Wiley-Blackwell; 2019. p. 231–56.
91. Griffin JS, Scott DW, Miller WH, et al. An open clinical trial on the efficacy of cetirizine hydrochloride in the management of allergic pruritus in cats. Can Vet J 2012; 53(1):47–50.
92. Denenberg S, editor. Small animal veterinary psychiatry. 1st edition. CAB International; 2020.
93. Landsberg GM, Wilson AL. Effects of clomipramine on cats presented for urine marking. J Am Anim Hosp Assoc 2005;41(1):3–11.
94. Seksel K, Lindeman M. Use of clomipramine in the treatment of anxiety-related and obsessive-compulsive disorders in cats. Aust Vet J 1998;76(5):317–21.

95. Martin KM. Effect of clomipramine on the electrocardiogram and serum thyroid concentrations of healthy cats. J Vet Behav 2010;5(3):123–9.

96. Pfeiffer E, Guy N, Cribb A. Clomipramine-induced urinary retention in a cat. Can Vet J 1999;40(4):265–7.

97. Chew DJ, Buffington CA, Kendall MS, et al. Amitriptyline treatment for severe recurrent idiopathic cystitis in cats. J Am Vet Med Assoc 1998;213(9):1282–6.

98. Dantas LM de S, Crowell-Davis, Sharron L. Miscellaneous Serotonergic Agents. In: Veterinary psychopharmacology. 2nd edition. Wiley-Blackwell; 2019. p. 129–46.

99. Daniels JT, Busby D, Chase-Topping M, et al. I wish he'd listen: Client-centered interviewing approaches are associated with higher compliance with behavioral modification advice in pet dog owners. J Vet Behav 2023;63:22–30.

Behavior and Cognition of the Senior Cat and Its Interaction with Physical Disease

Sagi Denenberg, DVM, MRCVS[a],*, Karen L. Machin, DVM, PhD[b],
Gary M. Landsberg, DVM[c]

KEYWORDS

• Cat • Cognitive dysfunction • Behavior • Treatment

KEY POINTS

- Elderly cats suffer from the same emotional disorders as younger cats but prevalence increases with age and deteriorating health.
- Cognitive dysfunction syndrome (CDS) in cats is similar to Alzheimer disease in humans. It is characterized by the accumulation of amyloid beta plaques and tau (hyperphosphorylated tau) protein, reduced cerebrovascular blood flow, mitochondrial dysfunction, and oxidative brain injury and inflammation leading to neuronal death.
- Age-related pathologic condition can complicate the diagnosis of CDS and contribute to the decline in elderly cats. Diagnosis is made through the exclusion of medical conditions.
- Behavior associated with CDS can be summarized with the acronym VISHDAAL: Vocalization, alterations in Interactions, Sleep–wake cycle changes, House-soiling, Disorientation, Activity level alterations, Anxiety, and Learning or memory deficits.
- Management and treatment of CDS can be accomplished through pharmacologic, diet and nutritional supplementation, and environmental enrichment aimed at slowing disease progression.

AGING IN CATS

Aging is a gradual deterioration in physiologic integrity resulting in functional and anatomic decline and increased susceptibility to pathologic conditions and eventual death.[1] Aging can vary, and the rate is influenced by breed, genetics, nutrition, environmental, and pathologic conditions.[2] Differentiating life stages into kitten (birth: 1 year), young adult (1–6 years), mature (7–10 years), senior (>10 years), and end of life (which can occur at any age), could help veterinarians target specific physical and behavioral

[a] North Toronto Veterinary Behaviour Specialty Clinic, 8705 Yonge Street, Richmond Hill, Ontario L4C 6Z1, Canada; [b] Department of Veterinary Biomedical Sciences, Western College of Veterinary Medicine, University of Saskatchewan, 52 Campus Drive, Saskatoon, Saskatchewan S7N 5B4, Canada; [c] CanCog Inc, Fergus, Ontario, Canada
* Corresponding author.
E-mail address: sagidvm@gmail.com

Vet Clin Small Anim 54 (2024) 153–168
https://doi.org/10.1016/j.cvsm.2023.09.001
0195-5616/24/© 2023 Elsevier Inc. All rights reserved.

changes and medical needs.[3] These changes can have both positive and negative influences on the owner. Age-related behavioral and medical problems can influence the human–animal bond, the owner's willingness to seek veterinary care and commitment to following veterinary recommendations.[4]

DETERIORATED HEALTH LEADING TO BEHAVIORAL CONCERNS

With the advancement of veterinary medicine and improved nutrition, domestic cats live longer lives.[5] However, with aging, there is an increased prevalence of medical health issues, including osteoarthritis, organ decline, and cognitive dysfunction, for which behavioral signs may be the first or sole sign. Moreover, any dermatologic, metabolic, infectious, or pain-related condition may play a significant role as a primary or contributing factor (**Table 1**).[2,6–8] The most reported signs are changes in activity, appetite, litter box use, sleep–wake cycles, temperament and social relationships, and cognitive ability, learning and memory.[7,8]

HEALTH AND WELFARE SCREENING

Because cats may hide physical ailments, and their life span is several times shorter than humans, semiannual veterinary visits are recommended in senior cats (more frequently if health issues are suspected or diagnosed). The senior veterinary visit should include a comprehensive physical examination, including neurologic, sensory, and orthopedic assessment and blood pressure measurement, and collection of the medical and behavioral history with cognitive dysfunction screening. Laboratory analysis should include hematology, biochemistry, and thyroid panels, urinalysis, and further diagnostics as determined by the clinical presentation.[5,9–11] One recent study found that of 206 cats aged older than 9 years, only 24% of cats had no physical health changes.[7] When screening 100 apparently healthy mature (6–10) and senior cats (>10), 72% had gingivitis, 25% or more with submandibular lymphadenopathy, elevated creatinine, proteinuria, or hyperglycemia; 14 were FIV positive; 11 presented heart murmurs; 8 increased blood pressure; and 3 elevated thyroxine.[12] Veterinarians must also consider that elderly cats may simultaneously have concurrent diseases leading to behavioral signs and that a greater number of behavior changes are observed in cats with more than one physical health condition.[13]

Timely recognition and reporting of behavioral changes are essential to early diagnosis and treatment. Owners may not notice or report mild or subtle signs or may assume that these changes are normal or untreatable. They may even become frustrated with their cat's behavior, leading to a delay in diagnosis, suboptimal care, and reduced quality of life.[3,14] Similarly, owners may not report problems because of concerns about euthanasia recommendations by their veterinarians.[9,15] Because owners are likely to report concerns when prompted; screening questionnaires can be invaluable diagnostic tools.[16]

Chronic pain is often underdiagnosed. Several studies have demonstrated that osteoarthritis has been estimated to affect between 40% and 92% of all cats, with prevalence increasing with age.[3,17,18] Osteoarthritis can lead to pain, reduced mobility, gait abnormalities, reduced self-maintenance behaviors, irritability and aggression, reduced appetite, altered social interactions, increased sleeping and vocalization, and house-soiling.[6,8,17] Cats with osteoarthritis may experience discomfort accessing the litter box, or experience litter box aversion and its location, or even aversion to the substrate if they are painful during elimination. Inappropriate elimination may continue after the medical problem and pain are resolved because of the expectation (anxiety) of discomfort associated with elimination and the litter box.[19]

Table 1
Behavioral changes in elderly cats

Mechanism of Disease	Etiology	Behavior
Neurologic	Frontal lobe trauma Intervertebral disc disease Hydrocephalus Infectious Toxicity	House-soiling Aggression/docility Erratic behaviors Altered social interactions Excessive vocalization Confusion, disorientation, and cognitive deficits Hyperesthesia Irritability Altered sleep–wake cycles Appetite

Neoplastic	Lymphoma
	Meningioma
	Pituitary: functional
	  endocrine tumors
		Sensory or motor deficits
		Aggression, agitation, lethargy,
		  anorexia, altered cognition,
		  consciousness/sleep–wake cycles,
		  altered social interactions, and
		  vocalization

Infectious	FIP/FIV/feline leukemia virus (FeLV)	Aggression Avoidance: altered social interactions Excessive vocalization

Dermatologic/
  Integument
	Sebum production
	  changes, scaly skin,
	  dandruff, and matting
	Hyperesthesia
	Allergies
		Reduced grooming
		Excessive grooming/self-trauma
		Hyperesthesia and aggression/
		  irritability
		House-soiling

Musculoskeletal/Pain	Osteoarthritis (pain)
	Feline knees and teeth
	  syndrome
		Changes in mobility
		Decreased activity
		House-soiling
		Sleep–wake cycle changes
		Vocalization
		Reduced appetite
		Altered social interactions
		Aggression/irritability
		Restlessness increased or
		  decreased grooming
		Altered response to stimuli
		Self-trauma

Dental	Periodontal disease Dental/oral pain	Changes in appetite and eating behavior Licking Decreased sociability Decreased grooming Increased sleeping
Gastrointestinal	Altered motility Constipation Parasites	House-soiling Aggression Licking, pica, and polyphagia Inappetence/anorexia Altered sleep Increased vocalization Restlessness

(continued on next page)

Table 1 *(continued)*		
Mechanism of Disease	**Etiology**	**Behavior**

Sensory	Reduced vision
	Hearing
	Smell or taste
		Aggression and irritability
		Agitation and avoidance
		Confusion/disorientation
		Reduced grooming
		Increased vocalization
		Sleep–wake cycle changes
		Altered social interactions
		Decreased responsiveness to
		  stimuli/verbal interactions
		House-soiling
		Changes in eating habits—decreased
		  appetite—more likely to eat certain
		  foods based on their aroma[29]

Urogenital	Chronic renal failure
	Urinary tract infection
	Lower urinary tract
	  disease/idiopathic
	  cystitis
		House-soiling
		Excessive vocalization
		Waking at night
		Aggression/irritability
		Increased sleeping
		Altered sociability

Systemic hypertension		Confusion Vocalization Agitation
Endocrinological	Hyperthyroidism Diabetes mellitus	Excessive vocalization House-soiling Aggression Irritability Sleep–wake cycle changes Altered activity Confusion/mental dullness

Chronic renal disease may be associated with increased sleeping, vocalization, and irritability, altered sociability, and urination outside the litter box.[6,8] A study reports that the prevalence of chronic renal disease in cats aged older than 15 years is nearly 81% and that there is an association between chronic renal disease and degenerative joint disease in cats, suggesting a possible underlying inflammatory or immune shared process.[20] Other maladies related to urinating outside the litter box include diabetes mellitus and insipidus; hyperthyroidism; neurologic conditions affecting control of urination; and urinary tract disorders including cystitis, urethritis, and urolithiasis. Possible rule-out diagnoses for defecation outside the litter box should also include pain, hyperthyroidism, colitis, causes of diarrhea or constipation, and gastrointestinal parasites.[21]

Elderly cats may be more prone to obesity due to reduced activity and poorer metabolism.[22] Obesity can influence the ability to perform normal behaviors such as grooming and running.[23] Obesity-related metabolic disturbances and chronic inflammation are associated with lameness, osteoarthritis and other musculoskeletal diseases, dermatologic conditions, cardiovascular and respiratory conditions, lower urinary tract conditions (especially idiopathic cystitis), neoplasia, and diabetes mellitus.[22] Maladies causing pain or discomfort may alter behavior. Conversely, senior and geriatric cats may lose weight and body condition because of underlying disease.

Increased blood urea nitrogen and creatinine may indicate protein breakdown rather than renal disease.[21]

Endocrine disruption is more common in aging animals and can significantly affect the central nervous system and behavior.[24,25] Elderly cats can experience diabetes mellitus, diabetes insipidus, insulinoma, hypoadrenocorticism, hyperadrenocorticism, hypothyroidism, and hyperthyroidism.[25] The most common endocrinopathy in the cat is diabetes mellitus,[25] which may be a function of aged cats being predisposed to the dysfunctional secretion of insulin and insulin resistance.[26] Hyperthyroidism is geriatric cats' most common endocrine disease and may be associated with aggression and increased vocalization.[6,8,24] The brain is a target organ for thyroid hormone[25,27] and plays a critical role in motor speed, mood, and cognition.[28]

Impaired hearing and vision may contribute to increased anxiety, agitation and confusion, increased or disrupted sleep, increased vocalization, altered social interactions, house-soiling, altered responses to stimuli, and withdrawn as navigating their familiar environment and routine becomes more difficult.[6,8] Changes in taste and smell may also occur in aging pets, potentially leading to altered food preferences and a decline in appetite. Reduction or loss of olfaction in cats is especially important because willingness and interest to eat are closely dependent on odor, whereas warming canned food to approximate body temperature may promote food consumption by increasing the attractiveness of aroma and taste.[15,29,30]

BEHAVIOR PROBLEMS IN ELDERLY CATS

Elderly cats suffer from the same emotional disorders as younger cats, and although the prevalence of behavioral problems varies among reports, they increase with age.[13,26,31] Aggression, agitation, or avoidance are nonspecific signs of disease.[32] Elderly cats may demonstrate personality changes, such as increased attention-seeking, restlessness, or sleep–wake cycle changes.[21] Onset of sensory changes (eg, decreased hearing or vision), hypothalamic-pituitary-adrenal-axis disorders, encephalopathy (hepatic or uremic), central nervous system disorders,[21,33] or pain[34] can occur later in life and must be investigated before reaching a diagnosis of cognitive dysfunction syndrome (CDS).

COGNITIVE DECLINE AND DYSFUNCTION

As cats age, owners may expect age-related changes. Aging is not a pathologic condition but will lead to deterioration in function and morphology of the body systems.[35] For example, with age, bone may shrink and lose density and muscles may lose strength and flexibility, so cats cannot jump as high as before. The iris pigmentation may change, and the pupil may become more dense (due to the development of fibrotic tissues) but these changes should not affect the cat's vision. Other changes may include reduced efficiency in glomerular filtration, cardiac output, and energy conversion from food intake but these changes should not lead to a disease or pathologic condition.

By age 10 years, elderly cats may start experiencing sensory (eg, vision and heading), cognitive and motor decline, and brain atrophy, which contribute to behavioral changes.[31,36,37] In a study screening 154 cats aged 11 to 21 years for signs of cognitive dysfunction, overall prevalence was 36%, ranging from 28% in cats 11 to 14 years to 50% in cats 15 years, with 19 cats diagnosed as having concurrent health problems.[38] Although previously described by the acronym DISHAA (Disorientation, changes in Interactions, Sleep-wake cycle changes, House-soiling, Activity level alteration, and Anxiety),[3,8,14,39,a] these behaviors might be better summarized by the acronym VISHDAAL, which lists the most common signs in order of prevalence:

Vocalization; alterations in Interactions, Sleep–wake cycle changes, House-soiling, Disorientation, Activity level alterations, Anxiety, and Learning and memory deficits.[9,15,40] One study of 37 cats with CDS documented increased vocalization during the day (64%) and during the night (67%). Cats with increased vocalization were reported to be more affectionate with owners and have increased signs of disorientation, altered sleep–wake cycles, decreased grooming, and house-soiling.[9,15] Owners attributed the main cause of the vocalization to attention seeking (40.5%), disorientation (40.5%), followed by resource (food) seeking (16.2%), and pain (2.7%).[15] Increased vocalization was most commonly associated with kidney disease, blindness, deafness, arthritis, and hyperthyroidism.[8]

Anatomic and physiologic changes affecting information processing, including sensory, learning, and memory, are related to changes in the caudate nucleus. Damage in this area can produce hyperactivity, fine motor coordination deficits, reactivity to auditory stimuli[31] and a decreased ability to habituate.[1] However, elderly cats are better able to recall some tasks reinforced or learned previously,[31,41] suggesting that some brain areas may be more resistant to age-related alterations.[42] Owners' schedule and environmental changes can have a greater influence as the cat ages,[14] which may be associated with caudate area damage.[43]

CDS in cats is an age-related decline in learning and memory, similar to Alzheimer disease in humans.[44] Alzheimer disease is characterized by the pathologic accumulation of protein aggregates, including amyloid beta (Aβ) peptide senile plaques and neurofibrillary tangles composed of hyperphosphorylated tau (pTau) protein.[45] These accumulations contribute to progressive neuronal dysfunction and loss and cognitive dysfunction.[46] Cats with Aβ deposition are more likely to display excessive vocalization, confusion, and wandering.[45] The presence pTau formation in cat brains is similar to humans with Alzheimer disease.[47] In cats older than 14 years, neuronal loss in the hippocampus was most severe when both Aβ plaques and pTau deposits were present, possibly contributing to CDS.[44]

The cause of CDS in cats is unknown; however, oxidative damage, vascular pathologic condition, and compromised cerebrovascular blood flow are thought to be involved.[9] With a high lipid content, limited repair mechanisms, and high demand for oxygen, the brain is more susceptible than other organs to damage.[8] Oxidative damage occurs in cats, dogs, and other species, including humans. Aged mitochondria experience oxidative damage, have less-efficient energy production, and release more free radicals such as hydrogen peroxide, superoxide, and nitric oxide.[48] Although free radicals are usually removed by antioxidant processes and free radical scavengers, the balance between production and removal can be influenced by aging, disease, and stress. Excess free radicals lead to cellular damage, dysfunction, and mutation in the brain.[2,9,14,49]

As cats age, they may experience brain hypoxia because of decreased cardiac output, systemic hypertension, anemia, altered blood viscosity, or platelet hypercoagulopathy.[9] Cerebral blood flow may also be altered by vascular and perivascular changes producing microhemorrhages or infarcts of the periventricular vessels and nonlipid atherosclerosis, Aβ deposition, vessel wall fibrosis, and endothelial proliferation and mineralization.[9,10]

In humans, cholinergic dysfunction has been linked with cognitive decline.[50–52] High densities of cholinergic synapses are found in the thalamus, striatum, limbic system, and neocortex, suggesting that cholinergic transmission is important in attention, learning, and higher order cognitive processing.[1] Myelin disruption, axonal degeneration, and decreased dendritic size and length of cholinergic neurons in the locus coeruleus important in the sleep–wake cycle are greater in cats aged 15 to 18 years compared with young cats aged 2 to 3 years, possibly causing sleep–wake cycle changes.[2] Similar to humans, elderly cats demonstrate altered sleeping patterns as a function of age with a decline in rapid eye movement (REM) sleep and an increase in brief awakenings and non-REM sleep.[53]

Laboratory studies assessing executive function, attention, and memory impairment have documented cognitive function decline in cats using a neuropsychological test apparatus.[54–57] These tests also provide a mechanism for assessing the effects of therapeutic agents on several different cognitive domains. In fact, although owners most commonly begin to recognize and report signs associated with CDS at 9 to 11 years and older[5,9,38] using a standardized test apparatus, an age-related decline in cognitive function has been demonstrated in cats as early as 6 to 7 years of age.[54,55] This age correlates with functional changes beginning at 6 to 7 years of age in the neurons of the caudate nucleus in cats.[9,31,42]

Typically, a diagnosis of CDS is made by ruling out potential causes of behavior changes (**Box 1**). However, elderly cats may have concomitant maladies that may exacerbate CDS. Therefore, it is important to identify all contributing conditions to intervene and improve welfare. Veterinarians must collect a minimum database, including the onset and progression of clinical signs, changes in mobility, possible toxin exposure, and routine and environmental changes. Any pathologic condition diagnosed should be treated before or concurrently with addressing CDS. Furthermore, monitoring the therapeutic response is not only essential to the pet's health and well-being but may be a component of the diagnostic process.

Owners should monitor behavior changes over time by keeping a diary or using a VISHDAAL assessment (**Table 2**). Progression of clinical signs can be tracked and aid in diagnosis by repeating the assessment 2 to 3 months apart. Owners should be instructed not to look at their first assessment until after they have completed their second assessment to avoid any bias.

Cognitive dysfunction and associated behavior changes influence the cat's quality of life and the cat-owner bond. Owners may become distressed by the cat's disorientation, confusion, and night activity (increased vocalization, activity, or attention seeking), particularly when it influences their own sleep.[9] Early diagnosis and treatment are important for both the cat and the owner.

Selegiline and propentofylline are licensed in some countries for CDS in dogs and can be used in cats.[9–11,32,39,58–61] Although the majority of studies demonstrate the

---

Box 1
Differential diagnoses for signs similar to cognitive dysfunction

Pain (any source including osteoarthritis, musculoskeletal problems, gastrointestinal, pancreatic, dental, and so forth)

Chronic disease (eg, liver or kidney failure)

Endocrine disorders (eg, hyperthyroidism, diabetes mellitus, and diabetes insipidus)

Hypertension

Infectious diseases (eg, toxoplasmosis, FIV, FeLV)

Urinary tract inflammation (eg, feline idiopathic cystitis) or infection

Neoplasia (eg, frontal lobe tumor, meningioma, and so forth)

Other inflammatory diseases

Other behavioral problems (eg, separation distress)

Table 2 Behavior signs of cognitive dysfunction syndrome in cats		
Behavior/Changes	Observations	Score (0–3)[a]
Disorientation	Difficulty navigating obstacles or getting stuck in one place Stares blankly at walls, floors, or into space Less responsive to stimuli Getting lost in the home	
Social interactions	Increased sociability/attention-seeking Less sociable, more fearful, avoidant, or aggressive	
Sleep–wake cycle	Increased pacing, restlessness, and waking at night Sleeps more during the day Increased vocalization (night)	
House-soiling	Soiling outside litterbox with urine, feces, or both	
Activity levels	Decrease in exploration or play. Decreased interest, willingness to go outside Decreased grooming Increased activity, including aimless pacing or wandering Repetitive behaviors such as pacing, licking, excessive grooming	
Anxiety	Agitation Increased restlessness when separated from owners More fearful of visual signs and auditory (sounds) stimuli Increased vocalization (day)	
Learning and memory	Less able to learn new tasks or to respond to previously learned commands or name Difficulty getting the cat's attention and increased distraction Decreased focus	

This assessment tool can be used for screening for signs and documenting changes occurring over time. The checklist incorporates both the DISHAA[b] questionnaire and VISHDAAL for cats.[10] It has not been validated.[10] and should not be relied on for diagnosis.

[a] Score 0 = none, 1 = mild, 2 = moderate, 3 = severe.

[b] Landsberg G. Cognitive Dysfunction Evaluation Tool (DISHAA). Available at https://www.purinainstitute.com/sites/default/files/2021-04/DISHAA-Assessment-Tool.pdf Accessed August 22, 2023.

efficacy of selegiline in dogs, it has been used anecdotally in cats (2.5–5 mg/cat q24 h) to improve disorientation and interactions with family members and reduce vocalization and restless or repetitive activities.[61] The monoamines neurotransmitters are degraded in the presynaptic neuron by the enzyme monoamines oxidase A (primarily active in the intestinal tract) and B (mostly active in the brain) in a process called deamination. Monoamine Oxidase Inhibitors (MAOIs) are medications that inhibit this enzyme. Selegiline is a MAOI with a greater affinity for MAO-B than MAO-A. It is commonly used for treating Alzheimer[62] and Parkinson[63] diseases in humans. Selegiline enhances antioxidant enzymes, reduces age-related neuronal loss, and reverses memory and learning deficits in rats.[64,65] The neuroprotective and antiaging effects are related to its ability to promote lipid peroxidases that remove oxygen-free radical species in the brain, counteract free radicals and stabilize membranes.[66] Selegiline also enhances the secretion of trophic factors from astrocytes, promoting neurons' growth, and survival.[67]

Selegiline inhibits presynaptic reuptake of dopamine, noradrenaline, and serotonin; increases the turnover of dopamine; reduces oxidative stress caused by dopamine degradation; and potentiates neural responses to dopamine.[59] Selegiline has 3 primary metabolites that may also function as sympathomimetics and contribute to its effects.[68] Owing to its stimulatory effect, selegiline should be given in the morning.[69] Selegiline should not be combined with tricyclic antidepressants (eg, clomipramine, amitriptyline, and TCAs), selelctive serotonin reuptake inhibitors (eg, fluoxetine, paroxetine, and sertraline), or serotonin and norepinephrine reuptake inhibitors (venlafaxine) because there is the risk of serotonin syndrome. Other possible drug interactions can occur with any MAOIs, alpha2-agonists, meperidine, metronidazole, prednisone, and trimethoprim sulfa.[59] Cats treated with up to 10 times the therapeutic dose of selegiline have not demonstrated toxicity.[69]

Propentofylline (5–15 mg/cat q24 h) has been used anecdotally in cats with some positive results.[9,32] It is a neuroprotectant that increases extracellular adenosine concentration in ischemic brains, inhibits platelet and neutrophil activation, promotes vasodilation, stimulates nerve growth factor production, and inhibits free radical production. Propentofylline may increase blood supply to the brain without increasing oxygen demand and improve glucose metabolism in the brain.[70]

Medications such as fluoxetine and sertraline that lack anticholinergic effects (eg, amitriptyline, clomipramine, and paroxetine), as well as benzodiazepines, clonidine, buspirone, trazodone, gabapentin, and pregabalin, have been used anecdotally for feline CDS.[9,10,32,39] One study in mice demonstrated that fluoxetine improved spatial learning and memory, reduced soluble Aβ and amyloid plaques in the hippocampus, and prevented dendritic spine synapse decline.[71] Care should be taken with the use of benzodiazepines because they may contribute to cognitive decline, although the correlation between benzodiazepine therapy and cognitive decline in elderly human patients is not conclusive. Stronger evidence of cognitive decline is associated with longer acting benzodiazepines and with longer durations of use.[72] Benzodiazepines are more frequently used to attenuate anxiety and night waking. Preference may be given to lorazepam and oxazepam, which have no intermediate metabolites.[32]

As alpha-adrenergic systems contribute to cognitive function, clonidine (no established dose but used anecdotally at 0.025–0.1 mg/cat q12 h) may be a useful adjunct medication. Aged rhesus monkeys with memory impairments treated with clonidine have improved spatial working memory.[73] Gabapentin and pregabalin may be useful in decreasing anxiety, providing analgesia for pain, and improving sleep–wake cycles. They should be used cautiously because some studies demonstrate decreases in cognitive function after administration.[74,75] Neurotrophins and their receptors modulate axonal and dendritic networks and synaptic plasticity.[76] Recently, a study investigated LM11A-31, a nonpeptide ligand that mimics the actions of a neurotrophin and targets the p75 neurotrophin receptor in feline immunodeficiency virus (FIV) infected cats. Infected cats demonstrated a neural decline in T-maze testing and novel object recognition within 12 to 18 months postinfection. In contrast, FIV-infected cats that were treated with LM11A-31 demonstrated cognitive improvements suggesting that LM11A-31 was able to alleviate cognitive decline. In addition, the behavior in some cats normalized to the level of uninfected cats, suggesting a potential reversal of deficits.[77] Although LM11A-31 has not been used specifically for CDS, given the minimal side effects,[77] further investigations may be warranted.

Environmental enrichment has been demonstrated to be neuroprotective in Alzheimer and other degenerative brain diseases in rodent models.[78] As in human and animal models, poor environmental stimulation is suspected to increase the risk of developing CDS later in life.[9] Access to novel and complex environments, including access to toys, social interactions with owners, food-hunting tasks, and a diet rich in antioxidants, is thought to have a synergetic action in improving cognitive function.[10] However, sudden environmental, diet, and routine changes can affect an aging cat experiencing CDS and potentially exacerbate behavioral problems leading to increased hiding, house-soiling, and anorexia.[9,79] Changes should be as gradual as possible and assessed.

Lowering resting places and providing low-sided litter boxes can help cats with musculoskeletal disorders and pain.[9] An automatic feeder, scatter feeding, or food toys to provide small meals during the night may reduce nighttime vocalization. It may be beneficial to set up a separate room to provide food, a litter box, and resting areas in a smaller space for cats that are easily disoriented.[5,9,40] Adding a nighttime routine involving a meal (the use of warmed canned food may stimulate appetite),[30] warm bedding, and affection from the owner may improve sleep. Some authors advocate responding to attention-seeking and vocalization to help reassure the cat. Punishment such as yelling and isolation are more likely to worsen vocalization and stress experienced by the cat.[9] Although no specific studies evaluate the use of feline facial pheromones synthetic analog (eg, Feliway) for CDS, studies demonstrated beneficial effects and decreased anxiety in unfamiliar surroundings, including hospitalization,[80] and transport.[81] Therefore, providing a pheromone diffuser in the environment may be beneficial.

Diet is a potential risk factor for cognitive decline in humans, and animal models indicate that gut microbiota composition and function can be involved in the pathophysiology and progression of Alzheimer disease.[82] Diets enriched with antioxidants and other compounds, including vitamin E, β-carotene, and essential fatty acids, are believed to reduce oxidative damage and Aβ production, and improve cognition. Other compounds that improve cell membrane health and mitochondrial function, such as alpha-lipoic acid, L-carnitine, and omega-3 fatty acids, have a positive effect.[83] There are no commercial feline diets specifically formulated for CDS. One study evaluated a diet supplemented with antioxidants, arginine, B vitamins, and fish oil and found that cats aged 5.5 to 8.7 years had a better cognitive ability.[55] An owners' survey by Hill's Pet Nutrition found that 70% of cats fed a diet containing antioxidants, essential fatty acids, chondroprotectants, L-carnitine, and lysine reduced CDS signs.[9]

There is a plethora of literature on the positive effects of long-chain n-3 polyunsaturated fatty acids (ie, PUFAs; omega 3) on improving or preventing cognitive decline and dementia in people.[84–86] Diets containing fish oil or supplemented with eicosapentaenoic acid (EPA) and docosahexaenoic acid (DHA) demonstrate improved cognition in healthy adults with mild cognitive decline.[87,88] Both EPA and DHA can generate neuroprotective metabolites and prenatal and postnatal brain development,[89] and EPA is thought to influence behavior and mood.[90] In dogs, high DHA from fish oil vitamin E, taurine, choline and L-carnitine was associated with improved neurocognitive development, including memory, psychomotor, immunologic, and retinal function and other measures of development.[91] It is thought that DHA suppresses insulin/neurotropic factors, neuroinflammation, and oxidative damage that contribute to synaptic loss and neuronal dysfunction in dementia. In addition, DHA increases neuroprotective neurotropic factor and reduces omega-6 fatty acid-related inflammatory products that are implicated in promoting Alzheimer disease.[85]

Diets formulated to reduce anxiety may provide some benefit to cats experienced CDS. Feline Mature Adult 7+ from Hills Pet Nutrition and Nestle Purina Pro Plan Age 7+ from Nestle Purina Petcare contain antioxidants, including omega-3 fatty acids, improved longevity in senior cats compared with those fed control diets. However, neither CDS nor behavior was evaluated.[92,93] Although diets with high medium chain triglycerides may benefit cats, they may be unpalatable.[9]

There has been considerable interest in dietary supplementation in the treatment of CDS. Many supplements have been tested in dogs with CDS and demonstrate some positive effects, although there is less evidence of efficacy in cats despite recommendations for use in cats.[9,88] S-adenosylmethionine (SAMe) stabilizes cell membranes and enhances antioxidant (glutathione) production. A study in aged cats given SAMe demonstrated improvement in cats with mild impairment but not the most impaired cats.[56] Nutraceutical supplementation including Senilife (CEVA Animal Health, Lenexa, KS, USA)[94] containing phosphatidylserine, Ginkgo biloba, vitamin E, and pyridoxine and Aktivait (VetPlus, Lytham, UK)[95] containing omega-3 fish oils, vitamin C and E, L-carnitine, and alpha-lipoic acid have demonstrated some positive effects in dogs but not in cats. The dog version of Aktivait contains alpha-lipoic acid but not in the cat product because alpha-lipoic acid is toxic to cats.[9]

CLINICS CARE POINTS

- Using questionnaires to screen senior cats for cognitive decline during routine veterinary visits can increase detection.
- Addressing signs of cognitive decline and other behavioral problems should be done as soon as the owner voices a concern.
- Appropriate screen for concurrent physiological and pain-related problems is imperative for successful managemet.

DISCLOSURE

None of the authors has any conflict of interest or received any funding for the purpose of this article.

REFERENCES

1. López-Otín C, Blasco MA, Partridge L, et al. The hallmarks of aging. Cell 2013; 153:1194–217.
2. Bellows J, Center S, Daristotle L, et al. Aging in cats: Common physical and functional changes. J Feline Med Surg 2016;18:533–50.
3. Quimby J, Gowland S, Carney HC, et al. 2021 AAFP-AAHA Feline Life Stages Guide. J Feline Med Surg 2021;23:211–33.
4. Lue TW, Pantenburg DP, Crawford PM. Impact of the owner-pet and client-veterinarian bond on the care that pets receive. J Am Vet Med Assoc 2008; 232:531–40.
5. Gunn-Moore DA. Cognitive Dysfunction in Cats: Clinical Assessment and Management. Top Companion Anim Med 2011;26:17–24.
6. Sordo L, Breheny C, Halls V, et al. Prevalence of disease and age-related behavioural changes in cats: Past and present. Vet Sci 2020;7:85.
7. Hajzler I, Nenadović K, Vučinić M. Health changes of old cats. J Vet Behav 2023; 63:16–21.
8. Bellows J, Center S, Daristotle L, et al. Evaluating aging in cats: How to determine what is healthy and what is disease. J Feline Med Surg 2016;18(7):551–70.

9. Sordo L, Gunn-Moore DA. Cognitive Dysfunction in Cats: Update on Neuropathological and Behavioural Changes Plus Clinical Management. Vet Rec 2021;188: 30–41.
10. Gunn-Moore D, Moffat K, Christie LA, et al. Cognitive dysfunction and the neurobiology of ageing in cats. J Sm An Pract 2007;48:546–53.
11. Ray M, Carney HC, Boynton B, et al. 2021 AAFP Feline Senior Care Guidelines. J Feline Med Surg 2021;23:613–38.
12. Paepe D, Verjans G, Duchateau L, et al. Routine Health Screening: Findings in apparently healthy middle-aged and old cats. J Feline Med Surg 2013;15:8–19.
13. Landsberg GM, Malamed R. Clinical picture of canine and feline cognitive impairment. In: Landsberg G, Madari A, Zilka N, editors. Canine and feline dementia: Molecular Basis, diagnostics and therapy. Cham (Switzerland): Springer; 2017. p. 1–11.
14. Landsberg GM, Denenberg S, Araujo JA. Cognitive dysfunction in cats. A syndrome we used to dismiss as "old age.". J Feline Med Surg 2010;12:837–48.
15. Cerna P, Gardiner H, Sordo L, et al. Potential causes of increased vocalisation in elderly cats with cognitive dysfunction syndrome as assessed by their owners. Animals 2020;10:1–15.
16. Duxbury MM, Sobcynski HJ, Flynn K, et al. Identifying behavior problems in veterinary primary care: the effectiveness of a screening questionnaire. Proc Am College Vet Behav 2023;23.
17. Slingerland LI, Hazewinkel HAW, Meij BP, et al. Cross-sectional study of the prevalence and clinical features of osteoarthritis in 100 cats. Vet J 2011;187:304–9.
18. Lascelles BDX, Henry JB, Brown J, et al. Cross-Sectional Study of the Prevalence of Radiographic Degenerative Joint Disease in Domesticated Cats. Vet Surg 2010;39:535–44.
19. Advances in Understanding and Treatment of Feline Inappropriate Elimination. Top Companion Anim Med 2010;25:195–202.
20. Marino CL, Lascelles BDX, Vaden SL, et al. Prevalence and classification of chronic kidney disease in cats randomly selected from four age groups and in cats recruited for degenerative joint disease studies. J Feline Med Surg 2014; 16:465–72.
21. Stelow E. Behavior as an Illness Indicator. Vet Clin NA: Sm An Pract. 2020;50: 695–706.
22. Teng KT, McGreevy PD, Toribio JALML, et al. Associations of body condition score with health conditions related to overweight and obesity in cats. J Sm An Pract 2018;59(10):603–15.
23. Laflamme DP. Nutrition for aging cats and dogs and the importance of body condition. Vet Clin North Am Small Anim Pract 2005;35(3):713–42.
24. Roberts C, Gruffydd-Jones T, Williams JL, et al. Influence of living in a multicat household on health and behaviour in a cohort of cats from the United Kingdom. Vet Rec 2020;187:27.
25. Scott-Moncrieff JC. Thyroid Disorders in the Geriatric Veterinary Patient. Vet Clin North Am Small Anim Pract 2012;42(4):707–25.
26. Camps T, Amat M, Manteca X. A review of medical conditions and behavioral problems in dogs and cats. Animals 2019;9:1133.
27. Samuels MH. Psychiatric and cognitive manifestations of hypothyroidism. Curr Opin Endocrinol Diabetes Obes 2014;21:377–83.
28. He XS, Ma N, Pan ZL, et al. Functional magnetic resource imaging assessment of altered brain function in hypothyroidism during working memory processing. Eur J Endocrinol 2011;164:951–9.

29. Pires KA, Miltenburg TZ, Miranda PD, et al. Factors affecting the results of food preference tests in cats. Res Vet Sci 2020;130:247–54.
30. Eyre R, Trehiou M, Marshall E, et al. Aging cats prefer warm food. J Vet Behav 2022;47:86–92.
31. Levine MS. Neurophysiological and morphological alterations in caudate neurons in aged cats. Ann N Y Acad Sci 1988;515:314–28.
32. Denenberg S, Landsberg G. Current pharmacological and non-pharmacological approaches for therapy of feline and canine dementia. In: Landsberg G, Madari A, Zilka N, editors. Canine and feline dementia: Molecular Basis, diagnostics and therapy. Cham (Switzerland): Springer; 2017. p. 129–43.
33. Landsberg GM, Denenberg S. Behaviour Problems in the Senior Pet. In: Horwitz DF, Mills DS, editors. BSAVA Manual of canine and feline Behavioural medicine. 2nd edition. Waterwells: BSAVA; 2012. p. 127–35.
34. Bennett D, Morton C. A study of owner observed behavioural and lifestyle changes in cats with musculoskeletal disease before and after analgesic therapy. J Feline Med Surg 2009;11:997–1004.
35. Goldston RT. Introduction and overview of geriatrics. In: Goldston RT, Hoskins JD, editors. Geriatrics and gerontology of the dog and cat. Philadelphia: WB Saunders; 1995. p. 1–8.
36. Tipold A, Mogicato G, Nationale Vétérinaire de Toulouse E, et al. Age-related brain atrophy in cats without apparent neurological and behavioral signs using voxel-based morphometry. Front Vet Sci 2022;9:1071002.
37. Harrison J, Buchwald J. Auditory brainstem responses in the aged cat. Neurobiol Aging 1982;3:163–71.
38. Moffat K, Landsberg G. An investigation of the prevalence of clinical signs of cognitive dysfunction syndrome (CDS) in cats. J Am Anim Hosp Assoc 2003; 39:512.
39. Karagiannis C, Mills D. Feline cognitive dysfunction syndrome. Vet Focus 2014; 24:42–7.
40. MacQuiddy B, Moreno J, Frank J, et al. Survey of risk factors and frequency of clinical signs observed with feline cognitive dysfunction syndrome. J Feline Med Surg 2022;24:e131–7.
41. McCune S, Stevenson J, Fretwell L, et al. Ageing does not significantly affect performance in a spatial learning task in the domestic cat (Felis silvestris catus). Appl Anim Behav Sci 2008;112:345–56.
42. Levine MS, Lloyd RL, Fisher RS, et al. Sensory, motor and cognitive alterations in aged cats. Neurobiol Aging 1987;8:253–63.
43. Villablanca JR, Olmstead CE, Levine MS, et al. Effects of caudate nuclei or frontal cortical ablations in kittens: Neurology and gross behavior. Exp Neurol 1978;61: 615–34.
44. Chambers JK, Tokuda T, Uchida K, et al. The domestic cat as a natural animal model of Alzheimer's disease. Acta Neuropathol Commun 2015;3:78.
45. Head E, Moffat K, Das P, et al. β-Amyloid deposition and tau phosphorylation in clinically characterized aged cats. Neurobiol Aging 2005;26:749–63.
46. Klug J, Snyder JM, Darvas M, et al. Aging pet cats develop neuropathology similar to human Alzheimer's disease. Aging Pathobiol Ther 2020;2:120–5.
47. Poncelet L, Ando K, Vergara C, et al. A 4R tauopathy develops without amyloid deposits in aged cat brains. Neurobiol Aging 2019;81:200–12.
48. Shigenaga MK, Hagen TM, Ames BN. Oxidative damage and mitochondrial decay in aging. Proc Natl Acad Sci U S A 1994;91:10771–8.

49. Kandlur A, Satyamoorthy K, Gangadharan G. Oxidative Stress in Cognitive and Epigenetic Aging: A Retrospective Glance. Front Mol Neurosci 2020;13:41.

50. Araujo JA, Studzinski CM, Milgram NW. Further evidence for the cholinergic hypothesis of aging and dementia from the canine model of aging. Prog Neuro-Psychopharmacol Biol Psychiatry 2005;29:411–22.

51. Hampel H, Mesulam MM, Cuello AC, et al. The cholinergic system in the pathophysiology and treatment of Alzheimer's disease. Brain 2018;141:1917–33.

52. Zhang JH, Sampogna S, Morales FR, et al. Age-related changes in cholinergic neurons in the laterodorsal and the pedunculo-pontine tegmental nuclei of cats: A combined light and electron microscopic study. Brain Res 2005;1052: 47–55.

53. Bowersox SS, Baker TL, Dement WC. Sleep-wakefulness patterns in the aged cat. Electroencephalogr Clin Neurophysiol 1984;58:240–52.

54. Milgram NW, Landsberg GM, De Rivera C, et al. Age and cognitive dysfunction in the domestic cat. Proceedings of the Am College Vet Behav/Assoc Vet Soc An Behav Symp 2011;28–9.

55. Pan Y, Araujo JA, Burrows J, et al. Cognitive enhancement in middle-aged and old cats with dietary supplementation with a nutrient blend containing fish oil, B vitamins, antioxidants and arginine. Br J Nutr 2013;110:40–9.

56. Araujo JA, Faubert ML, Brooks ML, et al. NOVIFIT® (NoviSAMe®) tablets improve executive function in aged dogs and cats: Implications for treatment of cognitive dysfunction syndrome. Int J Appl Res Vet Med 2010;10:90–8.

57. Mongillo P, Landsberg GM, Araujo JA, et al. Validation of a cognitive test battery for cats. Vet Behav 2010;5:32.

58. Hammerle M, Horst C, Levine E, et al. 2015 AAHA Canine and Feline Behavior Management Guidelines. J Am Anim Hosp Assoc 2015;51(4):205–21.

59. de Souza Dantas LM, Crowell-Davis SL. Monoamine oxidase inhibitors. In: Crowell-Davis SL, Murray TF, de Souza Dantas LM, editors. Veterinary Psychopharmacology: an evidence-Based Approach. 2nd edition. Incorporated: John Wiley & Sons; 2019. p. 185–99.

60. Pittari J, Rodan I, Beekman G, et al. American Association of Feline Practitioners. Senior Care Guidelines. J Feline Med Surg 2009;11:763–78.

61. Landsberg G. Therapeutic options for cognitive decline in senior pets. J Am Anim Hosp Assoc 2006;42:407–13.

62. Alafuzoff I, Helisalmi S, Heinonen EH, et al. Selegiline treatment and the extent of degenerative changes in brain tissue of patients with Alzheimer's disease. Eur J Clin Pharmacol 2000;55:815–9.

63. Rinne UK. Deprenyl (selegiline) in the treatment of Parkinson's disease. Acta Neurol Scand 1983;68:103–6.

64. Kiray M, Bagriyanik HA, Pekcetin C, et al. Deprenyl and the relationship between its effects on spatial memory, oxidant stress and hippocampal neurons in aged male rats. Physiol Res 2006;55:205–12.

65. Amenta F, Bongrani S, Cadel S, et al. Influence of treatment with l-deprenyl on the structure of the cerebellar cortex of aged rats. Mech Ageing Dev 1994;75:157–67.

66. Subramanian MV, James TJ. Age-related protective effect of deprenyl on changes in the levels of diagnostic marker enzymes and antioxidant defense enzymes activities in cerebellar tissue in Wistar rats. Cell Stress Chaperones 2010; 15:743–51.

67. Seniuk NA, Henderson JT, Tatton WG, et al. Increased CNTF gene expression in process-bearing astrocytes following injury is augmented by R(−)-deprenyl. J Neurosci Res 1994;37:278–86.

68. Fozard JR, Zreika M, Robin M, et al. The functional consequences of inhibition of monoamine oxidase type B: comparison of the pharmacological properties of l-deprenyl and MDL 72145. Naunyn-Schmiedeberg's Arch Pharmacol 1985; 331(2–3):186–93.

69. Denenberg S. Ageing-related problems in cats and dogs. In: Denenberg S, editor. Small animal veterinary Psychiatry. Oxfordshire: CAB International; 2021. p. 411–33.

70. Parkinson FE, Rudolphi KA, Fredholm BB. Propentofylline: A nucleoside transport inhibitor with neuroprotective effects in cerebral ischemia. Gen Pharmacol 1994; 25:1053–8.

71. Zhou C, Chao F, Zhang Y, et al. Fluoxetine delays the cognitive function decline and synaptic changes in a transgenic mouse model of early Alzheimer's disease. J Comp Neurol 2019;527:1378–87.

72. Picton JD, Brackett Marino A, Lovin Nealy K. Benzodiazepine use and cognitive decline in the elderly. American J Health Syst Pharm 2018;7:e6–12.

73. Arnsten AF, Goldman-Rakic PS. Noradrenergic mechanisms in age-related cognitive decline. J Neural Transm Suppl 1987;24:317–24.

74. Hosseini-Sharifabad A, Rabbani M, Sheikh-Darani A. The effect of long-term pregabalin administration on memory of rat in object recognition task. J Isfahan Med Sch 2016;38:325–31.

75. Lantz N, Beyea A. downward spiral: Dementia or drugs? J Am Geriatr Soc 2018; 66:S2.

76. Longo FM, Massa SM. Small-molecule modulation of neurotrophin receptors: A strategy for the treatment of neurological disease. Nat Rev Drug Discov 2013; 12:507–25.

77. Fogle JE, Hudson L, Thomson A, et al. Improved neurocognitive performance in FIV infected cats following treatment with the p75 neurotrophin receptor ligand LM11A-31. J Neurovirol 2021;27:302–32.

78. Nithianantharajah J, Hannan AJ. The neurobiology of brain and cognitive reserve: Mental and physical activity as modulators of brain disorders. Prog Neurobiol 2009;89(4):369–82.

79. Landsberg GM, DePorter T, Araujo JA. Clinical signs and management of anxiety, sleeplessness, and cognitive dysfunction in the senior pet. Vet Clin North Am Small Anim Pract 2011;41:565–90.

80. Griffith CA, Steigerwald ES, Buffington CAT. Effects of a synthetic facial pheromone on behavior of cats. J Am Vet Med Assoc 2000;217:154–1156.

81. Shu H, Gu X. Effect of a synthetic feline facial pheromone product on stress during transport in domestic cats: a randomised controlled pilot study. J Feline Med Surg 2022;24:691–9.

82. Ticinesi A, Mancabelli L, Carnevali L, et al. Interaction between diet and microbiota in the pathophysiology of Alzheimer's disease: Focus on polyphenols and dietary fibers. J Alzheimer's Dis. 2022;86:961–82.

83. Kaur H, Agarwal S, Agarwal M, et al. Therapeutic and preventative role of functional foods in the process of neurodegeneration. Int J Pharm Sci Res 2020;11: 8823222–9.

84. Salem N, Vandal M, Calon F. The benefit of docosahexaenoic acid for the adult brain in aging and dementia. Prostaglandins Leukot Essent Fatty Acids 2015; 92:15–22.

85. Cole GM, Frautschy SA. DHA may prevent age-related dementia. J Nutr 2010; 140:869–74.

86. Cole GM, Ma QL, Frautschy SA. Omega-3 fatty acids and dementia. Prostaglandins Leukot Essent Fatty Acids 2009;81:213–21.
87. Marszalek JR, Lodish HF. Docosahexaenoic acid, fatty acid-interacting proteins, and neuronal function: Breastmilk and fish are good for you. Annu Rev Cell Dev Biol 2005;21:633–57.
88. Tynes VV, Landsberg GM. Nutritional management of behavior and brain disorders in dogs and cats. Vet Clin North Am Small Anim Pract 2021;51:711–27.
89. Heinemann KM, Waldron MK, Bigley KE, et al. Long-chain (n-3) polyunsaturated fatty acids are more efficient than α-linolenic acid in improving electroretinogram responses of puppies exposed during gestation, lactation, and weaning. J Nutr 2005;135:1960–6.
90. Kidd PM. Omega-3 DHA and EPA for cognition, behavior, and mood: Clinical findings and structural-functional synergies with cell membrane phospholipids. Altern Med Rev 2007;12:207–27.
91. Zicker SC, Jewell DE, Yamka RM, et al. Evaluation of cognitive learning, memory, psychomotor, immunologic, and retinal functions in healthy puppies fed foods fortified with docosahexaenoic acid-rich fish oil from 8 to 52 weeks of age. J Am Vet Med Assoc 2012;241:583–94.
92. Cupp CJ, Kerr WW, Jean-Philippe C, et al. The role of nutritional interventions in the longevity and maintenance of long-term health in elderly cats. Int J Appl Res Vet Med 2008;6:69–81.
93. Cupp CJ, Jean-Philippe C, Kerr WW, et al. Effect of nutritional interventions on longevity of senior cats. Int J Appl Res Vet Med 2007;5:133–49.
94. Araujo JA, Landsberg GM, Milgram NW, et al. Improvement of short-term memory performance in aged beagles by a nutraceutical supplement containing phosphatidylserine, Ginkgo biloba, vitamin E, and pyridoxine. Can Vet J 2008;49: 379–85.
95. Heath SE, Barabas S, Craze PG. Nutritional supplementation in cases of canine cognitive dysfunction-A clinical trial. Appl Anim Behav Sci 2007;105:284–96.

The Interaction Between Behavioral and Physical Health in Rabbits

Valarie V. Tynes, DVM

KEYWORDS

- Anxiety • Fear • Pain • Aggression • Stress • Behavior

KEY POINTS

- Behaviroal and physical health are interconnected.
- The average pet rabbit likely lives wth a great deal of fear, anxiety and stress.
- Rabbits are highly social animals that should not live without a conspecific.
- Chronic pain or stress can result in the worsening of many medical conditions.

INTRODUCTION

Understanding the interaction between behavioral and physical health requires that one first understand the need to move past the belief that medical and behavioral health are somehow 2 separate entities. Medical conditions lead to changes in behavior, and in fact, recognizing subtle changes in behavior can be one of the most valuable tools we have to assess health and welfare. Some problem behaviors (those that are unacceptable to the owner) may represent an animal's attempt to adapt to an environment when adaptation may not be completely possible.[1] These behaviors may be referred to as maladaptive. Other problem behaviors reflect a dysregulation or dysfunction at the neurophysiological level, and these may be considered truly malfunctional. These behaviors have no functional value in any context. They are a result of neural pathology.[1] Determining which of these 2 categories any given problem behavior represents may not always be possible, but having an awareness that you simply cannot refer to an animal's problem as behavioral OR medical is critical to client education and to the long-term success of treatment. Essentially, all behaviors occur as a result of neurochemical activity in the brain, so it is not appropriate to consider a problem as medical/physical OR behavioral. Anxiety is just one example of a behavioral health condition that occurs because of neurophysiologic changes in the brain and that can negatively affect multiple body systems and thus contribute to many medical conditions. As one can see, this complex relationship between physical and behavioral

SPCA of Texas, 2400 Lone Star Drive, Dallas, TX 75212, USA
E-mail address: vtynes@spca.org

Vet Clin Small Anim 54 (2024) 169–179
https://doi.org/10.1016/j.cvsm.2023.08.001
0195-5616/24/© 2023 Elsevier Inc. All rights reserved.

vetsmall.theclinics.com

health often results in a cause-and-effect dilemma similar to the "chicken and egg" question. Answering which came first may not be as critical as simply recognizing the complexity of the intertwining relationship between the 2 and approaching treatment using both medicine and environmental and behavioral management.

Rabbits are susceptible to many health conditions that develop due to inadequate husbandry and most of these result in changes in behavior. To further complicate matters, rabbits are prey animals and as such are evolutionarily "programmed" to hide any illness or weakness for as long as possible. Nevertheless, changes in behavior can be excellent signs of illness when we use astute observation skills to recognize these signs before illness progresses to a critical state. The behavior of rabbits has also been demonstrated to change when an observer is present, as they are more likely to "freeze" than many other species when observed. So, the clinician must keep this in mind when attempting to interpret the behavior of a rabbit or assess pain.[2,3] In addition, chronic, unrecognized, and untreated pain may lead to fear and anxiety that will result in behavior changes, including but not limited to aggression. The average rabbit owner is often not completely familiar with normal rabbit behavior, and therefore, the practitioner may need to provide some education for them to learn how to recognize subtle signs of behavioral change that may indicate a problem.

DISCUSSION

Many different physical diseases in the rabbit can result in behavior changes. These diseases include but are not limited to dental problems such as malocclusion and abscesses, gastrointestinal stasis, arthritis, urinary calculi, and *Encephalitozoon cuniculi* infection. In addition, anxiety, fear, stress, and distress can influence the behavior of rabbits in association with these different disease processes.

A normal, healthy rabbit should be alert, inquisitive, and constantly sniffing. They should appear well groomed and clean because rabbits are meticulous groomers. A rabbit's behavior can be drastically changed by being in a novel environment and being handled by unfamiliar individuals, especially if it has not been well socialized by the owners. Owners will need to be questioned regarding the rabbit's normal behavior at home, the social environment, and its interactions with novel people to recognize problems or changes in the context of a new environment. History should be collected while the rabbit is first observed moving around the examination room and before any handling or restraint is attempted. History taking should include questions regarding housing and the social grouping at home. Ill rabbits may move away from their conspecifics and avoid social interactions; this is something that the owner may not think is important unless asked. If a rabbit has been removed from conspecifics and placed in a novel environment, this separation might also result in behavior changes such as immobility and decreased interest in surroundings. If the practitioner is unaware of the rabbit's social bonds, this behavior can easily be mistaken for pain or illness. When it is possible, pet owners should be encouraged to bring a companion rabbit with the patient, assuming they are closely bonded, because the presence of the companion can promote the exhibition of normal behaviors and thus increase the likelihood of witnessing any pain-related behaviors.[4]

Pain

Pain can be defined as an unpleasant sensory and emotional experience associated with actual or potential tissue damage and should be expected in any animal subjected to any procedure or disease model that would be likely to cause pain in a human.[5] Physiologic signs of pain in rabbits include, as one might expect, changes in respiration, heart rate, body temperature, and blood pressure. However, these physiologic signs are not predictive of pain alone, as they can also be elevated with fear, anxiety, or stress, which can happen in the rabbit with handling and physical examination alone.

Recent research has demonstrated that observers tend to focus on the face of the rabbit when trying to assess pain,[6] but other very important subtle changes can be missed when we do this. Grimace scales have been developed for many species, including the rabbit, and can be very useful in a clinical setting.[7] These scales are reliable and relatively easy to use. However, they do not allow for the recognition of varying degrees of pain that is necessary for determining when and if more analgesia may be needed. More recently, a multidimensional pain scale (the Bristol Rabbit Pain Scale [BRPS]) has been developed and was shown to have good internal consistency.[8]

Although more work is needed to validate the BRPS and confirm its clinical usefulness, multiple studies have identified the varying behaviors that can be associated with pain in the rabbit. A painful rabbit may demonstrate any of the following behavior and attitude changes[4]:

- Decreased movement around the enclosure
- Decreased searching or exploration
- Upward arching of the back
- Abdomen pressed to the floor
- Teeth grinding
- Decreased food and water intake
- Vocalizations
- Reduced activity
- Decreased or absent self-grooming behavior
- Squinting eyes
- Attempting to hide
- Aggression
- Depression
- Anxiety
- Hypersensitivity
- Licking painful area
- Decreased rearing
- Increased shuffling movements (slow shuffling movements where the hind legs are moved one at a time)
- Writhing (contractions of the abdominal muscles)

Recent research has identified behaviors associated with pain that may be easily overlooked because they occur at a low frequency and are very brief in their expression.[6] These behaviors are more likely to be seen in the hours immediately following surgery and include the following:

- Flinching
- Wincing
- Twitching
- Staggering

Many different factors can alter a rabbit's expression of pain and must be kept in mind when attempting to identify pain in a rabbit. These factors include the following:

- Novel environments;
- Group dynamics—rabbits housed socially may be even more likely to hide signs of pain or illness so as not to draw attention to themselves[5];

- Presence of an observer, especially if an unfamiliar person;
- Cause of the pain—intense acute pain may result in different physiologic and behavioral changes compared with low-grade or chronic pain.[5]

Pain causes many adverse effects on multiple body systems including inflammation, suppression of the immune system, negative effects on the cardiovascular system, and activation of the sympathetic nervous system.[5] The presence of pain results in stress. Stress can result in cardiomyopathy and acute heart failure secondary to catecholamine release.[9] The glucocorticoid release associated with stress results in increases in gastric acidity that can lead to ulceration and changes in gut motility, which in turn can lead to gut stasis, resulting in more pain and illness.[10]

Fear, Anxiety, and Stress

Fear can be defined as an emotional state that results in an organism avoiding something that it perceives as being imminently dangerous. The key word here is "perceives." Pet owners often need to be taught that their presence or actions may be scary to the animal, even when they do not think so. What really matters is if the animal thinks that the context is scary, because that is what the animal will respond to, that is, their feelings of being threatened. It may be equally important to help the pet owner understand that fear is also not something that is within the animal's immediate control; this is just one reason why punishing the animal can be so dangerous. Punishment will only serve to increase the fear.

Anxiety is the emotional state associated with the *anticipation* of a threat. The threat is not immediately present. Signs of fear and anxiety can seem similar, and differentiating them may not always be clinically relevant but recognizing that they are 2 different emotional states is useful to understanding the behavior of rabbits in the clinical setting. When an animal lives with chronic fear and anxiety that it cannot avoid, it will experience stress and ultimately distress. Stress activates both the sympathoadrenal medullary (SAM) and the hypothalamic-pituitary-adrenal (HPA) axes. The subsequent release of adrenaline and glucocorticoids affects numerous body systems, resulting in increased susceptibility to infection, hepatic disease, and gastrointestinal ileus. Gastrointestinal ileus continues to be one of the leading causes of morbidity and mortality in rabbits,[11] and although this is often a result of poor husbandry and nutrition, it can be highly affected by stress especially if the stress is chronic. Adrenaline release also leads to tachypnea, tachycardia, and hypertension, and these changes have been documented to result in fatal arrhythmias.[12] Stress can lead to immunosuppression that can ultimately trigger clinical signs of latent infections, common to rabbits. These infections include E cuniculi, Pasteurellosis, or enterotoxemia. Stressful handling can be followed by acute neurologic signs of E cuniculi such as a head tilt or seizures.[13]

Prey species such as the rabbit, when kept captive, can spend much of their lives in a state of fear and/or anxiety. If their environment is not designed with adequate hiding spaces so that rabbits can feel safe or if other predatory species such as dogs and cats are allowed to roam freely around their environment, the rabbits will likely experience frequent fear and thus stress. Solitary living has been shown to be an important source of stress for rabbits. They are social creatures, and fecal corticosterone levels have been found to be higher in rabbits living alone, confirming the importance of social housing.[14]

The individual temperament of a rabbit can also affect how it responds to fear- or anxiety-inducing stimulus. The research into rabbit temperament is limited but suggests that similar to many animals, behavioral differences representative of personality or temperament can be identified. One study identified 3 personality dimensions in the rabbit: exploration, boldness, and anxiety.[15] Recognizing that a rabbit may have an anxious temperament can be an important part of the clinician's assessment, because it can affect so many other aspects of the rabbit's health and well-being. Krall (2019) developed a simple anxiety assessment template for rabbits that in one study demonstrated excellent interobserver agreement and acceptable internal consistency.[12] Although more research is needed on this subject, this simple test could be a good place for the clinician to begin in assessing the anxiety of their patients.

The signs of a scared rabbit and a stressed rabbit can look similar. A stressed rabbit may

- Crouch down and hold their head near to the ground
- Muscles will be tense
- Ears will be held apart and lie flat against the back
- Eyes may be wide with dilated pupils
- May vocalize by grinding teeth or grunting

The clinician should note that many of these signs can also appear in rabbits in pain.

Anxiety and Anesthesia

Rabbits are prone to complications from anesthesia, and the risk increases when they are already stressed or anxious. The release of adrenaline involved when the rabbit is frightened, anxious, or stressed plays an important role in these potential complications. Anxiety has been shown in humans to complicate anesthesia induction and maintenance.[12] Research about the association between anxiety and anesthesia complications in rabbits is limited but, because rabbits are prey animals, they tend to be considered more anxious than the average companion animal. At least one study has demonstrated that anxious rabbits exhibit an increased frequency of intraoperative apnea, suggesting that anxiety is what predisposes rabbits to anesthetic complications.[12] Until more is known about this association, clinicians are encouraged to be attentive to the fear, anxiety, and stress exhibited by their rabbit patients.

Handling

If the rabbit is not habituated to the presence of people and is handled in a way that makes it feel unsafe, then it will likely experience frequent fear in these circumstances. For many rabbits, handling is one of the most stressful events they face, particularly in the context of the veterinary examination. Frequent, gentle handling from an early age has been shown to reduce the fear of humans in rabbits.[16,17] Associating handling with a small, tasty treat such as a piece of apple or carrot can also aid in building the human-rabbit relationship through classical conditioning. Most importantly though, people must handle rabbits in a way that makes them feel safe. Lifting a rabbit from above is likely to be very terrifying for the rabbit because normally, only a predator lifts a rabbit. The interaction that owners have with the rabbit should be focused more on petting, scratching, or playing so as to build trust. The handler must pay attention to the response of the rabbit to petting and scratching. If the rabbit walks away after a couple of seconds of petting, this suggests that it did not enjoy the petting that much. If, however, the rabbit leans in and closes its eyes, this suggests it does like that form of touch. Rabbits that like to be petted will also often place their head under their owner's hand and nudge upward. Rabbits may also make soft purring and clicking sounds, assumed to be signs of contentment when interacting with humans in an environment in which they feel safe.

If the rabbit is to be lifted, it should be able to clearly see the approaching person, and the lifting must be done gently and slowly at first so as not to startle the rabbit. The rabbit must also be lifted while being well supported under both the hind limbs and the front end. If a rabbit feels insecure about being lifted or if lifting causes it pain, it may struggle and cause injury to itself in the process. Rabbits have a relatively light-weight skeletal system, representing only 7% to 8% of their body weight, when compared with the 50% of body weight comprised by the skeletal muscles; this results in a skeleton that can be easily fractured by sudden, uncontrolled movements. Once lifted, the rabbit should be held snugly against the handler's body. The handler should then move to a location as quickly as possible where they can sit and allow the rabbit freedom to move around them. Lifting and holding or carrying the rabbit for longer than necessary is not recommended. Pet owners should be encouraged to train rabbits to enter and exit their habitats so that the need to lift and carry the rabbit is limited. Rabbits can also be taught a cue word that signifies they are going to be lifted. By making lifting predictable and rewarding (again by reinforcing with small bites of treats), it will be much less stressful for the rabbit.

Tonic immobility is a form of handling or restraint that has been recommended for rabbits in the past. Laying a rabbit on its back and stroking it can cause it to become still and apparently relaxed; this is an evolutionarily adaptive predator-avoidance response that is used as a method of "last resort" to avoid predation. By "playing dead," a prey animal may get one last chance to escape predation when the predator relaxes its grip. Studies have found that physiologic and behavioral indicators demonstrate that this is a highly stressful experience for the rabbit and the signs of stress remain for as much as 15 minutes posthandling.[18,19] Although this form of restraint may be acceptable for brief periods of handling and nonpainful procedures such as nail trimming, pet owners should be educated about the stressful nature of this type of handling.

Rabbits can discriminate between individuals,[20,21] and this can often result in different responses to different people depending on the rabbit's experience with those individuals. Rabbits are often acquired as pets for children and when handled carelessly, can quickly learn to struggle, bite, and scratch when reached for by the individual that they have learned to fear. Rabbits should only be acquired for children old enough to learn how to properly lift and handle the rabbit so as not to cause it fear or pain.

Trazodone hydrochloride, a serotonin antagonist and reuptake inhibitor, has been shown to be a safe and effective medication in dogs and cats for relieving anxiety. Although more research is needed in the rabbit, at least one study has demonstrated trazodone's safety when used in the rabbit at a dose of 40 mg/kg.[22] When rabbits have not been habituated to handling by humans and they seem to be stressed by veterinary visits, trazodone should be considered as a previsit medication.

Environment

Living in an inappropriate environment can also be extremely stressful for the rabbit. Examples of inadequate environmental features include but are not limited to the following:

- Solitary living—rabbits in the wild live in large groups. Research has suggested that rabbits value social contact as much as food and will work to access it.[23] Group living likely allows them to feel safer because more individuals are alert for predators. A rabbit living alone is going to be required to always be on alert for predators, resulting in some degree of chronic stress. Rabbits engage in social grooming; this helps to establish and maintain social bonds that also contributes to good mental health. Rabbits can also help maintain comfortable body temperatures by huddling together in cool temperatures. Research has shown that rabbits living alone are more likely to exhibit depressionlike behaviors, have lower body temperatures, and have poor emotional well-being.[23,24] It has even been suggested that solitary living decreases life span,[24] just one more example of the important relationship between physical and mental health.

- Inadequate space—rabbits are active animals that need enough space to run, hop, and dig. Guidelines for rabbit housing have been set[24,25] and suggest that a pair of rabbits should have a run size of at least 10 feet by 6 feet and a height of at least 3 feet. The rabbit needs to be able to stand up fully and take at least 3 full hops in one direction.
- Inability to exhibit a range of normal behaviors—rabbits are burrowing animals that also need to feel safe from predators. Other aspects of a habitat that helps to ensure good welfare include substrate to burrow or dig in, hiding places and elevated places for monitoring their environment. Rabbits should be able to express natural foraging behaviors for finding food, and they should be able to mark their territory effectively with chin secretions, urine, and fecal pellets.

In order to have good physical and mental health, and ultimately good welfare, a rabbit must have access to all of the aforementioned features in its environment.

Medical Conditions Associated with Behavior Changes

Gastrointestinal stasis is a condition that provides an excellent example of the relationship between physical and mental health. The rabbit has a unique form of gastrointestinal physiology that allows them to eat a diet high in poorly digestible roughage but still have a rapid gut transit time. This gut physiology allows for efficient fermentation and then reingestion in the form of caecotrophs. A high-fiber diet is necessary for this system to function efficiently. It also supports a healthy gut microbiome. Diets low in fiber and high in carbohydrates can lead to gut hypomotility and gastric stasis. Rabbits experiencing gut stasis will be anorexic, consume less water, and may be depressed and painful. This discomfort can lead to aggression. Conversely, if the rabbit is experiencing chronic stress, the activation of the stress systems (SAM and HPA) also results in changes in gut motility and gut permeability, both of which can further complicate the problem of gastrointestinal stasis in the rabbit.

Many medical conditions can result in pain and subsequently an aggressive response in the rabbit. These conditions include gastrointestinal disease as well as dental disease. Rabbit dentition is well adapted to their high-fiber diet. When rabbits are not fed a diet high in adequate roughage, they develop abnormal tooth wear, which leads to malocclusion and dental abscesses. Dental disease can lead to pain when chewing and subsequently anorexia and weight loss.

Trauma resulting in fractures and dislocations can also occur in the rabbit, and in some cases the only notable change may be an increase in aggression. For this reason, the first step any time there is a sudden appearance of aggressive behavior in the rabbit should be to perform a thorough physical examination.

Several neurologic diseases are common to pet rabbits. These diseases can result in changes in behavior such as a head tilt, tremors, ataxia, paresis, paralysis, and seizures.

Reproductive and urinary tract diseases can include neoplasia and urolithiasis, resulting in pain-related behaviors. Urinary incontinence can be caused by spinal fractures, dislocations, or central nervous system lesions due to E cuniculi infection.

Polyuria and polydipsia can occur secondary to many urinary tract diseases, but psychogenic polyuria and polydipsia have also been diagnosed in rabbits and may occur secondary to stress. When presented with a rabbit exhibiting polyuria/poly-dipsia, other systemic illnesses such as urinary tract disorders, metabolic diseases, and infections must first be ruled out. If psychogenic disease is suspected, all aspects of husbandry and environment, including the social environment, must be carefully investigated.

Rabbits are also subject to a variety of different dermatologic conditions caused by viral, bacterial, fungal, and parasitic conditions. Alone, these may not cause much change in behavior, but pain should still always be considered as a possible sequalae, and thus pain-related changes in behavior may be present. In addition, pruritis can also lead to discomfort that could potentially result in behavior change. The important role of pruritus in behavior change in dogs is just now being recognized,[26] but more research is needed to confirm that this may occur in rabbits.

Clinicians should also be aware that grooming is a common displacement behavior. Displacement behaviors are behaviors that may occur when an animal is motivated to perform a behavior but for some reason it is restricted from doing so. In those cases, another behavior that seems out of context for the situation is often seen and should be considered a sign of frustration or conflict; this can result in overgrooming and hair loss. A case of what seemed to be acral lick dermatitis has been documented in the rabbit and resolved with multimodal therapy including environmental enrichment. Hair pulling or barbering, as some people refer to it, has also been described in rabbits; this was suggested to occur as a result of a dominant rabbit barbering a subordinate rabbit. However, more recent research has confirmed that this behavior is seen in singly housed rabbits as well and may in fact be more common in them than in group-housed or pair-housed rabbits[27]; this supports the idea that barbering may occur secondary to the stress of social isolation. When presented with a rabbit with hair loss, once all likely infectious and neoplastic processes have been ruled out, the environment and history should be closely examined for causes of fear, anxiety, and stress.

Hair loss and self-mutilation have also been shown to occur in rabbits. In at least one case, self-mutilation occurred in a rabbit after receiving an intramuscular injection of ketamine and xylazine in the thigh.[28] In this case, the self-mutilation was thought to result from perineural drug infiltration around the sciatic nerve that resulted in dysesthesia. Rabbits are also known to overgroom skin over painful areas. Pain and altered sensation (dysesthesia, paresthesia, allodynia, and so on) should always be considered when faced with a rabbit that is excessively grooming one area.

BEHAVIOR PROBLEMS

The most commonly reported behavior problems in rabbits include the following.

- Aggression
- Elimination problems such as urine spraying or not using the litter tray
- Chewing of nonfood items and destruction in the home

Many of these behavior problems can have multiple causal factors including pain, fear, and frustration as described previously. Aggression is a common sequala to pain and discomfort, including that associated with poor handling technique. Rabbits can also learn to use aggression to avoid handling, especially when they have had handling in the past that hurt or frightened them. Elimination problems such as urine spraying can also be a result of pain, fear, or anxiety and in some cases medical conditions associated with the urogenital tract. Destructive behavior that occurs in the home is usually just a result of the attempts of a rabbit to exhibit its species-typical behaviors of chewing and digging. Owners need to be educated on how to prevent access to inappropriate items and provide the rabbit with appropriate items for using these highly motivated behaviors. When not allowed to perform these species typical behaviors, rabbits may also be more likely to engage in repetitive behaviors such as bar biting, pica, barbering, and fur chewing.[29,30] Providing the rabbit with a high-fiber diet in such a way that it must forage for its food by using "activity feeders" and similar devices will keep the animal mentally occupied and help prevent many unwanted behaviors, while also improving the rabbit's welfare.

If aggression toward people becomes a problem, the first instruction to the pet owner should be to stop lifting the rabbit if possible. Desensitizing and counterconditioning the rabbit is then initiated, so that the rabbits' associations with people are improved; this is most easily done with tiny bites of special treats. The rabbit should be coaxed into entering a carrier (again, treats may be useful) for moving it from one place to another, so that lifting can be avoided. Handling should occur mostly in the mornings and evenings, the time at which rabbits are naturally most active.

SUMMARY

The domestic rabbit still exhibits much of the behavioral repertoire of its wild ancestor. As a prey species, the rabbit is subject to a life filled with anxiety, fear, and stress, especially if it is not provided with a safe and appropriate habitat for the species, which must include freedom from exposure to predators, a habitat that allows freedom of movement, and the ability to express normal species-typical behaviors. Social housing is also critical to the rabbit's welfare. When not provided with these things, stress can become chronic and cause or contribute to a variety of different physical illnesses. In addition, certain physical health problems, such as those causing pain can contribute to chronic anxiety and stress, resulting in a cycle of illness/pain → stress → more illness. Pain is easily overlooked in the rabbit and can lead to significant behavior changes including aggression. A thorough physical examination to rule out underlying medical conditions must always be performed when a rabbit is presented for acute behavior change. Any physical disease will need to be treated, and at the same time, the husbandry of the rabbit must be corrected if needed and environmental needs met in order to ensure good physical and behavioral health for the rabbit.

CLINICS CARE POINTS

- Physical and behavioral health are complexly interrelated in most animals, including the rabbit.

- Fear, anxiety, and stress can lead to illness, and chronic illness, especially that causing pain, can result in stress.

- Meeting the environmental needs for safety, freedom of movement, freedom to express species typical behaviors, and appropriate nutrition are all equally critical to the behavioral and physical health of rabbits.

- The keeping of single rabbits should be avoided whenever possible. The rabbit is a highly social animal whose welfare is compromised by social isolation.

- Any rabbit presented for a behavior problem should first have a complete physical examination and history collected to include information about all aspects of husbandry and environment.

DISCLOSURE

The author has no conflict of interest to disclose.

REFERENCES

1. Mills DS. Medical paradigms for the study of problem behaviour: a critical review. Appl Anim Behav Sci 2003;81:265–77.
2. Dobromylskyi P, Flecknell PA, Lascelles BD, et al. Pain assessment. In: Flecknell P, Waterman-Pearson A, editors. Pain management in animals. London: WB Saunders; 2000. p. 53–80.
3. Leach MC, Allweiler S, Richardson CA, et al. Behavioural effect of ovariohysterectomy and oral administration of meloxicam in laboratory housed rabbits. Res Vet Sci 2009;87(2):336–47.
4. Miller AL, Leach MC. Pain recognition in rabbits. Vet Clin Exot Anim 2023;26: 187–99.
5. Kohn DF, Martin TE, Foley PL, et al. Guideines for the assessment and management of pain in rodents and rabbits. J Am Assoc Lab Anim Sci 2007;46(2): 97–108.
6. Leach MC, Coulter CA, Richardson CA, et al. Are we looking in the wrong place? Implications for behavioural-based pain assessment in rabbits (*Oryctolagus cuniculi*) and beyond? PLoS One 2011;6(3):e13347.
7. Keating S, Thomas AA, Flecknell PA, et al. Evaluation of EMLA cream for preventing pain during tattooing in rabbits: Changes in physiological, behavioural and facial expression responses. PLoS One 2012;7(9):e44437.
8. Benato L, Murrell J, Knowles, et al. Development of the Bristol Rabbit Pain Scale (BRPS): A multidimensional composite pain scale specific to rabbits (*Oryctolagus cuniculus*). PLoS One 2021;16(6):e0252417.
9. Weber HW, Van der Walt JJ. Cardiomyopathy in crowded rabbits. Recent Adv Stud Cardiac Struc Metab Rec Adv Study 1975;6:471–7.
10. Thompson L. Recognition and assessment of pain in small exotic mammals. In: Egger CM, Love L, Doherty T, editors. Pain management in veterinary practice. Oxford: Wiley Blackwell; 2014. p. 391–8.
11. Paul-Murphy J. Critical care of the rabbit. Vet Clin North Am Exotic Anim Pract 2007. https://doi.org/10.1016/j.cvex.2007.03.002.
12. Krall C, Glass S, Dancourt G, et al. Behavioral anxiety predisposes rabbits to intraoperative apnoea and cardiorespiratory instability. Appl Anim Behav Sci 2019; 221. https://doi.org/10.1016/j.applanim.2019.104875.
13. Harcourt-Brown FM. Critical Care in rabbits. Harrogate, UK: World small animal veterinary association world congress proceedings; 2010 [Paper presentation].
14. Lisiewicz NE, Water M, Jackson B. Social Stress in rabbits. In: Heath SE, editor. Proceedings of the 7th international behaviour meeting. Belgium: ESCVE; 2009. p. 85–9.
15. Andersson A, Laikre L, Bergvall U. Two shades of boldness: novel object and anti-predator behavior reflect different personality dimensions in domestic rabbits. J Ethology 2014;32:123–36.
16. Podberscek AL, Blackshaw JK, Beattie AW. The effects of repeated handling by familiar and unfamiliar people on rabbits in individual cages and group pens. Appl Anim Behav Sci 1991;28:273–365.
17. Csatádi K, Kustos K, Elben CS, et al. Even minimal human contact linked to nursing reduces fear responses toward humans in rabbits. Appl Anim Behav Sci 2005;95:123–8.

18. Farabollini F, Faccinetti F, Lupo C, et al. Time course of opiod and pituitary-adrenal hormone modifications during the immobility reaction in rabbits. Physiol Behav 1990;47(2):337–41.
19. McBride EA, Day S, McAdie T, et al. Trancing rabbits: Relaxed hypnosis or a state of fear?. In: Proceedings of the VDWE international congress on companion animal behaviour and welfare. Belgium: Vlaamse Dierenartsenvereniging, Sint-Niklaas; 2006. p. 135–7.
20. Davis H, Gibson JA. Can rabbits tell humans apart?: Discrimination of individual humans and its implications for animal research. Comp Med 2000;50(5):483–5.
21. Csatádi K, Ágnes B, Vilmos A. Specificity of early handling: Are rabbit pups able to distinguish between people? Appl Anim Behav Sci 2007;107:322–7.
22. Rickerl K, Reed J, Brundage C. Physiological effect of trazodone hydrochloride use for anxiety and sedation in rabbits (*Oryctolagus cuniculus*). FASEB Journal 2020;34:1–2.
23. Seaman SC, Waran NK, Mason G, et al. Animal economics: Assessing the motivation of female laboratory rabbits to reach a platform, social contact and food. Anim Behav 2008;75(1):31–42.
24. Schepers F, Koene P, Beerda B. Welfare assessment in pet rabbits. Anim Welf 2009;18:477–85.
25. Foote A. Evidence based approach to recognizing and reducing stress in pet rabbits. Veterinary Nursing Journal 2020;35(6):167–70.
26. Harvey D, Craigon PJ, Shaw SC, et al. Behavioral differences in dogs with atopic dermatitis suggest stress could be a significant problem associated with chronic pruritus. Animals 2019;9:813.
27. Reinhardt V. Hair pulling; a review. Lab Anim 2005;39(4):361–9.
28. Beyersd TM, Richardon JA, Prince MD. Axonal degeneration and self-mutilation as a complication of the intramuscular use of ketamine and xylazine in rabbits. Lab Anim Sci 1991;41:519–20.
29. Lidfors L. Behavioural effects of environmental enrichment for individually caged rabbits. Appl Anim Behav Sci 1997;52(1):157–69.
30. Hansen LT, Berthelsen H. The effect of environmental enrichment on the behaviour of caged rabbits (*Oryctolagus cuniculus*). Appl Anim Behav Sci 2000;68:163–78.

Sensory Processing Sensitivity and the Importance of Individuality and Personality in Veterinary Medicine

Maya Braem, Dr. med. vet.

KEYWORDS

- Sensory processing sensitivity • High sensitivity • Behavior problem
- Differential environmental susceptibility • Dog

KEY POINTS

- The personality trait "high sensitivity" or "canine sensory processing sensitivity" can be measured in dogs and shows parallels to high sensitivity in humans.
- High sensitivity in dogs affects how they are influenced by owner personality and communication.
- Considering high sensitivity in veterinary practice is likely to benefit all individuals, but especially high sensitive animals.

INTRODUCTION: INDIVIDUALITY AND PERSONALITY

To be yourself in a world that is constantly trying to make you something else is the greatest accomplishment.

(Ralph Waldo Emerson)

Ralph Waldo Emerson emphasized the importance of individuality already in the nineteenth century. He was, of course, referring to humans. "To be yourself in a world that is constantly trying to make you something else" —does this not apply to animals living in human society too? We expect such a great deal of adaptation to our ways of life, our language, even our moral and legal standards from our pets. Do we actually stop to see them as individuals, with their own personalities, subjective perceptions and experiences, individual needs and means of communication? Do we actually give them the opportunity to be themselves and thrive?

Veterinary hospital, University of Zürich, Winterthurerstrasse 260, CH 8057 Zürich, Switzerland
E-mail address: medvet@mayanimal.ch

Vet Clin Small Anim 54 (2024) 181–193
https://doi.org/10.1016/j.cvsm.2023.09.002
0195-5616/24/© 2023 Elsevier Inc. All rights reserved.

Our human world seems to be increasingly developing into a duality: focus on individuality on the one hand and more standardization on the other. These two aspects are not always easy to unite. This duality is equally developing in animal health, behavior, and welfare. In a world focused on economic growth, veterinarians are exposed to the pressure of standardization and efficiency. At the same time, knowledge and understanding of animal emotions, cognition, personality, and genetics is growing and with it the appreciation of the importance of considering the individual in veterinary medicine in general and veterinary behavior medicine in particular.

The Cambridge Dictionary defines individuality as "the qualities that make a person or thing different from others," that is, it requires the presence of several individuals and a comparison among these. One important aspect that contributes to individuality is personality. Personality encompasses individual differences in behaving, thinking, and feeling, which are stable over time and contexts.[1] Personality is therefore independent of how the individual compares to others, but although it can stand on its own, it can also be used to distinguish individuals from another. Several, individually more or less pronounced personality traits make up the whole of an individual's personality. Some of these traits have been studied and described in animals as well, for example, shyness–boldness,[2] impulsivity,[3] frustration[4] as well as the personality trait at the center of this article, sensory processing sensitivity (SPS).[5,6]

As veterinarians, we are confronted on a daily basis with the challenge of bridging the above-mentioned chasm: our approach is expected to be based on scientific evidence while considering at the same time the actual individual patient before us, who might not be behaving according to the statistically determined most likely norms.

The current state of our knowledge regarding SPS reflects this situation. Most of what we know about SPS stems from human research. Therefore, the information in this article concerning animals and SPS is in part extrapolated from human research and in part fed by the author's own empirical experience.

In the following text, paragraphs referring to literature about humans will be presented in a normal font, whereas those concerning animals (dogs in particular) will be presented in framed boxes.

WHAT DO WE KNOW ABOUT SENSORY PROCESSING SENSITIVITY?
Sensory Processing Sensitivity in Humans

Research into the personality trait of "Sensory Processing Sensitivity," also referred to as "high sensitivity" has grown rapidly since the term was first coined in 1997 by Aron and colleagues.[7] Fifteen to twenty percent of the human population carry this trait independent of gender or culture.[8] As with all personality traits, there is a normal distribution within the population and any specific individual lies on a spectrum of the trait that is more or less developed. Therefore, an individual is not either highly sensitive or not, but more or less so. Being a personality trait, it is part of what makes up the whole of this particular individual's personality and is not considered to be pathological. This implies that an individual cannot be "diagnosed" as being "highly sensitive," as little as introversion or extraversion can be diagnosed, but the trait is rather "measured" or described and considered to be part of the norm.

Simplified, individuals carrying this trait could be considered to have a "finer filter." Elaine Aron describes the following four main characteristics of SPS using the acronym DOES[9].

- D for Depth of processing: more highly sensitive individuals tend to want to understand and recognize associations; they typically collect and process information before they act, that is, show a "stop and watch behavior" and take their time to make decisions.[10]

- O for Overstimulation: individuals scoring higher on SPS are more easily overstimulated by external (eg, visual, acoustic, olfactory, tactile) as well as internal (eg, changes in self-perception, medication, physical health issues, pain) stimuli.[11]
- E for Emotional intensity: more highly sensitive individuals experience their own emotions intensely[12] and pick up on the emotions of others more easily.[13] They are often considered to be highly empathetic.
- S for Sensory Sensitivity: individuals scoring higher on SPS tend to be more attentive (or sensitive) to subtle exteroceptive[14–17] as well as interoceptive[18,19] stimuli.

Sensory Processing Sensitivity in Animals

The only scientifically based information to date focusing on SPS *sensu stricto* in another species apart from humans is our research on dogs.[5,20] However, possible relations to other traits or coping strategies have been suggested.[9] Duality in coping behaviors has been described in a variety of animal species ranging from fish to monkeys, for example, proactive/aggressive versus reactive/passive behaviors,[21–24] fast versus slow explorers,[25] shy versus bold individuals.[26,27] The direct correlation of these behaviors with SPS has not been investigated, however considering "only" the behavioral output aspect, the more reactive/passive/shy behaviors could represent or be related to the "stop and watch" behavior described for more highly sensitive humans by Aron and colleagues.[9] In order to survive, a population of social individuals must include a variety of personalities, for example, some individuals need to be more attentive to detail and warn the rest of the group of potential danger or notice subtle scents of food or water sources and weigh the pros and cons before acting. However, if the whole population consisted of only these more highly sensitive individuals, it would likely not last long, as gathering information and weighing all the options can be useful, but is of no help in the face of an immediate danger, such as a predator ready to attack. This is where less highly sensitive individuals are necessary, those who are quicker to make decisions and to act.

Canine Sensory Processing Sensitivity

The hypotheses and approach of our study looking into SPS in dogs were based on the knowledge acquired and shared in human psychology. The study consisted of a pilot phase designed to develop a questionnaire and a following international online survey to validate the questionnaire and to test the hypotheses proposed. For details of the studies please refer to the above-mentioned publications by Braem and colleagues.[5,20]

MEASURING HIGH SENSITIVITY
The Highly Sensitive Person Scale

Aron and colleagues, in their first study, developed and validated the "Highly Sensitive Person" (HSP)[7] scale. This original questionnaire—translated into several languages and adapted for children[28]—was unidimensional. The average of the 27 questions led to a single "HSP score" lying between 1 and 7, with 1 representing the lowest and 7 the highest degree of SPS.

Since then, further studies have diverged from this one-dimensionality and described sub-traits, which tease apart the characteristics associated with more "negative affect," such as being easily stressed and overwhelmed on the one hand, from those in relation to more "positive" aspects, such as being deeply touched by arts and music, noticing details, and picking up on emotions[29-31] on the other. Smolewska and colleagues[29] distinguish three sub-traits they refer to as ease of excitation, low sensory threshold, and esthetic sensitivity.

The Highly Sensitive Dog Scale

The results of our study on dogs revealed several parallels to SPS in humans.[5]

- The highly sensitive dog (HSD) scale: We were able to develop and scientifically validate an HSD scale consisting of 32 questions, which measures a trait that is comparable to SPS described in humans and to which we refer to as "canine Sensory Processing Sensitivity" (cSPS).
- Sub-traits of cSPS: A principal component analysis revealed three sub-traits comparable to those described by Smolewska and colleagues in humans,[29] representing aspects associated with more negative affect (termed "arousability" and "low sensory threshold") and those with more positive affect (referred to as "emotionality").
- Personality trait consistent over different contexts: The HSD score (the average of the 32 questions using a 1–7 Likert scale with 1 corresponding to low and 7 to high sensitivity) was greatly independent of factors described in the literature to influence behavior. These factors include dog (breed, sex, age, weight, physical health), owner (profession, SPS of owner, communication/training methods), and environmental (country of origin, living surroundings) factors.
- Personality trait consistent over time: Unpublished data from this author demonstrates a significant correlation of the cSPS score of puppies aged 9 to 12 weeks and the same dogs at 16 months of age ($P < .001$). This suggests stability over time and a predictive value of the questionnaire.

RELATION OF HIGH SENSITIVITY WITH OTHER PERSONALITY TRAITS

A common misconception in everyday life is that an individual is defined by only one personality trait. For example, the fact that a subject is "highly sensitive," "empathetic" or "introverted" is thought to explain why they behave in a certain way. Reality, as so often, is more complex: an individual's personality is the sum of the interaction of many traits. In addition, these traits may interact, increasing or decreasing a vulnerability for the development of psychological and/or physical health issues. It is therefore important to keep in mind throughout this article that we are only looking at one aspect, namely "high sensitivity," of the complex personality.

Sensory Srocessing Sensitivity and Fearfulness, Neuroticism, Shyness, Introversion, and Sensation Seeking

The original unidimensional approach of SPS[7] focused primarily on distinguishing high sensitivity from personality traits associated with negative affect, such as fearfulness, neuroticism, shyness, or introversion. Indeed, an overlap between these traits and SPS has been found, but they are not identical,[7,32] that is, a more highly sensitive individual is also more likely to be fearful, neurotic, shy, or introverted, but this does not have to be the case. Correlations with sensation seeking[33] have also been found, which poses a challenge within itself to find the appropriate balance of sensation while not being constantly overstimulated.

Canine sensory processing sensitivity and Fearfulness and Neuroticism

As our research built on the approach taken by Aron and colleagues in 1997, it was in a first step important to determine whether what was being measured by the developed questionnaire was distinct from the traits of fearfulness and neuroticism. Paralleling the findings in humans, cSPS overlapped with but was not identical to fearfulness and neuroticism. This means that a more HSD is also more likely to be fearful or neurotic, but this does not have to be the case.

DIFFERENTIAL SUSCEPTIBILITY

What makes one individual react more strongly to a particular situation or stressor than another? Personality seems to play an important role in the vulnerability to suffer from psychological and physical health issues. Considering the fine filter, deep processing of information and high emotionality related to SPS, it makes sense that more highly sensitive individuals would be more easily overwhelmed by more subtle and fewer stimuli than less highly sensitive individuals, that is, they are more easily stressed.

Even though everybody experiences it, stress itself is not a simple concept. It is in fact rather complex, consisting of a physical component on the one hand, which can be objectively "measured" or observed, such as changes in physiologic measures (eg, heart rate, temperature, and behaviors) and an emotional/psychological aspect on the other, which is subjective and not necessarily obvious to an "outsider." In addition, stress can be caused by a wide array of triggers, both on the physical as well as the psychological level. Stress, its perception, and tolerance play an important role in the development and persistence of both psychological and physical illnesses.

Vulnerability: Sensory Processing Sensitivity and Mental Health

It did not take long for research to focus on the interaction of SPS with stress, well-being, resilience, and various mental health problems in humans. Indeed, this personality trait has been correlated with a higher perception of stress,[11] decreased well-being,[34] and lower resilience[35] as well as a higher vulnerability to several mental health issues including anxiety, depression, and burnout.[36] Highly sensitive individuals seem to be particularly susceptible to the subjective component of stress.

Despite sharing some similar aspects, such as sensory sensitivity and attention to detail and correlation with specific sub-traints of SPS with some neurodevelopmental disorders such as attention-deficit hyperactivity disorder or autism spectrum disorders, SPS has been shown to be distinct from these.[37]

Differential Environmental Susceptibility: "for Better and for Worse"

For a long time, research has focused primarily on what is wrong, what renders individuals more vulnerable, what leads to stress, what signs indicate negative welfare and suffering, and what can be done to treat problems. In the 1990s, Seligman was one of the first psychologists to introduce the concept of "positive psychology"[38] in humans. In recent years, research in animal welfare has followed in these steps.[39]

Differential (environmental) susceptibility embraces both the vulnerability and the vantage sensitivity aspects (i.e., what advantages a particular personality trait might entail) and thereby recognizes that individuals with certain predispositions might be more susceptible to be affected by both negative AND positive experiences, that is, not only be more vulnerable but also show greater plasticity.[40]

SPS might just be one such a predisposing factor. More highly sensitive children who grew up in a negative, non-supporting environment were indeed more susceptible to developing mental health issues later on. However, more highly sensitive children whose environment was supportive and positive actually thrived more in life than their less highly sensitive peers.[41] Teenagers scoring higher on SPS responded better to antidepressant therapy than those scoring lower.[42] Broadening the view to not only focusing on potential faults but also including possible advantages and strengths involved with this trait opens a wide range of opportunities not only to better understand the needs of the individual and devise treatment plans but also to prevent the occurrence of psychological and physical problems as well as fulfilling the individual's potential.

Canine Sensory Processing Sensitivity: Behavior Problems in Dogs

The hypotheses of our study[5,20] were formulated bearing in mind the possible vulnerability to psychological and physical health problems as well as a higher susceptibility to environmental stimuli (in particular the interaction with the owner both on the level of personality as well as communication/training).

Again the results showed parallels to human psychology in that cSPS was positively correlated with the reported frequency of behavior problems, suggesting a possible vulnerability similar to that of SPS and mental health issues in humans.

Canine Sensory Processing Sensitivity and Differential Environmental Susceptibility

The concept of differential environmental susceptibility is of particular interest in the clinical context to understand symptoms, make diagnoses, develop treatment plans, and understand response to treatment, as well as prevent the development of problems.

In dogs too, high sensitivity seems to have a modulating effect on how environmental stimuli (owner personality (SPS), and communication/training methods in particular) affect the occurrence of behavior problems.

- *High sensitivity of dog and owner interact*: As hypothesized, the greater the difference between SPS of the owner and cSPS of the dog, the more behavior problems were reported for the dog. This was particularly the case if the dog was more highly sensitive than the owner. Formulated differently, the more similar dog and owner are in high sensitivity, the fewer behavior problems are reported, possibly suggesting a greater understanding of the dog's needs from the owner's side.
- *High sensitivity and positive punishment do not interact*: Based on the higher emotional intensity and deeper processing of information, we had hypothesized that the reporting of behavior problems would be higher in dogs scoring higher on cSPS when positive punishment (ie, the addition of something disagreeable, such as shouting at the dog or tugging on the lead) was used. This, however, was not confirmed: the reporting of positive punishment was correlated with more behavior problems independent of dog personality. Despite this result being correlational and not causal, placing this into the context of the existing literature and considering the clinical relevance, the potential important message is that positive punishment should be avoided in any dog, independent of its level of high sensitivity.
- *High sensitivity and negative punishment interact*: Somewhat surprisingly, but of no lesser practical relevance, negative punishment (ie, the withdrawal of something agreeable, such as attention or a reward) was found to interact with cSPS in regard to behavior problems. More behavior problems were reported for HSDs exposed to negative punishment than for less highly sensitive dogs exposed to negative punishment. Practically, this might suggest that more highly sensitive individuals might be more vulnerable to a lack of information.

High Sensitivity and Physical Health

As understanding of the complexity of the body and mind connection grows, the concept of psychosomatic illness or—using a more medical term—psychoneuroendocrinoimmunology and the contribution of stress on physical illness in medicine is appreciated.

With their higher subjective perception of stress, it is not farfetched to expect more highly sensitive individuals to also be more affected by physical illnesses for which stress is a relevant trigger, such as epilepsy or inflammatory-immunological diseases. On the other hand, individuals scoring higher on SPS tend to show more interoception, which might lead to them perceiving more subtle physical changes within their bodies and reacting more strongly to these.

In humans, several studies report results that suggest that differential susceptibility of highly sensitive individuals extends to some physical illnesses as well, such as chronic pain, gastrointestinal symptoms, and immune-mediated diseases including inflammatory bowel disease and Type I diabetes.[11,37,43–46]

Within the framework of our study, we collected data regarding health issues and found a tendency for physical health issues being reported more frequently in more HSDs; however, the effect was not as strong as for behavior problems (data not yet published).

There was, however, a significant positive correlation of behavior problems and health issues independent of personality, further solidifying the hypothesis of a psychological–physical association in dogs.

GENETIC CORRELATES

Aron and colleagues suggested that SPS was a "genetically determined trait." In the following years, several studies have investigated possible genetic associations, particularly regarding the metabolism of dopamine[47,48] and serotonin.[49,50]

There has been to date no research that has looked into a potential genetic basis of high sensitivity in dogs.

WHAT DOES THIS MEAN IN EVERYDAY LIFE AND CLINICAL PRACTICE?

- There are more and less highly sensitive dogs that react differently to environmental and, quite possibly, to internal stimuli. This means that they are likely to be more susceptible to influences and changes than less highly sensitive individuals are.
- High sensitivity in dogs can be measured using the validated HSD questionnaire.
- At least some of what we know from humans applies to dogs as well, that is, in practice, the acronym of DOES (ie, Depth of processing, Overstimulation, Emotional Intensity, Sensory Sensitivity) can be applied to dogs to gauge their sensitivity.

APPROACHING AND TREATING THE HIGHLY SENSITIVE VETERINARY PATIENT

Life is not about how fast you run or how high you climb, but how well you bounce
(Vivian Komori)

Grasping an animal's personality as a whole could be one possible stepping stone to bridging the gap discussed earlier between a systematic scientific approach and the individuality of an actual patient. Based on the above-mentioned findings in humans and dogs as well as own empirical experience, the following are suggestions of how—not exclusively, but particularly—more highly sensitive animals may benefit from veterinarians, especially behaviorists,recognizing and integrating this personality trait into their diagnostic process, handling, treatment as well as prevention plans. Despite the lack of solid scientific evidence to date, working by this assumption can only potentially benefit all individuals and would not do harm to any, and in the best case, it would help the individual to "bounce."

Applying the Basic Characteristics Described by DOES to Canine Sensory Processing Sensitivity in Dogs

- D as in Depth of Processing: As more highly sensitive patients process information perceived by all sense organs more deeply, this implies that on the one hand, they need to receive information and on the other they need to be provided enough time to process it.
- O as in Overstimulation/arousal: Although all animals are confronted with many stimuli in a veterinary setting, the likelihood of a more highly sensitive individual being overwhelmed is greater. This is especially the case if there is a lack of information, there is a quick and intense physiologic and emotional response and there is no time to process.
- E as in Emotional intensity: Remember that these individual not only experience their own emotions intensely but are also particularly fine-tuned to pick up on the emotions and moods of their surroundings. This includes a potentially anxious or nervous owner or a stressed or insecure staff member. Any stress-related, emotional, mental, or physical health issues of the owners (or veterinary staff) are more likely to contribute to the stress levels of these patients.
- S as in Sensory sensitivity/Interoceptive sensitivity: Highly sensitive patients not only are more likely to be aware of react more strongly to visual, acoustic, tactile, olfactory and gustatory stimuli but are probably also more interoceptive. They might perceive and react more strongly to more subtle changes within their bodies, such as a subtle pinch of a nerve in a specific situation, a slight change in perception due to focal epileptic seizures, a hint of feeling nauseated or dizzy or feeling "different" in response to medication, which in a less highly sensitive individual might not lead to an emotional reaction, arousal, or change in behavior. This physical discomfort might only be expressed as changes in behavior rather than obvious physical symptoms, for example, increased rest-lessness at night, sudden fear of being touched or going on walks or going into the yard, development/aggravation of fear of sounds and so forth. Regarding treatment, this may imply that the more highly sensitive patient shows more side effects or stronger effects of medication, necessitating lower doses, slower increases or weaning off of medication, or adaptation of choice of medication. Their sensitivity can lead to these patients responding more favorably to physical treatment techniques, such as osteopathy or acupuncture, Tellington Touch, Canine Bowen Technique or, on the other hand, to them being more easily overwhelmed, especially initially, by physical touch.

What We Can Do to Help Our Highly Sensitive Veterinary Patients

- Give them time: The need to understand and collect information takes time, which is often not provided to our pets in our fast-paced lives. Moreover, because we integrate our animals into our lives, they often have no opportunity or way of communicating when they actually need a break or more time to process. Often, the only way possible for such an individual to convey this is by "behaving" differently, and often in ways that either are not recognized (eg, subtle signs of stress or anxiety such as yawning, slowing down their pace, panting or breathing more shallowly) or actually bother the human surroundings (eg, by refusing to cooperate, stopping completely, being highly reactive, or aggressive). If they are not given this time or rest, this can lead to a state of chronic stress associated with more overt signs of psychological suffering, such as aggressive or "hyper" behaviors, as well as aggravation of physical symptoms such as excessive self-directed behaviors, interstitial cystitis, gastrointestinal symptoms, or immune-mediated diseases. Highly sensitive patients therefore need (more) time and more breaks both on a daily basis and during veterinary visits.

- Optimize stimulation: More highly sensitive individuals need or even seek information, are aware of details and process information more deeply. This process in itself has the potential of leading to intense emotions and quickly being over-stimulated and overwhelmed (also typical characteristics of more highly sensitive individuals). The challenge for the environment is to find the right amount and type of stimulation and the balance of stimulation and rest for the particular individual, especially in everyday situations. This is also a central aspect that needs to be considered in preventive work and treatment of highly sensitive patients, especially those showing behavior problems. If we can manage to optimize stimulation and experiences for the particular individual, we might be able to help this animal thrive as opposed to him or her being overwhelmed. This can mean that, for example, puppy classes are individually adapted because uncontrolled social interactions and play might not be suitable for every puppy. Exposing puppies to a whole range of possible stimuli during this socialization phase might actually be counterproductive for some individuals, while promoting curiosity, individuality and allowing choice as opposed to focusing on complete obedience might in the long-term promote psychological health and the human–animal bond, especially in the HSD. In the context of a veterinary visit, reduction of fear, anxiety, and stress applies to all animals independent of their personality. More highly sensitive individuals, however, might especially benefit from these measures.
- Provide information and a sense of control: Unpredictable and uncontrollable situations and interactions have the potential of increasing anxiety, fear, and stress in any individual. Considering differential susceptibility, however, individuals scoring higher on cSPS might be more affected by a lack of as well as an increase of predictability and controllability, in a negative and positive way, respectively, both in daily life and in the veterinary context.
- Promote relaxation: Stress reduction not only involves optimizing stimulation to the animal's need but also included active encouragement of relaxation, especially by tapping into the sensory sensitivity and emotional intensity aspects of cSPS. Some animals respond well to physical therapies such as osteopathy or Tellington Touch, others to relaxing odours, for example, lavender or valerian essential oils, some to calming sounds such as classical music, and others just need a calm, peaceful environment in the presence or absence of the owner.
- Offer emotional support: Allowing the owner to be present as an emotional support system for the animal can help, as long as the owner is not overly anxious him or herself. If additional anxiety issues are present in the veterinary context, use pre-veterinary anxiolytic medication. Again, this can help animals of all personalities, but highly sensitive and anxious individuals may especially benefit.
- Be aware of your own behaviors and emotions: The highly sensitive patient is also especially aware of your body language, your emotions, your own stress and anxiety levels. It is important to stop and watch, even just for a moment

and even if it does not correspond to your own personality, to subtly observe the patient, take a deep breath and adapt your way of communicating with the animal and its owner, if necessary.

- Internal support: SPS in humans is accompanied by an increased vulnerability to develop mental health problems. We also need to keep in mind that cSPS is not the only personality trait that defines the individual and other traits present in dogs, such as anxiety, may predispose to mental health problems as well. Therefore, psychoactive medication can be indicated in as needed situations or on a daily basis, both in patients suffering from primarily psychological as well as physical illnesses with a potentially high psychological stress component, such as epilepsy[51] or interstitial cystitis.[52,53] Keeping in mind the potential higher interoceptive sensitivity of highly sensitive patients, it is wise to start these individuals on lower doses and to gradually increase these if necessary and to generally adapt a slow weaning process of medication when possible.

One could conclude—in the sense of the Emerson quote presented at the beginning—that one of the greatest responsibilities of the (behavior) veterinarian is exactly this: to help create an environment, in which the individual animal can be itself.

CLINICS CARE POINTS

- Time and patience.
- Optimize stimulation.
- Provide information.
- Offer a sense of control, give them a choice and thereby a voice.
- Actively promote relaxation.
- Offer emotional support.
- Be aware of your own behaviors and emotions.
- Introduce changes gradually, including drug dosages.

DISCLOSURE

The author declares that she has no relevant or material financial interests that relate to the research described in this paper.

REFERENCES

1. Stamps J, Groothuis TGG. The development of animal personality: relevance, concepts and perspectives. Biol Rev 2010;85(2):301–25.
2. Svartberg K. A comparison of behaviour in test and in everyday life: evidence of three consistent boldness-related personality traits in dogs. Appl Anim Behav Sci 2005;91(1–2):103–28.
3. Wright HF, Mills DS, Pollux PMJ. Behavioural and physiological correlates of impulsivity in the domestic dog (Canis familiaris). Physiol Behav 2012;105(3): 676–82.
4. McPeake KJ, Collins LM, Zulch H, et al. The canine frustration questionnaire—Development of a new psychometric tool for measuring frustration in domestic dogs (Canis familiaris). Front Vet Sci 2019;6(MAY):152.

5. Braem M, Asher L, Furrer S, et al. Development of the "Highly Sensitive Dog" questionnaire to evaluate the personality dimension "Sensory Processing Sensitivity" in dogs. PLoS One 2017;12(5):e0177616.
6. Braem MD, Mills DS. Factors affecting response of dogs to obedience instruction: A field and experimental study. Appl Anim Behav Sci 2010;125(1–2):47–55.
7. Aron EN, Aron A. Sensory-processing sensitivity and its relation to introversion and emotionality. J Pers Soc Psychol 1997;73(2):345–68.
8. Aron A, Ketay S, Hedden T, et al. Temperament trait of sensory processing sensitivity moderates cultural differences in neural response. Soc Cogn Affect Neurosci 2010;5(2–3):219–26.
9. Aron EN, Aron A, Jagiellowicz J. Sensory processing sensitivity: a review in the light of the evolution of biological responsivity. Pers Soc Psychol Rev 2012;16(3):262–82.
10. Acevedo BP, Santander T, Marhenke R, et al. Sensory processing sensitivity predicts individual differences in resting-state functional connectivity associated with depth of processing. Neuropsychobiology 2021;80(2):185–200.
11. Benham G. The highly sensitive person: stress and physical symptom reports. Pers Indiv Differ 2006;40:1433–40.
12. Jagiellowicz J, Aron A, Aron EN, et al. High sensitivity: major differences in emotion and cognition processing. American Psychological Association Convention Presentation 2010. https://doi.org/10.1037/e614632010-001.
13. Acevedo BP, Aron EN, Aron A, et al. The highly sensitive brain: an fMRI study of sensory processing sensitivity and response to others' emotions. Brain Behav 2014;4(4):580–94.
14. Gerstenberg FXR. Sensory-processing sensitivity predicts performance on a visual search task followed by an increase in perceived stress. Pers Indiv Differ 2012;53(4):496–500.
15. Jagiellowicz J, Xu X, Aron A, et al. The trait of sensory processing sensitivity and neural responses to changes in visual scenes. Soc Cogn Affect Neur 2011;6(1):38–47.
16. Schaefer M, Kühnel A, Gärtner M. Sensory processing sensitivity and somatosensory brain activation when feeling touch. Sci Rep-uk 2022;12(1):12024.
17. Wallisch A, Little LM, Bruce AS, et al. Oral Sensory Sensitivity Influences Attentional Bias to Food Logo Images in Children: A Preliminary Investigation. Front Psychol 2022;13:895516.
18. Poerio GL, Mank S, Hostler TJ. The awesome as well as the awful: Heightened sensory sensitivity predicts the presence and intensity of Autonomous Sensory Meridian Response (ASMR). J Res Pers 2022;97. 104183.
19. Schredl M, Blamo AE, Ehrenfeld F, et al. Dream Recall Frequency and Sensory-Processing Sensitivity. Dreaming 2022;32(1):15–22.
20. Bräm M, Asher L, Würbel H, et al. Parallels in the interactive effect of highly sensitive personality and social factors on behaviour problems in dogs and humans. Sci Rep 2020;10(1):1–9.
21. Bolhuis JE, Schouten WGP, Schrama JW, et al. Individual coping characteristics, aggressiveness and fighting strategies in pigs. Anim Behav 2005;69(5):1085–91.
22. Suomi SJ. How Gene-Environment Interactions Shape Biobehavioral Development: Lessons From Studies With Rhesus Monkeys. Res Hum Dev 2004;1(3):205–22.
23. Benus RF, Bohus B, Koolhaas JM, et al. Behavioural strategies of aggressive and non-aggressive male mice in active shock avoidance. Behav Process 1989;20(1):1–12.

24. Coppens CM, Boer SFD, Koolhaas JM. Coping styles and behavioural flexibility: towards underlying mechanisms. Philos Trans R Soc Lond B Biol Sci 2010; 365(1560):4021–8.
25. Carere C, Drent PJ, Privitera L, et al. Personalities in great tits, Parus major: stability and consistency. Anim Behav 2005;70(4):795–805.
26. Carere C, Oers K van. Shy and bold great tits (Parus major): body temperature and breath rate in response to handling stress. Physiol Behav 2004;82(5):905–12.
27. Svartberg K. Shyness–boldness predicts performance in working dogs. Appl Anim Behav Sci 2002;79(2):157–74.
28. Pluess M, Assary E, Lionetti F, et al. Environmental sensitivity in children: Development of the highly sensitive child scale and identification of sensitivity groups. Dev Psychol 2017;54(1):51–70.
29. Smolewska KA, McCabe SB, Woody EZ. A psychometric evaluation of the Highly Sensitive Person Scale: The components of sensory-processing sensitivity and their relation to the BIS/BAS and "Big Five". Pers Indiv Differ 2005;40(6):1269–79.
30. Attary T, Ghazizadeh A. Localizing sensory processing sensitivity and its subdomains within its relevant trait space: a data-driven approach. Sci Rep-uk 2021; 11(1). 20343.
31. Evans DE, Rothbart MK. Temperamental sensitivity: Two constructs or one? Pers Indiv Differ 2007;44(1):108–18.
32. Aron EN, Aron A, Davies KM. Adult shyness: the interaction of temperamental sensitivity and an adverse childhood environment. Pers Soc Psychol Bull 2005; 31(2):181–97.
33. Acevedo BP, Aron EN, Aron A, et al. Sensory processing sensitivity and its relation to sensation seeking. Curr Res Behav Sci 2023;4. 100100.
34. Thomas H. Sensory Processing Sensitivity & Well Being within the Integral Community. Is there a vantage sensitivity. Integral Leadership Review 2015;22/1.
35. Gulla B, Golonka K. Exploring Protective Factors in Wellbeing: How Sensory Processing Sensitivity and Attention Awareness Interact With Resilience. Front Psychol 2021;12. 751679.
36. Costa-López B, Ruiz-Robledillo N, Ferrer-Cascales R, et al. Relationship between sensory processing sensitivity and mental health. J Clin Med 2021. https://doi.org/10.3390/ecerph-3-09064.
37. Damatac CG, ter Avest MJ, Wilderjans TF, et al. Sensory processing sensitivity associations with mental and somatic health in positive and negative environments: evidence for differential susceptibility. Published online 2023. doi:10.31234/osf.io/375gb.
38. Seligman MEP. Positive Psychology: A Personal History. Annu Rev Clin Psycho 2018;15(1):1–24.
39. Mellor D, Beausoleil N. Extending the 'Five Domains' model for animal welfare assessment to incorporate positive welfare states. Anim Welfare 2015;24(3): 241–53.
40. Belsky J, Pluess M. Beyond diathesis stress: Differential susceptibility to environmental influences. Psychol Bull 2009;135(6):885–908.
41. Keers R, Pluess M. Childhood quality influences genetic sensitivity to environmental influences across adulthood: A life-course Gene × Environment interaction study. Dev Psychopathol 2017;29(05):1921–33.
42. Pluess M, Boniwell I. Sensory-processing sensitivity predicts treatment response to a school-based depression prevention program: evidence of Vantage Sensitivity. Pers Indiv Differ 2015;82(C):40–5.

43. Koechlin H, Donado C, Locher C, et al. Sensory processing sensitivity in adolescents reporting chronic pain: an exploratory study. Pain Reports 2023;8(1):e1053.
44. Taghlidabad BG, Mashhadi RT. Investigating the Relationship Between Sensory Processing Sensitivity and Life Style With Stress in Patients With Irritable Bowel Syndrome. Pract Clin Psychol 2018;6(4):239–48.
45. Iimura S, Takasugi S. Sensory Processing Sensitivity and Gastrointestinal Symptoms in Japanese Adults. Int J Environ Res Pu 2022;19(16):9893.
46. Goldberg A, Ebraheem Z, Freiberg C, et al. Sweet and Sensitive: Sensory Processing Sensitivity and Type 1 Diabetes. J Pediatr Nurs 2018;38(C):e35–8.
47. Bakermans-Kranenburg MJ, Ijzendoorn MHV, Pijlman FTA, et al. Experimental evidence for differential susceptibility: Dopamine D4 receptor polymorphism (DRD4 VNTR) moderates intervention effects on toddlers' externalizing behavior in a randomized controlled trial. Dev Psychol 2008;44(1):293–300.
48. Chen C, Chen C, Moyzis R, et al. Contributions of dopamine-related genes and environmental factors to highly sensitive personality: a multi-step neuronal system-level approach. PLoS One 2011;6(7):e21636.
49. Homberg JR, Schubert D, Asan E, et al. Sensory processing sensitivity and serotonin gene variance: Insights into mechanisms shaping environmental sensitivity. Neurosci Biobehav Rev 2016;71:472–83.
50. Licht CL, Mortensen EL, Hjordt LV, et al. Serotonin transporter gene (SLC 6A4) variation and sensory processing sensitivity – comparison with other anxiety-related temperamental dimensions. Mol Genet Genom Med 2020;8:e1352.
51. Packer R, Hobbs SL, Veterinary EBF in. Behavioural interventions as an adjunctive treatment for canine epilepsy: a missing part of the epilepsy management toolkit? Frontiersin.org 2019. https://doi.org/10.3389/fvets.2019.00003.
52. Buffington C, Westropp J, Chew D, et al. Clinical evaluation of multimodal environmental modification (MEMO) in the management of cats with idiopathic cystitis. J Feline Med Surg 2006;8(4):261–8.
53. Westropp JL, Kass PH, Buffington CAT. Evaluation of the effects of stress in cats with idiopathic cystitis. American journal of veterinary research 2006;67(4):731–6.

Veterinary Psychopharmacology

Leticia M.S. Dantas, DVM, MS, PhD[a,b,*], Niwako Ogata, BVSc, PhD[a,c,*]

KEYWORDS

- Psychopharmacology • Veterinary psychiatry • Stress • Fear • Anxiety

KEY POINTS

- The stress response and the emotional states of fear and anxiety lead to neurotransmitter and hormonal changes that negatively affect multiple systems of the body.
- Psychopharmacology treatments can improve the quality of life and increase life span in veterinary patients.
- Clinicians need to understand mechanisms of action and drug associations to tailor care to each individual patient.

INTRODUCTION

The link between mental and behavioral problems in physical health is well-documented in human medicine, and a body of evidence has also grown in veterinary medicine.[1] The stress response, both acute and chronic, affects not just the central nervous system but multiple other systems in the body, such as cardiovascular, endocrine, gastrointestinal and the immune system.[2,3] Chronic mental and behavioral pathologies are associated with inflammation, dysfunctions in the immune response, and an increased risk for other chronic inflammatory and metabolic diseases.[4] Psychiatric treatments not only alleviate fear, stress, and anxiety, but also significantly increase qualify of life and increase lifespan for dogs and cats.[5]

It is important that clinicians understand the function of neurotransmitters and hormones on emotional processing, cognition and behavior, and drug mechanism of action so medication selection is appropriate. Drug selection should be based on each patient's individual's history, severity, and type of clinical signs, among other

Neither author has any commercial or financial conflicts of interest or any funding sources.
[a] American College of Veterinary Behaviorists, Certified Fear Free Professional; [b] Department of Biomedical Sciences, Behavioral Medicine Service, University of Georgia Veterinary Teaching Hospital, 501 D.W. Brooks Drive, Athens, GA 30602, USA; [c] Department of Clinical Sciences, Veterinary Behavior Medicine, Purdue University, 625 Harrison Street, West Lafayette, IN 47907, USA
* Corresponding authors. Department of Clinical Sciences, Veterinary Behavior Medicine, Purdue University, 625 Harrison Street, West Lafayette, IN 47907.
E-mail addresses: lsdantas@uga.edu; leticia.zoopsych@gmail.com (L.M.S.D.); nogata@purdue.edu; lsdantas@uga.edu; leticia.zoopsych@gmail.com (N.O.)

Vet Clin Small Anim 54 (2024) 195–205
https://doi.org/10.1016/j.cvsm.2023.07.003
0195-5616/24/Published by Elsevier Inc.

characteristics. Polypharmaceutical approaches are often more effective than single-drug treatments.[6]

MOST COMMONLY USED MEDICATION CLASSES IN VETERINARY PSYCHIATRY AND BEHAVIORAL MEDICINE
Selective Serotonin Reuptake Inhibitors

SSRIs mainly inhibit the reuptake of serotonin. This results in an increase in serotonergic neurotransmission by allowing serotonin molecules to act for extended periods of time. With prolonged use, there is a down-regulation of serotonin receptors. These medications can be effective for long term, chronic treatments, and are not appropriate for PRN or as needed administration. The only FDA-approved veterinary product is Reconcile (fluoxetine). Reconcile is licensed for an adjunct treatment with behavior modification for separation anxiety disorder in dogs. Two double-blind randomized placebo-controlled studies aimed to evaluate the effectiveness of fluoxetine in combination with behavior modification in dogs.[7,8] Simpson and colleagues (2007) resulted to enroll a total of 197 dogs, with 101 dogs receiving standardized behavior modification along with fluoxetine.[7] The study reported a significant improvement rate of 72% over the 8-week treatment period. In comparison, the remaining 96 dogs in the study were administered a placebo, resulting in a 50% improvement rate. Similarly, Landsberg and colleagues (2008) conducted a study involving 163 dogs, where 83 dogs received fluoxetine alone while 80 dogs received a placebo.[8] The study found a 65.1% improvement rate among the fluoxetine group over a 6-week treatment period, compared to a 51.3% improvement rate among the placebo group. Both studies emphasized the importance of combining behavior modification with fluoxetine to maximize treatment outcomes.

Other applications of treatments with SSRIs include several anxiety and fear-related problems, aggression, and obsessive-compulsive disorders in dogs and cats.[9] These medications are often augmented by other drugs for more effective treatment protocols. Most commonly used SSRIs in veterinary medicine are listed on the **Table 1** in the end of the text.

Tricyclic antidepressants

TCAs act as reuptake inhibitors of both serotonin and noradrenaline. They also have antihistaminic and anticholinergic effects and are α-1 adrenergic antagonists. The action on each of these four neurotransmitters varies widely among the different drugs belonging to this group. TCAs can be effective for long term, chronic treatments, and are not appropriate for as needed administration. Among TCAs, clomipramine is the drug with the highest serotonergic action. The brand name product, Clomicalm (clomipramine), is FDA approved as an adjunct treatment with behavior modification for separation anxiety in dogs. Other applications of clomipramine in dogs include anxiety and fear-related problems,[10] obsessive-compulsive disorder.[11-14] When it was used to treat aggression toward owners without behavior modification, no effects were observed comparing to placebo.[15] However, according to a case report,[16] when it was used to treat inter-dog aggression with environmental and behavior modification, the dog's behavior was improved.

Clomipramine has been used to treat feline behavioral problems, such as urine marking or psychogenic alopecia. In a meta-analysis of the use of clomipramine as a treatment for urine spraying in cats, Mills and colleagues (2011) found a significant association between clomipramine use and the number of cats that ceased urine spraying or decreased the behavior by 90%.[17] While in a prospective, double-blind, placebo-controlled, randomized trial, clomipramine was more effective than placebo in the

Table 1
Drug dosing and administration table

Medication Name/Class	Dog	Cat
Citalopram (SSRI)	0.5–1.0 mg/kg q24 h	-
Fluoxetine (SSRI)	1.0–2.0 mg/kg q24 h	0.5–1.5 mg/kg q24 h
Fluvoxamine (SSRI)	1–2 mg/kg q24 h	0.25–0.5 mg/kg q24 h
Paroxetine (SSRI)	1.0–1.5 mg/kg q24 h	0.5–1.5 mg/kg q24 h
Sertraline (SSRI)	0.5–4.0 mg/kg q24 h	0.5–1.5 mg/kg q24 h
Buspirone (Azapirone)	0.5–2.0 mg/kg q8–24h	2.5–7.5 mg/cat q12 h or 0.5–1.0 mg/kg q12 h
Trazodone (SARI)	1.7–19.5 mg/kg (q24 h or PRN) or 1.7–9.5 mg/kg PO q8-24h	50–100 mg per cat PRN or 10.6–33.3 mg/kg PRN
Venlavaxine (SNRI)	2.5 mg/kg q4h	0.9–1.9 mg/kg q24 h
Gabapentin (α2δ ligand)	2–20 mg/kg q8h 10–20 mg/kg (PRN)	3–10 mg/kg q8h 5–20 mg/kg (PRN)
Pregabalin (α2δ ligand)	2-4 mg/kg q 8–12h	1–2 mg/kg q12 h 5–10 mg/kg PRN
Clonidine (Alpha2 agonist)	0.01–0.05 mg/kg q 8–12h or PRN	Dose not published to this date
Dexmedetomidine oromucosal gel (Alpha2 agonist)	Follow Sileo® dosing table	1 dot/cat PRN
Alprazolam (benzodiazepine)	0.02–0.1 mg/kg q4h	0.0125–0.25 mg/kg q8h
Clonazepam (benzodiazepine)	0.1–0.5 mg/kg q8–12h	0.015–0.2 mg/kg q8h
Clorazepate (benzodiazepine)	0.5–2.0 mg/kg q4h	0.5–2.0 mg/kg q12 h
Lorazepam (benzodiazepine)	0.02–0.5 mg/kg q8–12h	0.03–0.08 mg/kg q12 h
Oxazepam (benzodiazepine)	0.04–0.5 mg/kg q6h	0.2–1.0 mg/kg q12–24h
Diazepam (benzodiazepine)	0.5–2.0 mg/kg q4h	0.1–1.0 mg/kg q4h
Amitriptyline (TCA)	1–6 mg/kg q12 h	0.5–2.0 mg/kg q12–24h
Clomipramine (TCA)	1.0–3.0 mg/kg q12 h	0.25–1.3 mg/kg q24 h
Doxepin (TCA)	3.0–5.0 mg/kg q8–12h	0.5–1.0 mg/kg q12 h
Imipramine (TCA)	0.5–2.0 mg/kg q8–12h	0.5–1.0 mg/kg q12–24h
Nortriptyline (TCA)	1.0–2.0 mg/kg q12 h	0.5–2.0 mg/kg q12–24h
Memantine (NMDA antagonist)	0.3–1 mg/kg q12 h	-
Huperzine-A (NMDA antagonist)	1 μg/kg q12 h	-

treatment of feline psychogenic alopecia.[18,19] Side effects reported from these studies are sedation, anorexia, and anticholinergic effects such as decreased frequency of urination and defecation. While clomipramine does not induce changes in EKG when it is used standard therapeutic doses in dogs and cats, sufficiently large doses can induce cardiotoxicity.[20,21] Clomipramine can decrease thyroid value, such as T4, fT4 in both dogs and cats, which may not present clinical signs of hypothyroidism.

Serotonin Noradrenaline (Norepinephrine) Reuptake Inhibitors

SNRIs inhibit the reuptake of both serotonin and noradrenaline. This increases the levels of these neurotransmitters in the extracellular space (synapses between neurons), which can lead to improved mood, reduced anxiety, and relief from chronic pain conditions.[22] Unlike SSRIs, which primarily affect serotonin levels, SNRIs also target noradrenaline, which is involved in the "fight or flight" or stress response. With prolonged use, SNRIs can lead to the down-regulation of both serotonin and noradrenaline receptors, which can contribute to their effectiveness as antidepressants and pain relievers. These medications can be effective for long term, chronic treatments, and are not appropriate for PRN or as needed administration. These medications are often augmented by other drugs for more effective treatment protocols.

SNRIs and TCAs have some similarities in their mechanism of action, however, TCAs also have additional effects on other neurotransmitters, which leads to additional side effects. In veterinary behavioral medicine, venlafaxine has been used to treat behavior problems related to anxiety, fear and aggression and possible underlying pain in cats.[22–25] It was originally published in a canine narcolepsy-cataplexy case report but it is current also used in dogs for similar anxiety and fear-related problems.[26]

Azapirones

Azapirones are partial agonists of 5HT1A receptors. Buspirone is the only azapirone that is commercially available in the United States. Buspirone can be used for a variety of anxiety disorders and behavioral responses secondary to anxiety and fear. It can also be used solo or, observing caution for the risk of serotonin syndrome, as an adjunct drug to treatments with antidepressants and other psychoactive medications in polypharmaceutical treatments.[27]

Buspirone is generally dosed two to three times a day and has delayed onset of action around 2 to 6 weeks after administration in cats.[28] Unlike benzodiazepines, buspirone does not cause dependency and serious side effects. The potential acute adverse effects of this drug such are sedation, aggression, and agitation in cats.[29] Due to poor bioavailability, transdermal administration is not recommended.[28,30]

Serotonin Antagonist and Reuptake Inhibitors

Trazodone is the most used SARI in veterinary medicine. It is an antagonist at 5HT 2A and 2C receptors and alpha 2 adrenoreceptor. It also stimulates 5-HT1A as serotonin reuptake inhibitor. Trazodone has a dose dependent effect where hypnotic effect is reported in low doses while anti-depressant effects are reported in the chronic administration of higher doses.[31] Similarly to buspirone, trazodone is used to treat fear, anxiety and several behavioral problems secondary to these emotional states. Trazodone can also be used by itself or with caution as an adjunct drug in polypharmaceutical treatments. This medication should not be combined with any MAOI.[27]

Adverse effects reported in human medicine includes nausea, vomiting, diarrhea, edema, drowsiness, dizziness, incoordination, sedation, lethargy, blurred vision, changes in weight, headache, muscle pain, dry mouth, bad taste in the mouth, stuffy nose, constipation, or change in sexual interest/ability. Additionally, tremors, seizures, mania, priapism, allergic reactions, suicidal behavior, QT prolongation, arrhythmias, hypotension, syncope, and sinus bradycardia have also been reported in humans. Low levels of potassium or magnesium in the blood can increase the risk of QT prolongation, so conditions that cause severe sweating, diarrhea, or vomiting and diuretics used together with trazodone may increase the risk in humans.[32,33] A case of acute hepatotoxicity in one dog treated with trazodone 4 mg/kg, q12 to 24h was reported.[34]

A randomized double-blind placebo-controlled studies with the mean dose of 15.13 ± 1.6 mg/kg/day (divided into twice-daily dosing) administration for up to

4 weeks post-surgery in dogs did not show differences in behavioral efficacy to placebo.[35] While Kim and colleagues (2022) reported trazodone administrating in the range of 9 to 12 mg/kg, 90 minutes before transport to the veterinary clinic reduced stress signs comparing to placebo.[36] Trazodone has only one double-blind placebo controlled study in cats with the administration of a single dose.[37] In this study, a single dose of 50 mg per cat (dose ranged from 7.7 mg/kg to 15.2 mg/kg) given 1 to 1.5 hours prior to the transport, reduced anxiety signs related to transport and veterinary examination scored by veterinarians and owners compared to placebo. The most common adverse reaction was sleepiness. When 50, 75 and 100 mg (doses were respectively 10.6–16.7 mg/kg, 16.0–25 mg/kg and 21.3–33.3 mg/kg) of single dose of trazodone was given, the lowest activity occurred at 2.5 h post-trazodone 100 mg but no other adverse effects.[38]

Alpha-2-delta Calcium Channel Ligands

Gabapentin

Gabapentin is a GABA analogue and binds with high affinity to α2-delta subunits of voltage-activated Ca2+ channels in the central nervous system and it reduces the release of neurotransmitters, such as substance P and excitatory amino acids.[39] It is used solo or as an adjunctive medication for seizures neuropathic pain and to treat anxiety and fear.

Pharmacokinetic studies in dogs have reported that maximum plasma concentration reached from 1.3 to 1.5 hours and half-life being 3.3 and 3.4 hours for oral doses of 10 to 20 mg/kg, respectively. There are two double-blind placebo controlled study in dogs. It is reported according to owner's observation, a single dose of gabapentin (25–30 mg/kg) appear to reduce the dog's fear response to storms.[40] Gabapentin was used in another study as pre-veterinary visit in healthy dogs with a single dose (50 mg/kg) and did not show significant behavior difference compared to placebo.[26] Both studies did not report major adverse effects but transient ataxia. Few dogs showed salivation, muscular fasciculation,[25] vomiting, and increased activity.[41]

Cats given 10 mg/kg dose exhibit high variation in absorption with mean peak levels being around 1.6 hours.[42,43] and the half-life being about 3 hours.[42] Several articles reported anxiolytic effects to alleviate the stress of veterinary visits in both healthy and unhealthy cats, such as hyperthyroid (tested dose was 20 mg/kg) and intradermal testing (25–35 mg/kg). Quimby and colleagues (2022) reported that gabapentin is primarily excreted by the kidneys and 50% or more dose reduction should be considered for renal patients.[44] Recently, based on the double-blind randomized placebo controlled study Eagan and colleagues, (2023) reported to use 10 mg/kg of liquid gabapentin BID improved signs of stress in cats at shelter.[45] It was beneficial in the behavioral modification progress during their stay in a shelter. That daily dose did not cause adverse effects during the treatment period for 4 to 51 days (median 11 days).

Pregabalin

Pregabalin is similar in mode of action to gabapentin, but it binds more potently to calcium channels and is faster acting. The half-life of pregabalin in dogs is 6.9 hours, and cats is 10.4 hours. Pregabalin has been known to be used for neuropathic pain in dogs.[46,47] One study published a single dose of pregabalin (5 mg/kg and 10 mg/kg) for a transport anxiety in cats suggested that it alleviated anxiety and fear associated with transportation.[48] Similarly to gabapentin, pregabalin can be used as a solo medication or in drug associations.

Alpha 2 Agonists

Stressors increase the responsivity of locus coeruleus neurons, which exaggerates noradrenaline reactivity. Therefore, pharmacologic agents, specifically target noradrenaline hyper-reactivity through these adrenergic receptors, alleviate stress responses. There are 4 subtypes, alpha2A, 2B, 2C, and 2D in alpha2 adrenergic receptors. Although its diversity, density, and locations among species appear to be different, in dogs alpha 2A receptors predominate in the central nervous system.[49]

Clonidine

Clonidine is a selective alpha2 adrenergic agonist with some alpha1 agonist activity. Clonidine binds to alph2 A, alpha2 B, and alpha2 C receptors as well as imidazoline receptors which are partially related to sedation and hypotensive.[50]

Ogata and Dodman (2011) studied clonidine for situational use with other anti-anxiety medications, such as TCAs or SSRIs, as a treatment of fear-based behavior problems and anxiety disorders (such as noise phobia, separation anxiety or fear/territorial aggression).[51] According to owners' report with the dose of 0.01 to 0.05 mg/kg oral administration, the reduction of fear-based behavior was observed 1.5 to 2 hours after the administration of clonidine and the effect waned after 4 to 6 hours. Although the study only reported increased noise sensitivity in one out of 22 dogs, dose-dependent adverse effects of hypotension, bradycardia, and sedation should be monitored.[50] No study using clonidine in cats has been published to this date, but clonidine is used as an antidiarrheal agent for inflammatory bowel disease in dogs and cats at 0.005 to 0.01 mg/kg BID-TID SC or PO.[52]

Dexmedetomidine

Dexmedetomidine oromucosal (OTM) gel form is FDA approved for the treatment of noise aversion in dogs. Time to maximum concentration, and bioavailability for dexmedetomidine OTM gel (Sileo) was 0.6 hour, and 28%, respectively and elimination half-life was 0.5 to 3 hours in the original study.[53]

Randomized double-blind placebo-controlled studies in dogs using dexmedetomidine OTM gel (Sileo) reported its effects to anxiety and fear related loud noises,[54] and during veterinary visits.[55,56] Two studies used the standard dose of 125 μg/m,[2,54,55] and the study used both 125 and 250 μg/m^2 doses[56] reported the higher dose was not necessary to enhance the treatment effect, yet mild bradycardia detected in the two out of 24 dogs with 250 μg/m^2 dose. Thus, the authors recommended to use the standard dose of 125 μg/m^2.

According to one pilot study by using 12 cats where Sileo(1 dot = 0.25 mL) OTM administration compared with 100 mg of oral gabapentin administration, and placebo, respectively for 10 minute-car ride anxiety, anxious behavior, such as lip licking, and cortisol response were significantly lower in Sileo and gabapentin treated felines compared with placebo. The cats with gabapentin treatment showed significantly lower respiratory rate post car ride compared with Sileo and placebo[57]

When thermal antinociception was compared between intramuscular and transmucosal administration of dexmedetomidine injectable form in cats, sedative and antinociceptive effects were similar. In both administration route high % of vomiting was observed within 10 minutes of the administration, which might have been prevented if the cats were fasted based on another study. Since the outcome is similar, the study concluded OTM route can be more tolerant route than IM in cats.[58]

Benzodiazepines

Benzodiazepines bind to $GABA_A$ receptors. These are DEA Schedule IV drugs and it should be prescribed carefully due to the potential for human abuse. Benzodiazepines can be prescribed to reduce anxiety, fear and panic, in which a rapid onset of action is desired. Examples of published use include specific phobias such as storm phobia or separation anxiety with panic attacks, and fear of people (without aggression) in dogs; urine marking, storm phobia, separation anxiety, and fearful behavior in cats.[59]

Benzodiazepines with active metabolites, especially diazepam, should be used with caution in cats because of the rare possibility of medication-induced hepatic necrosis.[60–63] Selection of benzodiazepines without active metabolites for cats is ideal.

The use of benzodiazepines in patients with the potential to display aggression is not advised, as there are reports of this group of medications increasing aggressive behavior. Benzodiazepines should be avoided or used with extreme caution in cases involving aggressive animals. It is essential that companion animal owners are educated about the potential risks if this medication is prescribed.[59] Selection of safer medications is advised.

Benzodiazepines have a wide variation in the optimum dose in patients. It is recommended that the pet owner gives the patient a test dose in the low range of the dosage schedule at a time when they will be home to watch the pet for several hours. It is also critical to inform clients for potential side effects, such as ataxia, incoordination and hyperphagia. Paradoxic excitement or sedation can also occur, and the dose needs to be adjusted accordingly or the medication should be discontinued. Additionally, benzodiazepines are known to potentially lead to tolerance and dependency. Tolerance is when a patient is on a benzodiazepine for an extended period, steadily greater doses may be eventually required to achieve the same behavioral effect.[64] Although dependency is not well documented in veterinary medicine, in humans it is associated with high dosage drug regimens, higher potency of benzodiazepines with the long duration of treatment.[65,66] Slow tapering off is recommended when discontinuing treatment. Abrupt discontinuation may result in rebound (resumption of symptoms that may be more intense than they were before treatment). All benzodiazepines have similar therapeutic effects, but its onset of action, duration, intensity and metabolisms vary.

N-methyl-D-aspartate Antagonists

Glutamate (or Glutamic acid) is an excitatory amino acid that works as the major neurotransmitter in the central nervous system, and NMDA receptor is one of the three ionotropic, ligand-gated, glutamate-sensitive neurotransmitter receptors. In veterinary medicine, NMDA antagonists, such as amantadine and ketamine, are primarily used for adjunctive analgesia to minimize the sensitization of the dorsal horn neurons.[67] Case reports using other NMDA antagonists, such as memantine[68] and Huperzine-A,[69] are also published. Memantine was used to treat obsessive-compulsive disorders in dogs, and the authors concluded that it may be an effective, well-tolerated option for the treatment of compulsive disorders in dogs either as a sole treatment or as an augmentation to fluoxetine. Huperzine A is a licensed drug to treat Alzheimer's disease (AD) in China and is classified as a dietary supplement by FDA in 1997 for memory impairment in humans. It is a reversible, potent, and selective acetylcholinesterase (AChE) inhibitor and a noncompetitive NMDA receptor antagonist.[70,71] A published case report using Huperzine A to treat putative complex partial seizures in dogs did not show any side effects during treatment[69]

SUMMARY

Often, veterinarians are still trained to understand the body as being composed of separate parts. The knowledge that the body is instead one integrated system, orchestrated by the brain's neurochemistry and endocrinology, should shed light to the fact that mental and behavioral health conditions not only effect the mind but also lead to systemic consequences.[3] This involves inflammation and negative impacts in the immune system, including the stress response which (especially when chronic) leads to co-morbidities and potentially decreased life span.[2] Treatment with psychopharmacology drugs can be lifesaving for patients whose behavioral problems put their lives at risk, and it is an integral part of wellness care.[5]

REFERENCES

1. Schneiderman N, Ironson G, Siegel SD. Stress and Heath: Psychological, Behavioral, and Biological Determinants. Annu Rev Clin Psychol 2005;1:607–28.
2. Fan Z, Bian Z, Huang H, et al. Dietary Strategies for Relieving Stress in Pet Dogs and Cats. Antioxidants 2023;12(3):545.
3. Seiler A, Fagundes CP, Christian LM. The Impact of Everyday Stressors on the Immune System and Health. In: Choukèr A, editor. Stress Challenges and Immunity in space. Cham: Springer; 2020. https://doi.org/10.1007/978-3-030-16996-1_6.
4. Zefferino R, Di Gioia S, Conese M. Molecular links between endocrine, nervous and immune system during chronic stress. Brain Behav 2020;11(2).
5. Dreschel N. The effects of fear and anxiety on health and lifespan in pet dogs. Appl Anim Behav Sci 2010;125(3–4):157–62.
6. Dantas LMS, Crowell-Davis SL, Ogata N. Combinations. In: Crowell-Davis SL, Murray T, Dantas LMS, editors. Veterinary psychopharmacology. 2nd edition. Hoboken, NJ: Wiley-Blackwell; 2019. p. 281–90.
7. Simpson BS, Landsberg GM, Reisner IR, et al. Effects of reconcile (fluoxetine) chewable tablets plus behavior management for canine separation anxiety. Vet. Ther. 2007;8:18–31.
8. Landsberg GM, Melese P, Sherman BL, et al. Effectiveness of fluoxetine chewable tablets in the treatment of canine separation anxiety. J Vet Behav Clin Appl Res 2008;3:11–8.
9. Ogata N, Dantas LMS, Crowell-Davis SL. Selective serotonin reuptake inhibitors. In: Crowell-Davis SL, Murray T, Dantas LMS, editors. Veterinary psychopharmacology. 2nd edition. Hoboken, NJ: Wiley-Blackwell; 2019. p. 103–28.
10. Crowell-Davis SL, Seibert LM, Sung W, et al. Use of clomipramine, alprazolam and behavior modification for treatment of storm phobia in dogs. J Am Vet Med Assoc 2003;222:744–8.
11. Goldberger E, Rapoport JL. Canine acral lick dermatitis-response to the antiobsessional drug clomipramine. J Am Anim Hosp Assoc 1991;27(2):179–82.
12. Moon-Fanelli AA. Dodman NH Description and development of compulsive tail chasing in terriers and response to clomipramine treatment. J Am Vet Med Assoc 1998;212(8):1252–7.
13. Overall KL, Dunham AE. Clinical features and outcome in dogs and cats with obsessive compulsive disorder: 126 cases (1989–2000). J Am Vet Med Assoc 2002;221(10):1445–52.
14. Rapoport JL, Ryland DH. Kriete M Drug treatment of canine acral lick: An animal model of obsessive-compulsive disorder. Arch Gen Psychiatry 1992;49:517–21.

15. White MM, Neilson JC, Hart BL, et al. Effects of clomipramine hydrochloride on dominance-related aggression in dogs. J Am Vet Med Assoc 1999;215(9): 1288–91.
16. Siracusa C. Status-related aggression, resource guarding, and fear-related aggression in 2 female mixed breed dogs. J. Vet. Behav. 2016;12:85–91.
17. Mills DS, Redgate SE, Landsberg GM. A meta-analysis of studies of treatments for feline urine spraying. PLoS One 2011;6(4):e18448.
18. Mertens PA, Torres S, Jessen C. The effects of clomipramine hydrochloride in cats with psychogenic alopecia: a prospective study. J Am Anim Hosp Assoc 2006;42:336–43.
19. Mertens P, Torres S. The use of clomipramine hydrochloride for the treatment of feline psychogenic alopecia. J Am Anim Hosp Assoc 2003;39:509–12.
20. Martin KM. Effect of clomipramine on the electrocardiogram and serum thyroid concentrations of healthy cats. J Vet Behav Clin Appl Res 2010;5:123–9.
21. Reich MR, Ohad DG, Overall KL, et al. Electrocardiographic assessment of anti-anxiety medication in dogs and correlation with serum drug concentration. J Am Vet Med Assoc 2000;216(10):1571–5.
22. Pflaum K, Bennett S. Investigation of the use of venlafaxine for treatment of refractory misdirected play and impulse-control aggression in a cat: A case report. J. Vet. Behav. 2021;42:22–5.
23. Hopfensperger MJ. Use of oral venlafaxine in cats with feline idiopathic cystitis or behavioral causes of periuria. Proceedings of the American College of Veterinary Behaviorists Annual Symposium; San Antonio, TX, USA, 2016, 13–17.
24. Katofiasc MA, Nissen J, Audia JE, et al. Comparison of the effects of serotonin selective , norepinephrine selective , and dual serotonin and norepinephrine re-uptake inhibitors on lower urinary tract function in cats. Life Sci 2002;71:1227–36.
25. Metz D, Medam T, Masson S. Double-blind, placebo-controlled trial of venlafax-ine to treat behavioural disorders in cats: a pilot study. J Feline Med Surg 2021. https://doi.org/10.1177/1098612X211036792.
26. Delucci L, Martino P, Baldovino A, et al. Use of venlafaxine in the treatment of a canine narcolepsy-cataplexy case. J Small Anim Pract 2010;51:132.
27. Dantas LMS, Crowell-Davis SL. Miscellaneous serotonergic agents. In: Crowell-Davis SL, Murray T, Dantas LMS, editors. Veterinary psychopharmacology. 2nd edition. Hoboken, NJ: Wiley-Blackwell; 2019. p. 129–46.
28. Chávez G, Pardo P, Ubilla MJ, et al. Effects on behavioural variables of oral versus transdermal buspirone administration in cats displaying urine marking. J Appl Anim Res 2016;44:454–7.
29. Hart BL, Eckstein RA, Powell KL, et al. Effectiveness of buspirone on urine spraying and inappropriate urination in cats. J Am Vet Med Assoc 1993;203(2):254–8.
30. Mealey KL, Peck KE, Bennett BS, et al. Systemic Absorption of Amitriptyline and Buspirone after Oral and Transdermal Administration to Healthy Cats. J Vet Intern Med 2004;18:43–6.
31. Settimo L, Taylor D. Evaluating the dose-dependent mechanism of action of trazodone by estimation of occupancies for different brain neurotransmitter targets. J Psychopharmacol 2018;32:96–104.
32. Al-Yassiri MM, Ankier SI, Bridges P Trazodone-. A new antidepressant. Life Sci 1981;28:2449–58.
33. Tarantino P, Appleton N, Lansdell K. Effect of trazodone on hERG channel current and QT-interval. Eur J Pharmacol 2005;510:75–85.
34. Arnold A, Davis A, Wismer T, et al. Suspected hepatotoxicity secondary to trazodone therapy in a dog. J Vet Emerg Crit Care 2020;1–5.

35. Gruen ME, Roe SC, Grif EH, et al. The use of trazodone to facilitate calm behavior after elective orthopedic surgery in dogs : Results and lessons learned from a clinical trial. J. Vet. Behav. 2017;22. https://doi.org/10.1016/j.jveb.2017.09.008.

36. Kim SA, Borchardt MR, Lee K, et al. Effects of trazodone on behavioral and physiological signs of stress in dogs during veterinary visits. J Am Vet Med Assoc 2022;260:876–83.

37. Stevens BJ, Frantz EM, Orlando JM, et al. Efficacy of a single dose of trazodone hydrochloride given to cats prior to veterinary visits to reduce signs of transport- and examination -related anxiety. J Am Vet Med Assoc 2016;249:202–7.

38. Orlando JM, Case BC, Thomson AE, et al. Use of oral trazodone for sedation in cats: a pilot study. J Feline Med Surg 2015;1–7. https://doi.org/10.1177/1098612X15587956.

39. Cunningham MO, Woodhall GL, Thompson SE, et al. Dual effects of gabapentin and pregabalin on glutamate release at rat entorhinal synapses in vitro. Eur J Neurosci 2004;20:1566–76.

40. Bleuer-Elsner S, Medam T, Masson S. Effects of a single oral dose of gabapentin on storm phobia in dogs: A double-blind, placebo-controlled crossover trial. Vet Rec 2021;1–7. https://doi.org/10.1002/vetr.453.

41. Stollar OO, Moore GE, Mukhopadhyay A, et al. Effects of a single dose of orally administered gabapentin in dogs during a veterinary visit: a double-blinded, placebo-controlled study. J Am Vet Med Assoc 2022;260:1031–40. https://doi.org/10.2460/javma.21.03.0167.

42. Pypendop BH, Siao KT, Ilkiw JE. Thermal antinociceptive effect of orally administered gabapentin in healthy cats. Am J Vet Res 2010;71:1027–32. https://doi.org/10.2460/ajvr.71.9.1027.

43. Siao KT, Pypendop BH, Ilkiw JE. Pharmacokinetics of gabapentin in cats. Am J Vet Res 2010;71:817–21.

44. Quimby JM, Lorbach SK, Saffire A, et al. Serum concentrations of gabapentin in cats with chronic kidney disease. J Feline Med Surg 2022. https://doi.org/10.1177/1098612X221077017.

45. Eagan B, van Hafted K, Protopopova A. Daily gabapentin improved behavior modification progress and decreased stress in shelter cats from hoarding environments in a double-blind randomized placebo-controlled clinical trial. JAVMA 2023. https://doi.org/10.2460/javma.23.01.0044.

46. Moore SA. Managing neuropathic pain in dogs. Front Vet Sci 2016;3:1–8. https://doi.org/10.3389/fvets.2016.00012.

47. Sanchis-mora S, Chang YM, Abeyesinghe SM, et al. Pregabalin for the treatment of syringomyelia-associated neuropathic pain in dogs : A randomised , placebo-controlled , double-masked clinical trial. Vet J 2019;250:55–62.

48. Lamminen T, Korpivaara M, Suokko M, et al. Efficacy of a Single Dose of Pregabalin on Signs of Anxiety in Cats During Transportation—A Pilot Study. Front Vet Sci 2021;8:1–8.

49. Schwartz DD, Jones WG, Hedden KP, et al. Molecular and pharmacological characterization of the canine brainstem alpha-2A adrenergic receptor. J. Vet. Pharmacol. Ther. 1999;22:380–6.

50. Ogata N, Dantas LMS. Sympatholytic agents. In: Crowell-Davis SL, Murray T, Dantas LMS, editors. Veterinary psychopharmacology. 2nd edition. Hoboken, NJ: Wiley-Blackwell; 2019. p. 157–69.

51. Ogata N, Dodman N. The use of clonidine in the treatment of fear-based behavior problems in dogs: An open trial. J. Vet. Behav. 2011;6:130–7.

52. Plumb DC. Veterinary drug Handbook. 8th edition. Hoboken, NJ: Wiley-Blackwell; 2015.
53. NADA 141-456, Sileo® package Insert, Zoetis Inc. Kalamazoo, MI 49007
54. Korpivaara M, Laapas K, Huhtinen M, et al. Dexmedetomidine oromucosal gel for noise associated acute anxiety and fear in dogs—a randomised, double-blind, placebo-controlled clinical study. Vet Rec 2017;180:356.
55. Hauser H, Campbell S, Korpivaara M, et al. In-hospital administration ofdexmedetomi- dine oromucosal gel for stress reduction in dogs during veteri- nary visits: a randomized, double-blinded, placebo-controlled study. J Vet Behav 2020;39: 77–85.
56. Korpivaara M, Huhtinen M, Aspegrén J, et al. Dexmedetomidine oromucosal gel reduces fear and anxiety in dogs during veterinary visits: A randomised, double-blind, placebo-controlled clinical pilot study. Vet Rec 2021;e832. https://doi.org/ 10.1002/vetr.832.
57. Landsberg G, Dunn D, Korpivaara M. Anxiolytic effect of dexmedetomidine oro-mucosal gel (Sileo®) and gabapentin in a csavel anxiety model. In: Proceedings of the 12th International Veterinary Behaviour Meeting. 2019: 94-95.
58. Slingsby LS, Taylor PM, Monroe T. Thermal antinociception after dexmedetomi-dine administration in cats: a comparison between intramuscular and oral trans-mucosal administration. J Feline Med Surg 2009;11:829–34.
59. Dantas LMS, Crowell-Davis SL. Benzodiazepines. In: Crowell-Davis SL, Murray T, Dantas LMS, editors. Veterinary psychopharmacology. 2nd edition. Hoboken, NJ: Wiley-Blackwell; 2019. p. 67–102.
60. Center SA, Elston TH, Rowland PH, et al. Fulminant hepatic failure associated with oral administration of diazepam in 11 cats. J Am Vet Med Assoc 1996; 209:618–25.
61. Hughes D, Moreau RE, Overall KL, et al. Acute hepatic necrosis and liver failure associated with benzodiazepine therapy in six cats, 1986–1995. J Vet Emerg Crit Care 1996;6:13–20.
62. Levy JK. Letters to the editor. J Am Vet Med Assoc 1994;205(7):966.
63. Levy JK, Cullen JM, Bunch SE, et al. Adverse reaction to diazepam in cats. J Am Vet Med Assoc 1994;205(2):156–7.
64. Danneberg P, Weber KH. Chemical structure and biological activity of the diaze-pines. Br J Clin Pharmacol 1983;16:231S–43S.
65. Brett J, Murnion B. Management of benzodiazepine misuse and dependence. Aust Prescr 2015;38:152–5.
66. Riss J, Cloyd J, Gates J, et al. Benzodiazepines in epilepsy: pharmacology and pharmacokinetics. Acta Neurol Scand 2008;118:69–86.
67. Lamont LA. Adjunctive Analgesic Therapy in Veterinary Medicine. Vet Clin North Am - Small Anim Pract 2008;38(6):1187–203.
68. Schneider BM, Dodman NH, Maranda L. Use of memantine in treatment of canine compulsive disorders. J Vet Behav Clin Appl Res 2009b;4:118–26.
69. Schneider BM, Dodman NH, Faissler D, et al. Clinical use of an herbal-derived compound (Huperzine A) to treat putative complex partial seizures in a dog. Ep-ilepsy Behav 2009a;15:529–34.
70. Tang XC, Han YF. Pharmacological Profile of huperzine A, a novel acetylcholines-terase inhibitor from chinese herb. CNS Drug Rev 1999;5(3):281–300.
71. Zhang HY, Zhao X-Y, Chen X-Q, et al. Spermidine antagonizes the inhibitory ef-fect of huperzine A on [3H]dizocilpine (MK-801)binding in synaptic memebrane of rat cerebral cortex. Neurosci Lett 2002;319:107–10.

9780443129971